T0263612

Cancer in Companion Animals

Editors

PHILIP J. BERGMAN
CRAIG A. CLIFFORD

VETERINARY CLINICS OF NORTH AMERICA: SMALL ANIMAL PRACTICE

www.vetsmall.theclinics.com

September 2019 • Volume 49 • Number 5

ELSEVIER

1600 John F. Kennedy Boulevard • Suite 1800 • Philadelphia, Pennsylvania, 19103-2899
http://www.vetsmall.theclinics.com

VETERINARY CLINICS OF NORTH AMERICA: SMALL ANIMAL PRACTICE Volume 49, Number 5 September 2019 ISSN 0195-5616, ISBN-13: 978-0-323-68220-6

Editor: Colleen Dietzler

Developmental Editor: Laura Kavanaugh

Veterinary Clinics of North America: Small Animal Practice (ISSN 0195-5616) is published bimonthly by Elsevier Inc., 360 Park Avenue South, New York, NY 10010-1710. Months of issue are January, March, May, July, September, and November. Business and Editorial Offices: 1600 John F. Kennedy Blvd., Ste. 1800, Philadelphia, PA 19103-2899. Customer Service Office: 3251 Riverport Lane, Maryland Heights, MO 63043. Periodicals postage paid at New York, NY and additional mailing offices. Subscription prices are $338.00 per year (domestic individuals), $662.00 per year (domestic institutions), $100.00 per year (domestic students/residents), $451.00 per year (Canadian individuals), $823.00 per year (Canadian institutions), $474.00 per year (international individuals), $823.00 per year (international institutions), and $220.00 per year (international and Canadian students/residents). To receive student/resident rate, orders must be accompained by name of affiliated institution, date of term, and the *signature* of program/residency coordinator on institution letterhead. Orders will be billed at individual rate until proof of status is received. Foreign air speed delivery is included in all *Clinics* subscription prices. All prices are subject to change without notice. **POSTMASTER:** Send address changes to *Veterinary Clinics of North America: Small Animal Practice*, Elsevier Health Sciences Division, Subscription Customer Service, 3251 Riverport Lane, Maryland Heights, MO 63043. Customer Service (orders, claims, online, change of address): Elsevier Periodicals Customer Service, Elsevier Health Sciences Division Subscription **Customer Service 3251 Riverport Lane Maryland Heights, MO 63043. Tel: 1-800-654-2452 (U.S. and Canada); 314-447-8871 (outside U.S. and Canada). Fax: 314-447-8029. E-mail: journalscustomerservice-usa@elsevier.com (for print support); journalsonlinesupport-usa@elsevier.com (for online support).**

Reprints. For copies of 100 or more of articles in this publication, please contact the Commercial Reprints Department, Elsevier Inc., 360 Park Avenue South, New York, NY 10010-1710. Tel.: 212-633-3874; Fax: 212-633-3820; E-mail: reprints@elsevier.com.

Veterinary Clinics of North America: Small Animal Practice is also published in Japanese by Inter Zoo Publishing Co., Ltd., Aoyama Crystal-Bldg 5F, 3-5-12 Kitaaoyama, Minato-ku, Tokyo 107-0061, Japan.

Veterinary Clinics of North America: Small Animal Practice is covered in *Current Contents/Agriculture, Biology and Environmental Sciences, Science Citation Index, ASCA, MEDLINE/PubMed (Index Medicus), Excerpta Medica, and BIOSIS.*

Contributors

EDITORS

PHILIP J. BERGMAN, DVM, MS, PhD
Diplomate, American College of Veterinary Internal Medicine (Oncology); Director, Clinical Studies, VCA, Adjunct Associate Faculty Member, Memorial Sloan Kettering Cancer Center, New York, New York, USA; Oncologist, Katonah-Bedford Veterinary Center, Bedford Hills, New York, USA

CRAIG A. CLIFFORD, DVM, MS
Diplomate, American College of Veterinary Internal Medicine (Oncology); Director, Clinical Studies, Hope Veterinary Specialists, Medical Oncology Service, Malvern, Pennsylvania, USA

AUTHORS

ALFONSO BALDI, MD
Department of Environmental, Biological and Pharmaceutical Sciences and Technologies, Campania University "Luigi Vanvitelli," Caserta, Italy

PHILIP J. BERGMAN, DVM, MS, PhD
Diplomate, American College of Veterinary Internal Medicine (Oncology); Director, Clinical Studies, VCA, Adjunct Associate Faculty Member, Memorial Sloan Kettering Cancer Center, New York, New York, USA; Oncologist, Katonah-Bedford Veterinary Center, Bedford Hills, New York, USA

SARAH E. BOSTON, DVM, DVSc
Diplomate, American College of Veterinary Surgeons (Small Animal); ACVS Founding Fellow in Surgical Oncology, ACVS Founding Fellow, Oral and Maxillofacial Surgery, VCA Canada, 404 Veterinary Emergency and Referral Hospital, Newmarket, Ontario, Canada

MATTHEW BREEN, PhD, C.Biol, FRSB
Oscar J Fletcher Distinguished Professor of Comparative Oncology Genetics, Department of Molecular Biomedical Sciences, College of Veterinary Medicine, North Carolina State University, Raleigh, North Carolina, USA

MELINDA CAMUS, DVM
Diplomate, American College of Veterinary Pathologists; Department of Pathology, College of Veterinary Medicine, University of Georgia, Athens, Georgia, USA

CRAIG A. CLIFFORD, DVM, MS
Diplomate, American College of Veterinary Internal Medicine (Oncology); Director, Clinical Studies, Hope Veterinary Specialists, Medical Oncology Service, Malvern, Pennsylvania, USA

WILLIAM T.N. CULP, VMD
ACVS Founding Fellow of Surgical Oncology, ACVS Founding Fellow, Minimally Invasive Surgery, Professor, Department of Surgical and Radiological Sciences, University of California, Davis, Davis, California, USA

TRACY L. GIEGER, DVM
Associate Clinical Professor, Radiation Oncology, Department of Clinical Sciences, College of Veterinary Medicine, North Carolina State University, Raleigh, North Carolina, USA

MAUREEN A. GRIFFIN, DVM
Resident, Veterinary Medical Teaching Hospital, University of California, Davis, California, USA

MEGAN GUTWILLIG
Graduate Student, Sackler School of Graduate Biomedical Sciences, Tufts University, Boston, Massachusetts, USA

CHAD M. JOHANNES, DVM
Diplomate, American College of Veterinary Internal Medicine (Small Animal Internal Medicine, Oncology); Assistant Professor, Department of Veterinary Clinical Sciences, Iowa State University College of Veterinary Medicine, Ames, Iowa, USA

ANNA KATOGIRITIS, DVM
EthosVeterinaryHealth LLC, Woburn, Massachusetts, USA; EthosDiscovery(501c3), Washington, DC, USA

CHAND KHANNA, DVM, PhD
Diplomate, American College of Veterinary Internal Medicine (Oncology); Diplomate, American College of Veterinary Pathologists (Hons); Chief Science Officer, EthosVeterinaryHealth LLC, Woburn, Massachusetts, USA; President, EthosDiscovery(501c3), Washington, DC, USA

DR. MED. VET. DR. HABIL. MATTI KIUPEL, BS, MS, PhD
Diplomate, American College of Veterinary Pathologists; Veterinary Diagnostic Laboratory, Department of Pathobiology and Diagnostic Investigation, College of Veterinary Medicine, Michigan State University, Lansing, Michigan, USA

JULIUS M. LIPTAK, BVSc, MVetClinStud
Fellow, Australian College of Veterinary Scientists, Diplomate, American College of Veterinary Surgeons (Small Animal); Diplomate, European College of Veterinary Surgeons; ACVS Founding Fellow, Surgical Oncology, VCA Canada, Alta Vista Animal Hospital, Ottawa, Ontario, Canada

PRIYA LONDHE, PhD
Postdoctoral Fellow, Tufts University School of Medicine, Boston, Massachusetts, USA

CHERYL LONDON, DVM, PhD
Anne Engen and Dusty Professor of Comparative Oncology, Cummings School of Veterinary Medicine and School of Medicine, Tufts University, Tufts University School of Medicine, Boston, Massachusetts, USA

CHRISTINE MULLIN, VMD
Diplomate, American College of Veterinary Internal Medicine (Oncology); Hope Veterinary Specialists, Medical Oncology Service, Malvern, Pennsylvania, USA

MARGARET L. MUSSER, DVM
Diplomate, American College of Veterinary Internal Medicine (Oncology); Assistant Professor, Department of Veterinary Clinical Sciences, Iowa State University College of Veterinary Medicine, Ames, Iowa, USA

MICHAEL W. NOLAN, DVM, PhD
Associate Professor, Radiation Oncology, Department of Clinical Sciences, College of Veterinary Medicine, North Carolina State University, Raleigh, North Carolina, USA

ENRICO PIERLUIGI SPUGNINI, DVM, PhD
Diplomate, American College of Veterinary Internal Medicine (Oncology); Diplomate, European College of Veterinary Internal Medicine-Companion Animals (Oncology); Biopulse srl, Naples, Italy

DOUGLAS H. THAMM, VMD
Diplomate, American College of Veterinary Internal Medicine (Oncology); Barbara Cox Anthony Professor of Oncology, Flint Animal Cancer Center, College of Veterinary Medicine and Biomedical Sciences, Colorado State University, Fort Collins, Colorado, USA

CLAIRE WILEY, VMD
Diplomate, American College of Veterinary Medicine (Small Animal Internal Medicine); Clinician Investigator, Department of Molecular Biomedical Sciences, College of Veterinary Medicine, North Carolina State University, Raleigh, North Carolina, USA

CATHERINE F. WISE, BS
Program in Environmental and Molecular Toxicology, Department of Biological Sciences, North Carolina State University, NC State College of Veterinary Medicine, Raleigh, North Carolina, USA

Contents

Preface: Recent Advancements in Veterinary Oncology xiii

Philip J. Bergman and Craig A. Clifford

Novel Noninvasive Diagnostics 781

Claire Wiley, Catherine F. Wise, and Matthew Breen

Molecular diagnostics have revolutionized human oncology to allow early detection, targeted therapy, monitoring throughout treatment, and evidence of recurrence. By identifying genetic signatures associated with cancers, liquid biopsy techniques have been developed to diagnose and monitor cancer in noninvasive or minimally invasive ways. These techniques offer new opportunities for improving cancer screening, diagnosis, and monitoring the impact of therapy on the patients over time. Liquid biopsy also drives drug development programs. Similar diagnostics hold promise for comparable results in the veterinary field. Several noninvasive/minimally invasive techniques have been described in veterinary medicine that could be referred to as liquid biopsy.

Nonselective Lymph Node Dissection and Sentinel Lymph Node Mapping and Biopsy 793

Julius M. Liptak and Sarah E. Boston

Clinical staging is important for determining the extent of disease in animals with malignant cancers. The status of the lymph node will help determine whether adjuvant treatment is indicated. Historically, the regional anatomic lymph node has been sampled to determine the presence or absence of metastatic disease, but there is increasing evidence that the regional anatomic lymph node is often different to the sentinel lymph node. As a result, several sentinel lymph node mapping techniques have been described for more accurate clinical staging of oncologic patients.

Towards the Delivery of Precision Veterinary Cancer Medicine 809

Anna Katogiritis and Chand Khanna

We introduce a next phase in the evolution of medicine affecting human and veterinary patients. This evolution, genomic cancer medicine (Pmed), involves expansion of genomic and molecular biology into clinical medicine. The implementation of these new technologies has already begun and is a commercial reality. We introduce the underpinnings for this evolution, and focus on application in complex disease states. Pet owners have begun requesting Pmed technologies. To meet this demand, it is important to be aware of the opportunities and obstacles associated with available Pmed offerings as well as the current state of the field.

Diagnosis and Prognosis of Canine Cutaneous Mast Cell Tumors 819

Matti Kiupel and Melinda Camus

Canine cutaneous mast cell tumors (MCTs) are among the most common canine cutaneous tumors, with highly variable biological behavior. This review describes in detail current approaches for cytologic and histologic diagnosis and prognosis, including advantages and limitations of cytologic and histologic grading and utilization of molecular markers, for example, Ki67, AgNORs, KIT expression, and c-Kit mutations, for a more accurate detection of aggressive MCTs. Furthermore, the current approach to evaluate surgical margins and spread to local lymph nodes is discussed.

Anorexia and the Cancer Patient **837**

Chad M. Johannes and Margaret L. Musser

Appetite influences perceived quality of life for a dog or cat with cancer. Inappetence often is multifactorial, complicating treatment. Cancer-related anorexia/cachexia syndrome is a metabolic, paraneoplastic syndrome characterized by decreased food intake, involuntary weight loss, and loss of fat and muscle. If weight loss/cachexia has an impact on canine and feline cancer patients as in humans, management may improve survival times and quality of life. The challenge is having effective, proved therapies available for clinical use. Recent Food and Drug Administration approvals for appetite stimulation have renewed interest and discussion and has the potential to alter the course of case management.

Histiocytic Sarcoma and Hemangiosarcoma Update **855**

Christine Mullin and Craig A. Clifford

Histiocytic sarcoma (HS) and hemangiosarcoma (HSA) are uncommon and aggressive neoplasms that develop much more frequently in dogs than in cats. Breed-specific predispositions have been identified for both cancers. The development of novel diagnostics is underway and may aid in earlier diagnosis. Therapeutic approaches to HS and HSA depend on the stage of disease and may include surgery, radiation therapy, and chemotherapy. Such interventions improve outcome; however, aside from a small number of clinical circumstances, both diseases are considered largely incurable. Continued efforts toward the identification of driver mutations and subsequent druggable targets may lead to improvements in long-term prognosis.

Cancer Immunotherapies **881**

Philip J. Bergman

The enhanced understanding of immunology experienced over the last 4 decades afforded through the tools of molecular biology has recently translated into cancer immunotherapy becoming one of the most exciting and rapidly expanding fields. Human cancer immunotherapy is now recognized as one of the pillars of treatment alongside surgery, radiation, and chemotherapy. The field of veterinary cancer immunotherapy has also rapidly advanced in the last decade with a handful of commercially available products and a plethora of investigational cancer immunotherapies that will hopefully expand the veterinary oncology treatment toolkit over time.

Novel Treatments for Lymphoma **903**

Douglas H. Thamm

Lymphoma is a common disease in companion animals. Although conventional chemotherapy has the potential to induce remission and prolong life, relapse is common, and novel treatments are needed to improve outcome. This review discusses recent modifications/adjustments to conventional standard of care therapy for canine and feline lymphoma, as well as cutting-edge immunotherapy and small-molecule-based approaches that are in varying stages of regulatory approval.

Targeted Therapies in Veterinary Oncology **917**

Priya Londhe, Megan Gutwillig, and Cheryl London

Advances in molecular biology have permitted a much more detailed understanding of cellular dysfunction at the molecular and genetic levels in cancer cells. This has resulted in the identification of novel targets for therapeutic intervention, including proteins that regulate signal transduction, gene expression, and protein turnover. In many instances, small molecules are used to disrupt the function of these targets, often through competitive inhibition of ATP binding or the prevention of necessary protein-protein interactions. More than 40 small molecule inhibitors are now approved to treat a variety of human cancers, substantially impacting patient outcomes.

Update in Veterinary Radiation Oncology: Focus on Stereotactic Radiation Therapy **933**

Michael W. Nolan and Tracy L. Gieger

Stereotactic radiotherapy (SRT) involves the precise delivery of highly conformal, dose-intense radiation to well-demarcated tumors. Special equipment and expertise are needed, and a unique biological mechanism distinguishes SRT from other forms of external beam radiotherapy. Families find the convenient schedules and minimal acute toxicity of SRT appealing. Common indications in veterinary oncology include nasal, brain, and bone tumors. Many other solid tumors can also be treated, including spinal, oral, lung, heart-base, liver, adrenal, and prostatic malignancies. Accessibility of SRT is improving, and new data are constantly emerging to define parameters for appropriate case selection, radiation dose prescription, and long-term follow-up."

Veterinary Clinics: Tumor Ablation **949**

William T.N. Culp and Maureen A. Griffin

Over the past decade, interventional oncology techniques have become integrated into the treatment plans of companion animals with cancer on a regular basis. Although procedures such as stenting are performed commonly, other less frequently utilized techniques for locoregional therapy, such as embolization and ablation, are emerging and demonstrating promise. Tumor ablation techniques are categorized into two subgroups: chemical ablation and energy-based ablation. Increased utilization of ablation will allow for the determination of specific indications and evaluation of outcomes for these techniques.

Electrochemotherapy in Veterinary Oncology: State-of-the-Art and Perspectives **967**

Enrico Pierluigi Spugnini and Alfonso Baldi

Tumor microenvironment represents a key obstacle for the effectiveness of anticancer drugs. Electrochemotherapy involves the systemic or local delivery of lipophobic drugs such as bleomycin and cisplatin, with the application of permeabilizing electric pulses having appropriate amplitude and waveforms. This greatly enhances the uptake of these drugs by an estimated factor of 700-fold for bleomycin and 4 to 8 times for cisplatin. Because of its efficacy and limited morbidity, this therapeutic option is becoming more and more available in veterinary oncology either as an adjuvant to surgery or as first line of treatment with palliative or curative purposes.

VETERINARY CLINICS OF NORTH AMERICA: SMALL ANIMAL PRACTICE

Preface

Recent Advancements in Veterinary Oncology

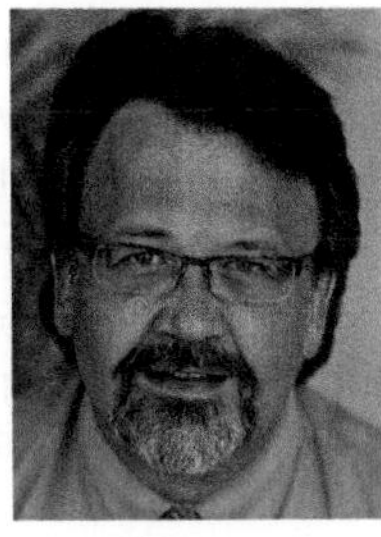

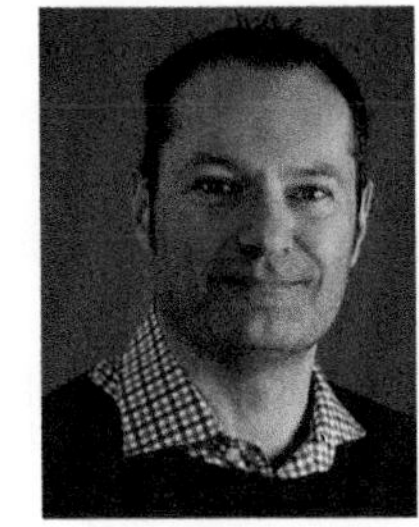

Philip J. Bergman, DVM, MS, PhD Craig A. Clifford, DVM, MS
Editors

We are entering an exciting time in veterinary oncology, whereby the seeds planted within the comparative oncology realm many years ago are now coming to bloom in the form of a greater molecular understanding of cancer in companion animals. The comparative animal model has garnered significant interest in both industry and academia, and the ensuing research has yielded breakthrough discoveries from advanced diagnostics to novel therapies, the sum of which provides opportunities to improve the longevity and quality of life of our patients.

We feel this issue of *Veterinary Clinics of North America: Small Animal Practice* highlights the wide breadth of advancements within our field. With diverse topics ranging from the first new conditionally approved chemotherapeutic for lymphoma, novel BRAF testing for canine urothelial carcinoma, updates in the new field of interventional radiology, review of current and future tyrosine kinase inhibitors, updates in stereotactic radiation, a review of the use of electrochemotherapy, updates on canine histiocytic sarcoma and hemangiosarcoma, a review of current and future immunotherapeutics, and discussions on histologic versus cytologic grading for canine mast cell tumors. We

Vet Clin Small Anim 49 (2019) xiii–xiv
https://doi.org/10.1016/j.cvsm.2019.06.001
0195-5616/19/© 2019 Published by Elsevier Inc.

hope the reader will share our outlook: that the future of veterinary oncology is very bright.

Philip J. Bergman, DVM, MS, PhD
VCA
Memorial Sloan Kettering Cancer Center
Katonah-Bedford Veterinary Center
546 Bedford Road
Bedford Hills, NY, 10507, USA

Craig A. Clifford, DVM, MS
Hope Veterinary Specialists
Malvern, PA 19355, USA

E-mail addresses:
Philip.Bergman@vca.com (P.J. Bergman)
Cliffdoc2000@yahoo.com (C.A. Clifford)

Novel Noninvasive Diagnostics

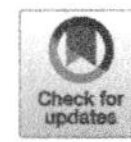

Claire Wiley, VMD[a], Catherine F. Wise, BS[b,c], Matthew Breen, PhD, C.Biol, FRSB[a,*]

KEYWORDS

• Canine • Cancer • Liquid biopsy • Bladder • Prostate • BRAF • Lymphoma

KEY POINTS

- A cancer signature is an indicator of the presence of a cancer, ideally with high sensitivity and specificity.
- A liquid biopsy allows for the detection of cancer cells, or cell remnants, from a tumor that are circulating in the blood or deposited into the urine of a patient.
- Early detection of a cancer has the potential to provide more time to intervene with appropriate therapy to help delay onset of clinical symptoms.

INTRODUCTION

Molecular diagnostics have revolutionized human oncology to allow early detection, targeted therapy, monitoring throughout treatment, and evidence of recurrence. By identifying genetic signatures associated with cancers, liquid biopsy techniques have been developed to diagnose and monitor cancer in noninvasive or minimally invasive ways.[1,2] These techniques offer new opportunities for improving cancer screening, diagnosis, and monitoring of the impact of therapy on the patients over time.[3,4] Liquid biopsy also drives drug development programs.[2] Similar diagnostics now hold promise for comparable results in the veterinary field.

Several noninvasive/minimally invasive techniques have been described in veterinary medicine that could be referred to as liquid biopsy. These include

---

Disclosure Statement: M. Breen is a founder and stockholder in Sentinel Biomedical, the company that developed the CADET range of laboratory molecular assays for use in veterinary medicine. C. Wise and C. Wiley have nothing to disclose.

[a] Department of Molecular Biomedical Sciences, College of Veterinary Medicine, North Carolina State University, CVM Research Building, 1060 William Moore Drive, Raleigh, NC 27607, USA; [b] Program in Environmental and Molecular Toxicology, Department of Biological Sciences, North Carolina State University, NC State College of Veterinary Medicine, CVM Research Building, 1060 William Moore Drive, Raleigh, NC 27606, USA; [c] NC State College of Veterinary Medicine, North Carolina State University, CVM Research Building, 1060 William Moore Drive, Raleigh, NC 27607, USA

* Corresponding author.

E-mail address: mbreen3@ncsu.edu

Vet Clin Small Anim 49 (2019) 781–791

https://doi.org/10.1016/j.cvsm.2019.05.002

vetsmall.theclinics.com

0195-5616/19/

CADET® *BRAF* and CADET® *BRAF*-PLUS assays for the diagnosis and monitoring of canine transitional cell carcinoma (TCC)/urothelial carcinoma (UC)
Cell block preparation for various cancers
Polymerase chain reaction (PCR) for antigen receptor rearrangement (PARR), flow cytometry for lymphoid malignancies
CADET® HM assay for diagnosing canine histiocytic malignancies

LIQUID BIOPSY

The use of fluids to detect cells and DNA released by tumors is referred to as liquid biopsy.[5] Circulating cell free nucleic acids (cfNAs) were first described almost 70 years ago, but the idea of liquid biopsies went undiscovered until 1994, when fragments of a driver oncogene (a mutant *RAS* gene) were identified in the blood of cancer patients.[5] More recently, advances in technology have allowed the detection of these types of mutant alleles with high specificity and sensitivity. Cancer patients have higher cfDNA concentrations than in normal/healthy controls, and metastases is generally associated with even higher levels.[1] The increased release of cfDNA from tumors is thought to be associated with the fast turnover of cells and resulting apoptosis.[5] Liquid biopsy was first described as the identification of neoplastic biological materials, such as circulating tumor cells or circulating cfDNA, in the peripheral blood.[2] More recently, this term has broadened to encompass all body fluids, including urine, cerebrospinal fluid, and cavitary effusions.[2]

In a recent study of human patients with solid tumors, the presence of tumor-associated cfDNA in the plasma varied with tumor type.[6] Patients with detectable plasma concentrations of tumor-associated cfDNA either had primary liver or ovarian cancer, or metastatic pancreatic, bladder, colon, stomach, breast, esophagus, liver, or other cancers of the head and neck.[6] In contrast, less than 50% of patients with medulloblastomas or metastatic cancers of the kidney, prostate, or thyroid, and less than 10% of patients with gliomas had detectable tumor-associated cfDNA in their plasma. These results suggest that urine may be a superior liquid matrix for monitoring renal, prostate, and bladder tumors, and such cancers are more readily identified using mutations detected from intact cells exfoliated into the urine.

Genotyping of human cancers is becoming a routine component of the diagnostic work-up and aids in differentiation, staging, and sometimes treatment. Genotyping of tumor-associated DNA and cfDNA obtained using a liquid biopsy offers the advantage of easy, rapid, and safe access to the tumor in contrast to traditional biopsies or fine needle aspirates. Liquid biopsies are also increasingly being used to monitor the mutation burden in patient specimens during treatment, as well as to identify residual disease and recurrence. There is strong evidence indicating that use of liquid biopsy approaches allows recurrence or metastasis to be detected earlier than with conventional methods.[3,4]

Liquid Biopsies for Transitional Cell Carcinoma/Urothelial Carcinoma

CADET® BRAF

The CADET® *BRAF* can be utilized in multiple clinical applications for canine TCC/UC: diagnosis, screening of high-risk breeds, monitoring, identification of metastasis, and targeted therapy. The foundation for the CADET® *BRAF* comes from 2 recent studies performed by research teams at North Carolina State University (NC State)[7] and the National Institutes of Health (NIH).[8] A single mutation in exon 15 of the canine *BRAF* gene was detected in pathology-verified tumor biopsy specimens of canine TCC/UC. The NC State team identified the mutation comparing the DNA sequences of all genes of the dog DNA isolated from TCC/UC tissue samples with those from non-neoplastic tissues. The NIH team identified the mutation by evaluating RNA sequences in affected tissues. The discovery of the same mutation independently by 2 groups using 2 different approaches provided cross-validation of the data. The result of this single mutation is 1 amino change (valine to glutamic acid) in the BRAF protein in the tumor cells. This change, located in the activation segment of the kinase domain of the gene, results in a mutated protein with increased kinase activity that signals the cells to proliferate, leading to the development of a tumor. The *BRAF* mutation has not been detected in numerous non-neoplastic bladder tissues, including inflammatory bladder tissue and polyps.[9]

In cases where a dog has a TCC/UC, cells from the mass, ranging from early to late in the course of disease, are shed into the urine and so contribute to the cells recovered. The NC State team developed a rapid and highly sensitive test to detect the presence of this mutation in cells shed into the urine[9] (**Fig. 1**). Further development by Sentinel Biomedical (Raleigh, NC) (www.SentinelBiomedical.com) led to the refinement and commercialization of the world's first liquid biopsy for a veterinary cancer in the form of the CADET® *BRAF*. CADET® *BRAF* analysis is based on identification and quantification of wild-type and mutated *BRAF* alleles recovered from cells exfoliated into the urine. A comparison between the level of *BRAF* wild type and *BRAF* mutant alleles provided a quantitative measure of cells recovered from the urine samples. Quantification is presented as a percent fractional abundance of mutant alleles. Most cells with the *BRAF* mutation are heterozygous, so the fractional abundance of the mutation typically does not exceed 50%.

CADET® *BRAF* analysis Liquid biopsy (urine sample) is added to a collection jar containing a preservative. Cellular DNA is isolated from the urine specimen using an optimized chemistry. Analytical reagents are mixed with the urine DNA, including 2 differentially labeled fluorescent DNA probes designed to detect the wild-type (green) and mutant (blue) *BRAF* sequences. The reaction mixture is partitioned in approximately 20,000 1 nL sized droplets, and the DNA in each droplet is allowed to bind to the sequence-specific fluorescent probes and amplify by PCR. Droplets containing amplicons where the *BRAF* sequence is wild type fluoresce green, and those that contain the mutant *BRAF* gene fluoresce blue. Each droplet is removed from the mixture and scored independently based on its fluorescence properties; green droplets are scored as *BRAF* wild type, and blue droplets are scored as *BRAF* mutant. These data are used to calculate the detection threshold for that specific sample, and, if a BRAF mutation is detected, the relative proportion of mutant alleles (fractional abundance). There are 2 possible outcomes from CADET® *BRAF* analysis; detected or undetected. If the sample is *BRAF* mutation detected, the fractional abundance is provided, which may be used as a baseline to monitor changes in urinary *BRAF* mutation levels during subsequent treatment. If the sample is *BRAF* undetected, the detection threshold indicates the technical sensitivity of the sample assessed and whether the specimen provided is eligible for analysis with CADET® *BRAF-PLUS*.

CADET® *BRAF-PLUS* analysis Fifteen percent of dogs with clinical signs of TCC/UC do not have *BRAF*-associated disease. Over two-thirds of these TCC/UC cases (when eligible for analysis) are detected with further analysis using CADET® *BRAF*-PLUS. The same DNA sample used for CADET® *BRAF* is used for this additional analysis. Analytical reagents are mixed with the urine DNA, including differentially labeled fluorescent DNA probes designed to detect the relative abundance of 3 specific regions of the canine genome. After partitioning into approximately 20,000 1 nL droplets, the

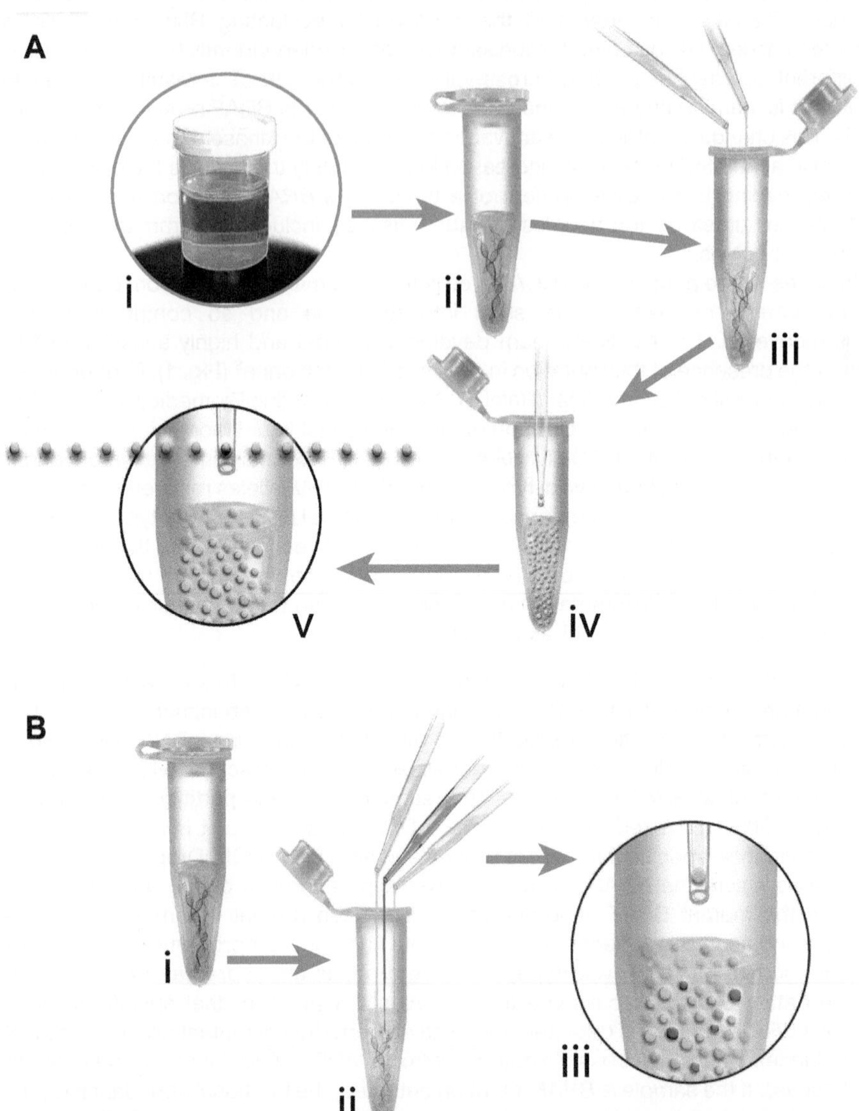

Fig. 1. Schematic representation of the analytical process for (*A*) CADET® *BRAF* and (*B*) *BRAF*-PLUS. Reproduced with permission of Sentinel Biomedical Inc.

DNA in each droplet is allowed to bind to these 3 sequence-specific fluorescent probes and amplified by PCR. The droplets are removed and evaluated individually for their fluorescence properties. The data are used to calculate the relative number of copies of each of the 3 target regions to determine if the DNA sample evaluated has signatures consistent with canine TCC/UC.

Diagnosis Conventionally, biopsy and histopathologic evaluation confirm a diagnosis of canine TCC/UC. Cytology is frequently used to support a diagnosis of TCC/UC through the identification of abnormal epithelial cells in urine sediment, or in samples obtained by traumatic catheterization, prostatic wash, and/or fine needle aspiration.[10–12] However, cytologic analysis of epithelial cells can be misleading, as benign epithelial cells can resemble malignant cells with variation in cell size.[13] Fine needle aspiration of potential tumor tissue in the bladder carries the risk of disseminating tumor cells along the needle tract and so should be performed with caution.[14,15] Further imaging and evaluation of local lymph nodes may be performed to assess for metastases.

The CADET® *BRAF* is a noninvasive tool to aid in the clinical diagnosis of TCC/UC. Overall biological sensitivity of CADET® *BRAF* to detect a canine TCC/UC in a free-catch urine specimen is 85%, and although technical sensitivity is sample dependent, this is typically over 99.9%. Although some other canine cancers do present with the same *BRAF* mutation at low frequency,[7] these have not yet been detected in urine specimens of such patients. The specificity to detect a canine TCC/UC is currently greater than 99%.

Importantly, in all cases that have had a biopsy of a visible mass for pathology evaluation, there is 100% concordance between the presence of a *BRAF* mutation detected in free-catch urine and subsequent confirmation of a TCC/UC in the biopsy of the mass. In contrast, false-positive results have not been identified to date; in studies of over 1000 controls, a *BRAF* mutation has not been detected in urine specimens from dogs that were shown not to have a TCC/UC. Unlike previous, and less discriminatory tests for canine TCC/UC, CADET® *BRAF* is unaffected by the presence of blood or bacteria in the urine. Although a positive test indicates the presence of *BRAF* mutation load being shed into the urine, the test does not indicate the location of the TCC/UC. Imaging of the region will help identify tumor location and might also contribute to decisions regarding the most appropriate clinical management.

Screening of high-risk breeds CADET® *BRAF* was designed specifically to identify cells in the urine that carry the *BRAF* mutation, and to do so with a forensic level of detection. As such, the assay can detect as few as 10 mutant bearing cells in a urine sample and so has the potential to identify TCC/UC cases at early, preclinical stages of the disease. This is a characteristic feature of an effective early screening assay; to detect the presence of an emerging cancer as early as possible in the course of the disease, with the aim of providing more time for the most appropriate intervention to combat the disease.

Most cases of TCC/UC present with lower urinary tract signs that are shared with several other conditions, including urinary infections, polyps, and bladder stones. Although prevalence of urinary tract infections (UTIs) is difficult to estimate, bacterial UTI is conservatively 25 times more common than TCC/UC.[16–20] When a dog first presents with lower urinary tract signs, veterinarians generally treat the most common cause and prescribe antibiotics or nonsteroidal anti-inflammatory drugs (NSAIDs) before evaluating for TCC/UC. Dogs may receive a series of therapies, sometimes over several months. During this time, however, while clinical signs may improve, a TCC/UC tumor can continue to develop into a more advanced state, become larger, potentially invading the muscle wall and having a greater chance of metastasis. When repeated treatments fail to fully resolve clinical signs, the dog is then evaluated for the presence of a TCC/UC, usually via urine cytology, abdominal ultrasound, and/or cystoscopy. With conventional approaches, at the time of diagnosis over 90% of dogs present with an intermediate- to high-grade invasive canine TCC/UC, and superficial, low-grade tumors are rare.[21] Metastasis is also common, present in approximately 20% of canine TCCs/UCs at the time of diagnosis.[22] The high predominance of advanced tumors detected by conventional means may reflect the prolonged time taken to diagnose the tumors in most cases.

CADET® *BRAF* provides a means to screen free-catch urine of healthy dogs from breeds with an increased risk of developing TCC/UC (eg, Beagle, Scottish terrier, Shetland sheepdog, or West Highland white terrier) (www.AKC.org). This enables owners of dogs that test positive at low levels to follow-up with their veterinarian and seek the most appropriate treatment early in the course of the disease. Earlier detection is expected to improve the quality and duration of the dogs' lives. However, early diagnosis can also be associated with unnecessary, harmful therapy and should be approached with caution. A clinical trial evaluating dogs with low levels of the *BRAF* mutation for histopathologic evidence of disease is underway. This study is recruiting over 1000 dogs, and data will be available in late 2019/early 2020. This first of its kind study will determine the time period between detection of a low urinary CADET® *BRAF* level and progression to develop clinical signs caused by TCC/UC.

Monitoring Once a dog has been diagnosed as positive for CADET® *BRAF* and shown to have a TCC/UC, repeat analysis may be used over time to monitor changing levels of the mutational load detected in free-catch urine during treatment. Early provisional data have shown that although NSAIDs such as piroxicam may have a minor impact on reducing the level of the CADET® *BRAF* mutation shed into urine, conventional chemotherapeutic agents such as mitoxantrone may be associated with a progressive and substantial reduction in the CADET® *BRAF* mutation levels over the course of treatment (Wiley and colleagues, unpublished data [manuscript in prep], 2019). Temporally matched ultrasonography of dozens of cases revealed a progressive reduction in the size of a bladder mass/wall thickness, and the clinical impact for the dog was alleviation of clinical signs (Wiley and colleagues, unpublished data [manuscript in prep], 2019). These data indicate that large changes in the CADET® *BRAF* mutational level detected in the urine over time may be used as an indicator of changes in tumor size and proliferation. Conversely, a marked increase in levels of the CADET® *BRAF* mutation over time during treatment might suggest that treatment is not curbing proliferation of TCC/UC (Wiley and colleagues, unpublished data [manuscript in prep], 2019). If the level of the CADET® *BRAF* mutation has substantially decreased during treatment and begins to increase after treatment, an increase in proliferation is suggested and indicates potential relapse. Serial monitoring of the CADET® *BRAF* mutation may also provide another metric for assessing chemotherapeutic efficacy when ultrasonography suggests stable disease. Although more studies are needed to confirm these findings, these combined data provide early insight into the use of this liquid biopsy as means to monitor residual disease in the patient, both during treatment and during remission.

Identification of metastases In dogs with TCC/UC harboring the CADET® *BRAF* mutation, metastases and neoplastic effusions also harbor the mutation (Wise and colleagues, unpublished data [manuscript in prep], 2019). Preliminary evaluation of metastases to various organs including lymph nodes, lungs, and adrenal glands in dogs with histologically confirmed diagnosis of metastatic TCC/UC demonstrates that metastases share similar genetic signatures, including genome-wide DNA copy number profiles and the CADET® *BRAF* mutation (Wise and colleagues, unpublished data [manuscript in prep], 2019). Furthermore, the *BRAF* mutation has been detected in neoplastic pleural effusion and peritoneal effusions. This provides opportunity to utilize the CADET *BRAF* to identify metastases in cases of ambiguous cytology or histopathology.

Targeted therapy Current treatment of canine TCC/UC includes the use of chemotherapy, cyclooxygenase inhibitors, radiation therapy, surgery, and combinations of these treatments. Where single agent therapy is used, the proportion of dogs entering remission is generally low (<20%), although this is increased to 35% to 50% with combined chemotherapy and cyclooxygenase inhibitors.[19] Dogs treated with single-agent NSAID therapy have a median survival time of approximately 6 to 7 months, whereas a combination of cytotoxic chemotherapy (typically mitoxantrone) and an NSAID yields median survival times closer to 10 months.[19] Although less common than drug-based intervention, surgery and radiation therapy are also used when appropriate. Addition of full-course intensity-modulated and image-guided radiation therapy is associated with a 60% response rate, and a median survival time of greater than 21 months.[23] Partial cystectomy offers similar results when combined with NSAID therapy, resulting in a median survival time of 25 months.[24]

The identification of the CADET® *BRAF* mutation in canine TCC/UC has led to the evaluation of a selective *BRAF* inhibitor in canine TCC/UC, and early results are encouraging. A phase 1/2 clinical trial of single-agent vermurafenib (Zelboraf, Genentech, San Francisco, CA) therapy for canine TCC/UC is still ongoing (Knapp, unpublished data, 2018). At the time of the writing of this article, in that trial, tumor responses were assessable in 31 dogs, noting a remission rate (≥50% decrease in tumor volume and no new tumor lesions) of 12 out of 31 (39%) dogs, stable disease (<50% change in tumor volume and no new tumor lesions) in 17 of 31 dogs (55%), and progressive disease (≥50% increase in tumor volume and no new tumor lesions) in 2 of 31 dogs (6%). The current median progression-free interval is 152 days (range 29 to 767 days), and the current median survival is 204 days (range 29 to 767 + days).[25] This remission rate is the highest achieved with single-agent therapy and is expected to increase with a combination of drug protocols.[19,25] Adverse events reported include mild-to-moderate anorexia and the development of cutaneous masses. Contrary to most cytotoxic cancer drugs, this targeted therapy did not result in any myelosuppression. This selective *BRAF* inhibitor shows promise to improve quality of life and survival of dogs with *BRAF* positive TCC/UC.

CADET® BRAF-PLUS

Further work by the authors' group at NC State identified that canine TCC/UC is also associated with highly recurrent DNA copy number aberrations involving segments of dog chromosomes 13, 19, and 36.[18] These data were used to develop a second molecular assay, CADET® *BRAF*-PLUS, that uses the same liquid biopsy processed for CADET® *BRAF*. Instead of detecting a mutant allele, however, this assay assesses specific DNA copy number aberrations through 2 relative ratios, comparing chromosome segments of both 36 and 13 independently to a segment of chromosome 19. This assay is recommended as an aid for diagnosis of TCC/UC in dogs with clinical signs, and is less useful as a preclinical screening assay. Analysis of thousands of urine specimens from dogs with and without TCC/UC indicated that the specific combination of these copy number changes could be detected in over two-thirds of cases of canine TCC/UC where the dog had clinical signs, but was not associated with the presence of a *BRAF* mutation. Because this population of dogs represents 15% of all cases of canine TCC/UC, CADET® *BRAF*-PLUS increases the combined biological sensitivity to detect a canine TCC/UC from a free-catch urine specimen to over 95%, and also has a specificity of greater than 99%.

Multipurpose Liquid Biopsy

Cell blocks

Bodily fluids can be converted into biopsies through the creation of a formalin fixed cell block. Several techniques have been described in veterinary medicine, including embedding specimens with paraffin,[26–28] HistoGel,[29] surgical gel foam,[30] or agarose.[28,31,32]

The fixation process maintains cell cluster architecture, facilitates immunohistochemistry, and preserves samples.

However, this strategy has a longer turnaround time for diagnosis than traditional cytology or other liquid biopsy techniques.

Because of its ease of preparation, the cell tube block technique has the potential for widespread application in private practice.[27] To prepare a cell tube block, plain type capillary tubes are filled with liquid samples and centrifuged in a microhematocrit centrifuge. Then, tubes are broken at the liquid-solid interface, fixed in formalin for 24 hours, and embedded in paraffin.[27] This process produces an enriched neoplastic cell layer, which has the benefits for immunohistochemistry and molecular characterization.[27]

Minimally Invasive/Liquid Biopsy for Lymphoid Malignancies

Polymerase chain reaction for antigen receptor rearrangement

Although the PCR for antigen receptor rearrangement (PARR) assay is primarily used for phenotyping lymphoma as B cell versus T cell, this test can confirm lymphoma or leukemia in samples with ambiguous cytologic or histologic morphology.[12] The PARR assay assesses clonality of the lymphocytes by using PCR to determine the length of the immunoglobulin genes in B cells or T-cell receptor genes in T cells.[33] The PARR assay is capable of detecting 1:100 neoplastic cells.[33] False-positive results are rare, but possible with some infectious diseases, such as *Ehrlichia canis* or Panola Mountain *Ehrlichia sp.*[33] Although sensitivity and specificity can vary with laboratories, a recent study of a large patient cohort of 271 dogs determined that the sensitivity and specificity of PARR for diagnosing canine lymphoma are 86.5% and 98.7%, respectively.[34] For this assay, DNA is first isolated from neoplastic cells obtained from blood, cytology samples, or tissue samples, including formalin-fixed paraffin-embedded tissues. PCR amplifies the variable region of T-cell receptor or immunoglobulin genes, and PCR products are separated by size.[12] Detection of a single-sized PCR product suggests clonality, whereas the detection of multiple PCR products supports a reactive process.[12]

Flow cytometry

Flow cytometry is another minimally invasive method used to diagnose and immunophenotype lymphoma or leukemia using liquid samples obtained from blood or fine needle aspirates injected into cell culture media.[12] Briefly, flow cytometry involves marking cells with antibodies conjugated to fluorescent proteins. A specific wavelength of light excites the fluorescent protein, and sophisticated imaging equipment sorts cells based on relative fluorescence. Multiple antibodies can be used with this versatile technology. Although some proteins, such as CD45, are expressed on the surface of all lymph cells, others are typically restricted to subpopulations of T cells (eg, CD3) and B cells (eg, CD79a, CD20). More specific reagents can also be used to determine the proportion of each subtype in a population of cells.[12]

Minimally Invasive Biopsy for Histiocytic Malignancies

CADET® HM

Histiocytic malignancies (HMs) share many cytologic and histologic features with other round cell neoplasia, and as many as 70% of cases initially diagnosed as HM may be misclassified.[35,36] Distinction between HM and plasma cell tumors can be particularly challenging. CADET® HM is a new molecular tool for facilitating a quick and accurate diagnosis of HM, potentially without the need for tissue biopsies. Small samples enriched for tumor cells, such as from effusions or fine needle aspirates, may be used to perform this assay, and of course histologic samples can also be used. The assay determines the number of copies of a region of the canine genome and is based on data indicating that reduction in copy number is consistent with a canine HM.[37] CADET® HM has been validated with over 500 unique, pathology-verified canine cancer specimens from HM and multiple other similar tumor types, including lymphoma, plasma cell tumors, hemangiosarcoma, amelanotic melanoma, and mast cell tumors. Use of this assay offers sensitivity of 78% and specificity of 95% to detect a canine HM. This genetic signature is a highly sensitive and accurate marker for distinction of canine HM from these other tumor types.

SUMMARY

With the advent of new advancements in molecular technologies, liquid biopsies and minimally invasive sampling techniques are starting to become available for veterinary medicine. Cell blocks, PARR, flow cytometry, and the CADET® assays are designed to complement other diagnostics. Noninvasive diagnostics are also being used as monitoring tools to assess changes in the level of mutant cells, which may be an indicator of the efficacy of therapy and a guide to aid identification of impending relapse. As in human medicine, it is expected that more noninvasive tests will soon be available to guide therapeutic choices in veterinary medicine.

ACKNOWLEDGMENT

The authors wish to thank the North Carolina State University Cancer Genomics fund for their generous financial support.

REFERENCES

1. Diaz LA Jr, Bardelli A. Liquid biopsies: genotyping circulating tumor DNA. J Clin Oncol 2014;32(6):579–86.
2. Neoh KH, Hassan AA, Chen A, et al. Rethinking liquid biopsy: microfluidic assays for mobile tumor cells in human body fluids. Biomaterials 2018;150:112–24.
3. Beaver JA, Jelovac D, Balukrishna S, et al. Detection of cancer DNA in plasma of patients with early-stage breast cancer. Clin Cancer Res 2014;20(10):2643–50.
4. Wimberger P, Roth C, Pantel K, et al. Impact of platinum-based chemotherapy on circulating nucleic acid levels, protease activities in blood and disseminated tumor cells in bone marrow of ovarian cancer patients. Int J Cancer 2011;128(11): 2572–80.
5. Siravegna G, Bardelli A. Genotyping cell-free tumor DNA in the blood to detect residual disease and drug resistance. Genome Biol 2014;15(8):449.
6. Bettegowda C, Sausen M, Leary RJ, et al. Detection of circulating tumor DNA in early- and late-stage human malignancies. Sci Transl Med 2014;6(224):224ra224.
7. Mochizuki H, Kennedy K, Shapiro SG, et al. BRAF mutations in canine cancers. PLoS One 2015;10(6):e0129534.
8. Decker B, Parker HG, Dhawan D, et al. Homologous mutation to human BRAF V600E is common in naturally occurring canine bladder cancer–evidence for a relevant model system and urine-based diagnostic test. Mol Cancer Res 2015; 13(6):993–1002.

9. Mochizuki H, Shapiro SG, Breen M. Detection of BRAF mutation in urine DNA as a molecular diagnostic for canine urothelial and prostatic carcinoma. PLoS One 2015;10(12):e0144170.
10. Bell F, Klausner J, Hayden D, et al. Clinical and pathologic features of prostatic adenocarcinoma in sexually intact and castrated dogs: 31 cases (1970-1987). J Am Vet Med Assoc 1991;199:1623–30.
11. Powe J, Canfield P, Martin P. Evaluation of the cytologic diagnosis of canine prostatic disorders. Vet Clin Pathol 2004;33:150–4.
12. Knapp D, McMillan S. Tumors of the urinary system. In: Withrow SJ, Vail DM, Rodney LP, editors. Withrow and MacEwen's small animal clinical oncology. 5th edition. St Louis (MO): Elsevier-Saunders; 2013. p. 572–82.
13. Zinkl J. Examination of the urinary sediment. In: Cowell R, Meinkoth J, Denicola D, editors. Diagnostic cytology and hematology of the dog and cat. 3rd edition. Maryland Heights (MO): Mosby; 2008. p. 350–68.
14. Higuchi T, Burcham GN, Childress MO, et al. Characterization and treatment of transitional cell carcinoma of the abdominal wall in dogs: 24 cases (1985-2010). J Am Vet Med Assoc 2013;242(4):499–506.
15. Nyland TG, Wallack ST, Wisner ER. Needle-tract implantation following us-guided fine-needle aspiration biopsy of transitional cell carcinoma of the bladder, urethra, and prostate. Vet Radiol Ultrasound 2002;43(1):50–3.
16. Bartges JW. Diagnosis of urinary tract infections. Vet Clin North Am Small Anim Pract 2004;34(4):923–33, vi.
17. American Veterinary Medical Association. U.S. pet ownership & demographics sourcebook. Schaumburg (IL): American Veterinary Medical Association; 2012.
18. Shapiro SG, Raghunath S, Williams C, et al. Canine urothelial carcinoma: genomically aberrant and comparatively relevant. Chromosome Res 2015;23(2):311–31.
19. Knapp DW, Ramos-Vara JA, Moore GE, et al. Urinary bladder cancer in dogs, a naturally occurring model for cancer biology and drug development. ILAR J 2014;55(1):100–18.
20. Fulkerson CM, Knapp DW. Management of transitional cell carcinoma of the urinary bladder in dogs: a review. Vet J 2015;205(2):217–25.
21. Patrick D, Fitzgerald S, Sesterhenn A, et al. Classification of canine urinary bladder urothelial tumours based on the World Health Organization/International Society of Urological Pathology consensus classification. J Comp Pathol 2006; 135:190–9.
22. Knapp D, Glickman N, Denicola D, et al. Naturally-occurring canine transitional cell carcinoma of the urinary bladder: a relevant model of human invasive bladder cancer. Urol Oncol 2000;5:47–59.
23. Nolan MW, Kogan L, Griffin LR, et al. Intensity-modulated and image-guided radiation therapy for treatment of genitourinary carcinomas in dogs. J Vet Intern Med 2012;26(4):987–95.
24. Marvel SJ, Seguin B, Dailey DD, et al. Clinical outcome of partial cystectomy for transitional cell carcinoma of the canine bladder. Vet Comp Oncol 2017;15(4): 1417–27.
25. Knapp DW. Antitumor effects, safety, and mechanisms of resistance of BRAF-targeted therapy in dogs with naturally-occurring invasive urothelial carcinoma. Paper presented at: American College of Veterinary Pathology Annual Meeting. Washington, DC, November 7, 2018.
26. Taylor BE, Leibman NF, Luong R, et al. Detection of carcinoma micrometastases in bone marrow of dogs and cats using conventional and cell block cytology. Vet Clin Pathol 2013;42(1):85–91.

27. Marcos R, Santos M, Marrinhas C, et al. Cell tube block: a new technique to produce cell blocks from fluid cytology samples. Vet Clin Pathol 2017;46(1):195–201.
28. Fernandes NC, Guerra JM, Ressio RA, et al. Liquid-based cytology and cell block immunocytochemistry in veterinary medicine: comparison with standard cytology for the evaluation of canine lymphoid samples. Vet Comp Oncol 2016; 14(Suppl 1):107–16.
29. Joiner KS, Spangler EA. Evaluation of HistoGel-embedded specimens for use in veterinary diagnostic pathology. J Vet Diagn Invest 2012;24(4):710–5.
30. Wallace KA, Goldschmidt MH, Patel RT. Converting fluid-based cytologic specimens to histologic specimens for immunohistochemistry. Vet Clin Pathol 2015; 44(2):303–9.
31. Zanoni DS, Grandi F, Cagnini DQ, et al. Agarose cell block technique as a complementary method in the diagnosis of fungal osteomyelitis in a dog. Open Vet J 2012;2(1):19–22.
32. Zanoni DS, Grandi F, Rocha NS. Use of the agarose cell block technique in veterinary diagnostic cytopathology: an "old and forgotten" method. Vet Clin Pathol 2012;41(3):307–8.
33. Burnett RC, Vernau W, Modiano JF, et al. Diagnosis of canine lymphoid neoplasia using clonal rearrangements of antigen receptor genes. Vet Pathol 2003;40(1): 32–41.
34. Waugh EM, Gallagher A, Haining H, et al. Optimisation and validation of a PCR for antigen receptor rearrangement (PARR) assay to detect clonality in canine lymphoid malignancies. Vet Immunol Immunopathol 2016;182:115–24.
35. Pazdzior-Czapula K, Otrocka-Domagala I, Rotkiewicz T, et al. Cytomorphometry of canine cutaneous histiocytoma. Pol J Vet Sci 2014;17(3):413–20.
36. Dervisis NG, Kiupel M, Qin Q, et al. Clinical prognostic factors in canine histiocytic sarcoma. Vet Comp Oncol 2017;15(4):1171–80.
37. Kennedy K, Thomas R, Durrant J, et al. Genome-wide DNA copy number analysis and targeted transcriptional analysis of canine histiocytic malignancies identifies diagnostic signatures and highlights disruption of spindle assembly complex. Chromosome Res 2019. https://doi.org/10.1007/s10577-019-09606-0.

Nonselective Lymph Node Dissection and Sentinel Lymph Node Mapping and Biopsy

Julius M. Liptak, BVSc, MVetClinStud, FACVSc[a,*],
Sarah E. Boston, DVM, DVSc[b]

KEYWORDS

• Lymph node • Sentinel lymph node • Indirect lymphography

KEY POINTS

- Lymph node staging is diagnostically and therapeutically important and is often important in determining the prognosis.
- For clinical staging purposes, the regional lymph node or nodes can be excised based on expected lymphatic drainage patterns or the sentinel lymph node can be identified and specifically excised.
- Peripheral lymph nodes are often excised based on the expected lymphatic drainage of the region and the accessibility of the lymph node and potential morbidity of lymph node excision.
- The sentinel lymph node is the first draining lymph node and is representative of the entire lymphatic bed, and the sentinel lymph node is frequently different to the regional anatomic lymph node because lymphatic drainage is variable and unpredictable.
- Sentinel lymph node mapping techniques include contrast-enhanced ultrasonography, lymphoscintigraphy, intraoperative peritumoral injection of blue dye, intraoperative peritumoral injection of a radiocolloid, and indirect lymphography.

INTRODUCTION

Lymph node evaluation is an important part of staging for neoplasia in human and veterinary patients and is an important predictor of prognosis in many tumor types.[1–3] Metastasis to the draining lymph node also may predict the potential for distant metastasis,[4] and lymph node removal may be therapeutic as well as diagnostic in some cases.[5–8] Clinical methods of lymph node evaluation include palpation and lymph node measurement, fine-needle aspiration, imaging with ultrasound or

Disclosure Statement: The authors have nothing to disclose.
[a] VCA Canada – Alta Vista Animal Hospital, 2616 Bank Street, Ottawa, Ontario K1T 1M9, Canada; [b] VCA Canada, 404 Veterinary Emergency and Referral Hospital, 510 Harry Walker Parkway South, Newmarket, Ontario L3Y 0B3, Canada
* Corresponding author.
E-mail address: animalcancersurgeon@icloud.com

Vet Clin Small Anim 49 (2019) 793–807
https://doi.org/10.1016/j.cvsm.2019.04.003 vetsmall.theclinics.com
0195-5616/19/

computed tomography (CT), and histopathology.[9–16] Several studies in the veterinary literature have shown that palpation characteristics and cytology alone lack sensitivity and specificity in the evaluation of patients for metastasis to the lymph nodes.[9,13,16,17] A recent study evaluating the clinical utility of lymph node cytology for staging solid tumors in dogs found that the sensitivity was low for sarcoma, melanoma, and mast cell tumors but high for carcinomas and other round cell tumors.[16] CT is often used clinically to evaluate lymph nodes for metastatic disease. This method has shown clinical utility in the evaluation of tracheobronchial lymph node metastasis in dogs with pulmonary carcinoma.[10,11] Abdominal ultrasound and CT are routinely used to assess for metastatic disease to the medial ilial and sacral lymph centers in dogs with apocrine gland anal sac adenocarcinoma (AGASAC) (**Fig. 1**).[18–20] A recent study evaluating the diagnostic accuracy of contrast-enhanced CT for assessment of lymph node metastasis in dogs with tumors of the head reported a sensitivity and specificity of 11.6% and 94.0%, respectively; a positive and negative predictive value of 41.7% and 74.3%, respectively; and an overall accuracy of 71.9% (**Fig. 2**).[15] Regardless, histopathology remains the gold standard for the assessment of lymph nodes for metastatic disease, and other methods of evaluation for metastatic disease may lack accuracy.

The surgical removal of the lymph nodes that drain the head has been described in dogs, with 3 reported approaches for elective lymph node dissection (**Fig. 3**).[14,21–23]

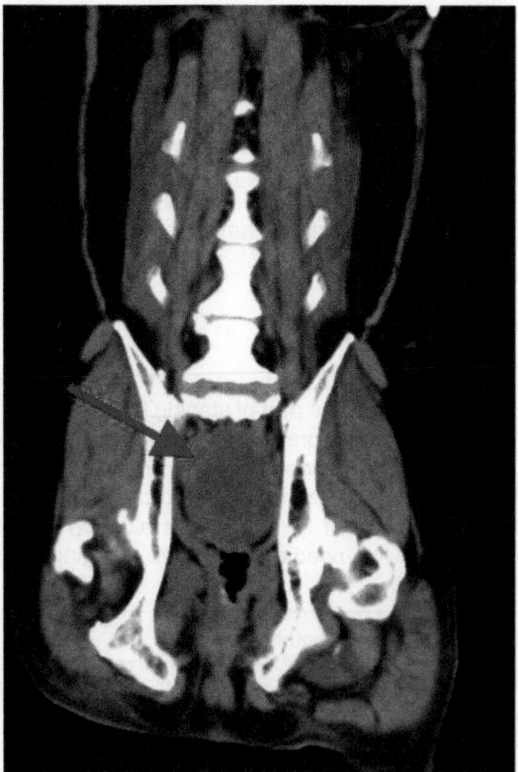

Fig. 1. CT scan of a dog with an apocrine gland anal gland adenocarcinoma and metastasis to the medial iliac lymph node (*arrow*). CT scan is more accurate for the detection of metastatic intraabdominal lymph nodes, especially sacral lymph nodes within the pelvic canal.

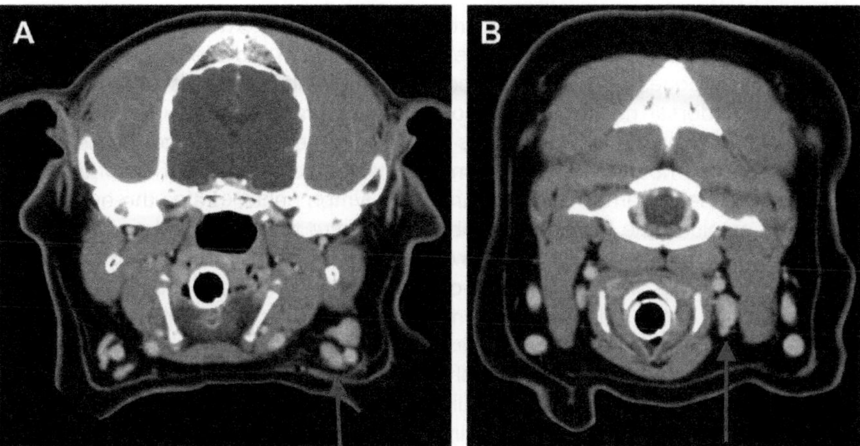

Fig. 2. CT of the skull of a dog showing (*A*) the mandibular lymph node (*arrow*) and (*B*) the medial retropharyngeal lymph node (*arrow*). Malignant tumors of the oral cavity and head most commonly metastasize to the mandibular and medial retropharyngeal lymph nodes.

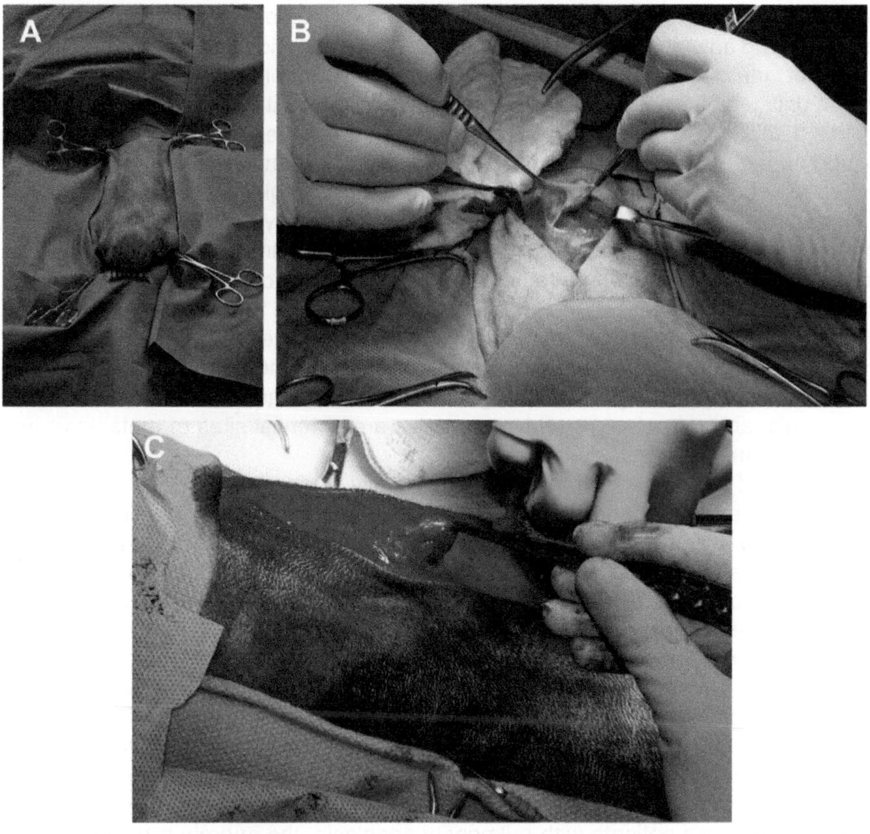

Fig. 3. (*A*) Positioning of a dog in dorsal recumbency before elective lymph node dissection for bilateral removal of the mandibular and medial retropharyngeal lymph nodes via a single incision. Elective extirpation of one of the (*B*) mandibular and (*C*) medial retropharyngeal lymph nodes via a single incision.

The lymph centers of interest are the parotid, mandibular, and medial retropharyngeal lymph centers.[24] The parotid lymph node drains the dorsal and lateral structures of the head, the dorsal bones of the skull, the contents of the orbit, the masticatory muscles, and the caudodorsal muzzle of the dog.[24] Consideration should be given to the removal of this lymph node for tumors that are in these regions of the head. The mandibular lymph nodes are most commonly sampled because of their peripheral location and ease of sampling. The mandibular lymph center drains the eyelids, the skin of the cranium, the temporomandibular joint, the tongue, the pharynx, and the floor of the oral cavity.[24] The lymphatics of the floor of the oral cavity cross at random points and may drain either ipsilaterally or contralaterally.[24] The medial retropharyngeal lymph center is not palpable and is more difficult to access surgically, but it is an important lymph center for clinical staging as it is one of the collecting centers of the head. The medial retropharyngeal lymph center drains the tongue; walls of the oral, nasal, and pharyngeal cavities; the salivary glands; the deep external ear; larynx; esophagus; and deep nasal cavity.[24] Importantly, it also receives lymph from the lateral retropharyngeal, parotid, and mandibular lymph centers.[24] It is important to consider the region of the head of interest when considering the most appropriate lymph node dissection technique.

One approach to lymph node dissection for tumors of the head describes the ipsilateral removal of the mandibular, parotid, and medial retropharyngeal lymph nodes.[21] The advantage to this approach is that the parotid lymph node is sampled. However, the disadvantage is that the contralateral lymph nodes are not sampled with a unilateral approach and hence sampling of the contralateral lymph nodes requires a second surgical approach. An alternative approach for the removal of the lymph nodes of the head and neck involves removal of the mandibular and medial retropharyngeal lymph nodes bilaterally through a single ventral incision.[14,22,23] This technique has several advantages, including the ability to evaluate the ipsilateral and contralateral lymph centers, the ability to place Rummel tourniquets via the same incision for cases where removal of the primary tumor may result in significant blood loss, and, in some cases, the patient may not need to be repositioned during the removal of the primary tumor.[14,22,23] A recent study evaluating the patterns of metastasis following the removal of the mandibular and retropharyngeal lymph nodes bilaterally in dogs with malignancies of the head showed that both the mandibular and retropharyngeal lymph nodes are potential sites of metastasis and that contralateral metastasis is common.[14]

Removal of a peripheral lymph node is generally straightforward. The approach to each of these lymph centers has been described.[25] In general, a skin incision is made directly over the lymph node and a combination of blunt dissection and electrocautery are used with a goal of remaining outside of the lymph node capsule.[25] The vasculature to the hilus of the lymph node can either be cauterized or be ligated.[25] Closure of the surgical site is routine.

The decision to remove suspected or confirmed metastatic lymph nodes from within a body cavity is more complicated compared with peripheral lymph node extirpation, and careful assessment of the potential morbidity, risks, and benefits of lymph node extirpation must be considered. For dogs with pulmonary carcinoma, tracheobronchial lymph node metastasis has been shown to be prognostic for survival,[26] and the tracheobronchial lymph nodes are routinely removed at the time of primary tumor removal. In human patients with pulmonary neoplasia, the approach to lymph node dissection is determined by the lung lobe affected and is a directed lymph node dissection.[27,28] In veterinary oncology, tracheobronchial lymph node removal is less precise and usually only accessible and/or enlarged tracheobronchial lymph nodes are extirpated.[3] Removal of the tracheobronchial lymph nodes via an open approach to the thorax is accomplished by palpation of the lymph node directly and blunt dissection about the lymph node. Care is taken to avoid damaging the structures in this area, notably the aorta, pulmonary vasculature, and bronchus (**Fig. 4**). If lung lobectomy is performed by thoracoscopy, one potential drawback is that lymph node removal is more complicated via this approach. However, removal of the tracheobronchial lymph nodes via thoracoscopy has been described.[29]

AGASAC in dogs will frequently metastasize to the iliosacral lymph centers.[5,6,18–20,30] Despite often substantial metastatic disease to the lymph nodes within the abdomen in dogs with AGASAC, removal of the primary mass and metastatic lymph nodes is recommended because this results in a significant improvement in survival times.[5,6] When the lymph nodes are grossly enlarged, the decision to extirpate the lymph nodes is straightforward, especially as the enlarged medial iliac lymph nodes may contribute to the clinical signs associated with rectal obstruction.[5,6,30] When the lymph nodes are not considered metastatic based on preoperative imaging, elective lymph node dissection is generally not performed primarily due to increased surgical time and patient morbidity without a documented clinical benefit. The use of laparoscopy to assess and remove these lymph nodes has been reported and may decrease the morbidity of this procedure.[31]

In human surgical oncology, there has been an increasing trend away from dissection of a specific lymph node or regional lymph node beds in preference for sentinel lymph node (SLN) mapping and biopsy.[32,33] There are several theoretic and practical drawbacks to nonselective lymph node dissection techniques, including incomplete staging with a risk of missing metastatic lymph nodes and a greater potential for postoperative morbidity and complications with no associated survival benefit.[32–34]

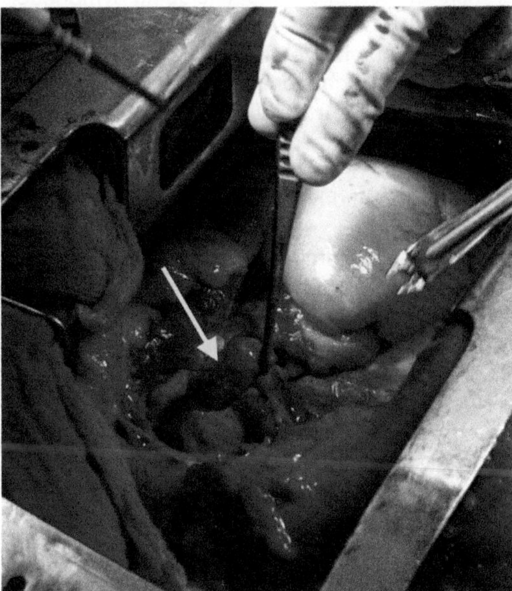

Fig. 4. Left lateral thoracotomy following lung lobectomy for a primary bronchoalveolar carcinoma (cranial is toward the left top corner of image). A tracheobronchial lymph node is being removed for clinical staging purposes (*arrow*).

One of the concerns with nonselective lymph node extirpation is that lymphatic drainage patterns are not uniform or predictable. Single afferent lymphatic vessels can drain into a single lymph node, multiple afferent lymphatic vessels can drain into a single lymph node, and single divergent or multiple afferent lymphatic vessels can drain into more than one lymph node.[35] In people, preoperative scintigraphy has identified aberrant lymphatic drainage in 48%, 23%, 12%, and 8% of patients with melanomas of the head and neck, trunk, upper extremities, and lower extremities, respectively.[35] A similar finding was reported in dogs with mammary tumors.[36] Furthermore, there is indirect evidence of a similar lack of uniformity in lymphatic drainage in other anatomic regions in dogs and cats. In veterinary medicine, the regional anatomic lymph node is often aspirated or biopsied to determine the absence or presence of metastatic disease; however, because of the possibility of aberrant lymphatic drainage from the tumor, the regional anatomic lymph node may not be the first draining lymph node (or SLN). In a study of 19 dogs with cutaneous mast cell tumors, 8 dogs (42%) had SLNs different to the regional anatomic lymph node.[37] As previously described, the regional lymph nodes for head tumors include the mandibular, parotid, and medial retropharyngeal lymph nodes; however, the parotid and medial retropharyngeal lymph nodes are not externally palpable. In one study, only 55% of 31 cats and dogs with oral tumors and metastasis to the regional lymph nodes had metastasis to the mandibular lymph nodes, with metastasis to the medial retropharyngeal and parotid lymph nodes in the remaining cases.[38] Hence, approximately 45% of animals with cutaneous mast cell tumors and oral tumors would have had the incorrect lymph node sampled and metastatic disease missed if only the regional anatomic lymph node was aspirated or biopsied.

Extensive nonselective lymph node dissections were commonly performed in women with breast, vulvar, cervical, and endometrial cancer for clinical staging purposes to avoid missing potential metastatic lymph nodes; however, this was associated with a higher risk of complications (including lymphedema, lymphocysts, wound dehiscence, nerve disruption, and chronic pain), longer hospitalization times, long-term morbidity, and no survival benefit.[39–45] As discussed earlier, similar approaches have been described in cats and dogs, especially with oral tumors.[14,21–23] Although the complication rate is not significantly greater with these more extensive lymph node dissections, each described approach has the potential to miss metastatic lymph nodes. The unilateral approach for extirpation of the ipsilateral mandibular, medial retropharyngeal, and parotid lymph nodes[21] misses metastasis to the contralateral lymph nodes, which has been reported in 62% of dogs with malignant oral tumors.[14] Dissection of the ipsilateral and contralateral mandibular and medial retropharyngeal lymph nodes has been described[14,22,23]; however, this approach does not include the parotid lymph nodes and metastasis to the parotid lymph node has been documented.[38] Furthermore, the buccal lymph node was identified as the SLN in a cat with a malignant melanoma of the lip by one of the authors (JML) (**Fig. 5**).

To minimize the risk of these less discriminate approaches, SLN mapping and biopsy techniques have been developed in human medicine for many different tumor types and are increasingly being adopted in veterinary medicine. The SLN is an important concept in surgical oncology and has been described as the "most pervasive innovation in surgical oncology."[32] The SLN concept is based on the theory that the metastatic process occurs in an orderly progression within the lymphatic system with tumor cells draining into a specific lymph node (ie, SLN) in a regional lymphatic field before draining into other regional lymph nodes.[41,46] The SLN has an important role as a filter and barrier for disseminating tumor cells.[46] Conceptually, distant metastasis should not be present if the SLN does not have evidence of a tumor

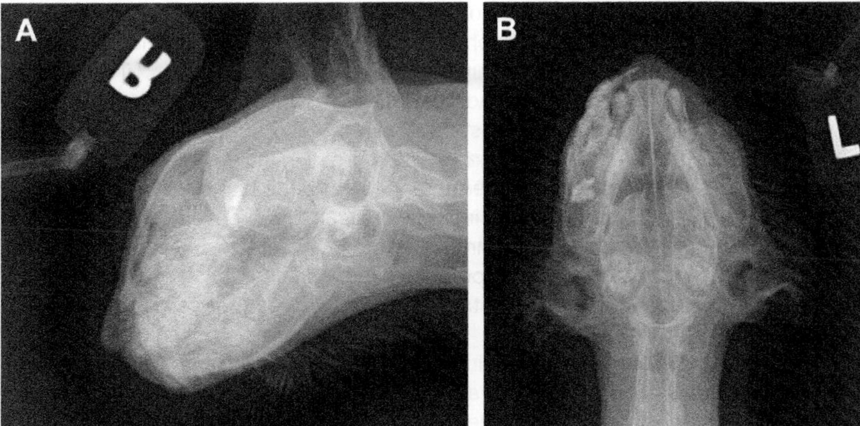

Fig. 5. Indirect lymphography with 4-quadrant peritumoral injection of Lipiodol in a cat with an incompletely excised malignant melanoma of the lip. Regional lateral (*A*) and ventrodorsal (*B*) radiographs of the head 24 hours post-Lipiodol injection show that the SLN is the buccal lymph node. This case illustrates the importance of SLN mapping in the clinical staging of patients with malignant tumors because the lymphatic drainage of malignant tumors is not predictable and routine sampling of the regional anatomic lymph node can miss potentially metastatic lymph nodes.

burden, but distant metastasis is possible if the SLN has histologic evidence of metastatic tumor cells. Hence, the status of the SLN may reflect the status of the entire regional lymphatic bed; the probability that a non-SLN is positive for metastatic disease when the SLN is free of tumor is less than 0.1%.[46,47] SLNs are successfully identified in more than 94% to 99% of women with breast cancer,[40,41,45,48] 97% of women with endometrial cancer,[49] 98% of people with squamous cell carcinoma of the tongue,[50] and 94% of patients with gastric cancer.[51,52] The SLN is not specific for tumor type or location, and it changes from patient to patient. In people, identification of the SLN is important in the diagnosis of lymph node metastasis, early identification of patients requiring additional therapeutic options to manage metastatic disease (such as more extensive lymph node dissection and adjuvant chemotherapy or radiation therapy), and establishing a prognosis.[40,41] Similarly, 42% of dogs with cutaneous mast cell tumors were offered additional treatments as a result of their SLN biopsy results that otherwise would not have been discussed.[37] In one study of nonselective bilateral mandibular and medial retropharyngeal lymph node extirpation in dogs with oral tumors, 31% of dogs had metastasis to all 4 extirpated lymph nodes[14]; theoretically, animals with metastatic SLNs would be candidates for more extensive dissections of the regional lymph node bed. Despite the importance of SLNs in numerous types of cancer in human oncology (including head and neck cancer, breast cancer, cutaneous melanoma, gastric carcinoma, colon cancer, and genitourinary cancers), this concept is just beginning to be investigated and accepted in veterinary medicine.

SLNs can be identified using several techniques, including contrast-enhanced ultrasonography; lymphoscintigraphy; peritumoral injection of blue dye or indocyanine green; and intraoperative cytology, histopathology, or one-step nucleic acid amplification.[40,41,45,53–55] The use of preoperative lymphoscintigraphy has been reported in both human and veterinary medicine. In human medicine, the advantages of preoperative lymphoscintigraphy include documentation of the lymphatic drainage pattern and the number of SLNs, and for surgical planning because the location of the SLN is known before surgery.[41] Lymphoscintigraphy using 99m-technetium dextran has been used to investigate mammary lymphatic drainage in dogs.[36] This showed a wide variety of lymphatic drainage and SLN locations with the first and second mammary glands draining into the cranial sternal, axillary, and superficial cervical lymph nodes, and the fourth and fifth mammary glands draining into the superficial inguinal and medial iliac lymph nodes.[36] Furthermore, 44% of dogs had communications between lymph nodes. Disadvantages include cost and decreased sensitivity when compared with an intraoperative gamma probe as radioactive SLNs are frequently identified in cases with negative preoperative lymphoscintigraphy scans.[41] In veterinary medicine, an additional disadvantage is the limited number of facilities with nuclear medicine capabilities.

In people, the most commonly used intraoperative SLN mapping techniques include peritumoral injections of a radioactive isotope and/or a blue dye, although near-infrared imaging with indocyanine green dye is becoming more popular.[45] The SLN mapping learning curve and identification rate are significantly improved when both techniques are used in combination.[40,41] Technetium 99m-labelled sulfur colloid is the preferred isotope for SLN mapping, although others have been described.[40,41] Successful identification of the radioactive isotope depends on isotope uptake from the peritumoral tissue by lymphatics and the transit time to the SLN.[40] Isotope uptake and transit time depend on the size of the isotope and the volume of the injection.[40] Uptake and transit time are quicker with smaller particulate size and larger volumes of injection. The transit of radiocolloids will often terminate in the first SLN, which ensures better identification of the SLN, whereas blue dyes have the potential to pass into secondary echelon lymph nodes.[40] There are several disadvantages with the use of radioactive isotopes, including legislation governing the administration of radiopharmaceuticals to patients and the handling of radioactive materials.[41,45] Furthermore, the use of radiocolloids results in radioactive contamination of all swabs and drapes used during surgery (and hence protocols need to be designed to appropriately deal with these waste materials), and surgeons and surgical staff need to be appropriately trained to manage waste.[41,45] Lastly, for veterinary medicine, these facilities are not widely available and the gamma probe used intraoperatively is expensive.

The peritumoral injection of a blue dye enables the surgeon to identify blue-stained lymphatic tracts draining from the tumor (**Fig. 6**) and, by following these tracts, allows identification of the SLN. Several dyes have been used for this purpose (such as patent blue dye, isosulphan blue, and methylene blue), and all have the common characteristic of weak binding to albumin, which permits their absorption into the lymphatics and delineation of the lymphatic drainage of tumors.[40,41,45] Patent blue dye and isosulphan blue can both result in allergies, ranging from skin rashes to life-threatening anaphylaxis, in 1% to 3% of people.[40,41,45] Methylene blue is associated with a lower risk of allergies but can induce an intense tissue reaction, which may result in skin necrosis if injected superficially.[40,41,45] The risks of allergies and tissue reactions have not been evaluated in cats and dogs. The injection of blue dye causes skin staining, which typically lasts several months, but may also cause permanent tattooing. The intraoperative evaluation of surgical margins can be difficult following peritumoral injection of blue dye (**Fig. 7**) and hence the marking of surgical margins with a sterile permanent marker pen is recommended before SLN mapping with a blue dye. All blue dyes enter the circulation, which may make patients seem cyanotic and interfere with pulse oximetry.[40,41,45] The blue dye is excreted in urine postoperatively and hence urine may seem discolored.[41]

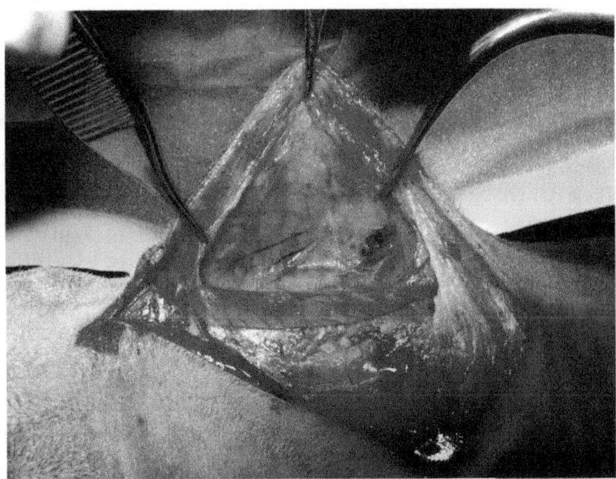

Fig. 6. Intraoperative image following 4-quadrant periturmoral injection of methylene blue. The afferent lymphatics draining the tumor and the SLN are discolored blue; this aides in identification of the SLN and, when used in combination with other techniques, increases the accuracy of identifying the SLN.

SLN identification using blue dye alone is a difficult technique to learn and requires a wider surgical exposure to trace the afferent lymphatics to the SLN.[41] Meta-analyses in human oncology shows that the SLN identification rate is lower, and the false-negative rate higher, when using either blue dye alone (86%) or radiocolloid alone

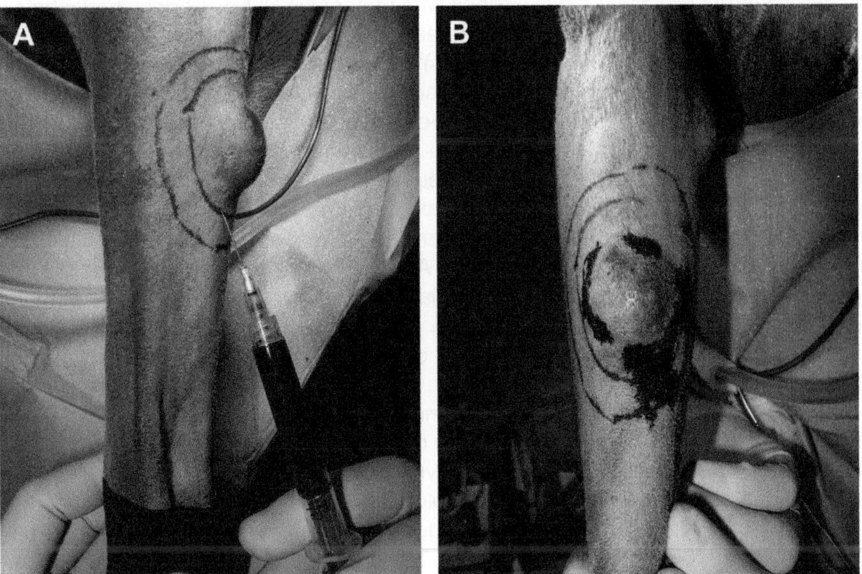

Fig. 7. (*A*) The planned 2 cm lateral surgical margins around a cutaneous mast cell tumor on the antebrachium of a dog are marked with a sterile marker pen and then methylene blue is injected in 4 quadrants peritumorally. (*B*) The methylene blue stains the skin and can make intraoperative identification of tumor margins difficult. Marking the surgical margins before peritumoral methylene blue injection improves identification of the lateral margins required for wide tumor resection.

(86%) compared with a combination of both techniques (96%).[45] In people, the preferred SLN mapping technique involves a combination of intraoperative blue dye and radioisotope as this is easier with a shorter learning curve, surgical dissection is less extensive, the SLN is more likely to be identified, and this is especially so for SLNs in an abnormal location.[41] This has been investigated in 24 dogs with various spontaneous tumors with 89% of SLNs identified using preoperative lymphoscintigraphy, 97% with an intraoperative gamma probe, and 77% with intraoperative blue dye.[56] One of the SLNs missed with the gamma probe was identified with intraoperative blue dye mapping. In a pilot study of 6 dogs, the tracheobronchial SLN was identified in 5 dogs using technetium sulfur colloid and in 3 dogs with isosulphan blue dye.[57] In a clinical study of 7 dogs with lung tumors, the SLN was identified in 5 dogs with a gamma probe and in 2 dogs with methylene blue.[3] The major obstacle to SLN mapping in veterinary medicine is the poor availability of the commonly used radioactive SLN techniques in human medicine, such as lymphoscintigraphy and intraoperative radiocolloids. For this reason, indirect lymphography has been an active area of research in veterinary oncology.

The 2 most common methods are the use of a water-soluble contrast agent (iopamidol) in combination with CT scan imaging[58–61] and the use of a lipid-soluble contrast agent (Lipiodol) in combination with regional radiographs 24 hours after contrast agent injection.[58,62] In one study of 33 dogs with mammary tumors, SLN mapping was performed with 4-quadrant peritumoral injection of 1 mL iopamidol (370 mg/ml).[59] A helical CT scanner was used to acquire 3 mm transverse images at 1 minute and 3 minutes postinjection. Three SLN patterns were identified: homogenous (uniform distribution of contrast agent), heterogenous (nonuniform distribution of contrast agent), and absent. Dogs with homogenous SLN pattern did not have evidence of metastatic nodal disease. Of the 16 dogs with metastatic SLNs, 13 dogs had a heterogenous SLN pattern. In addition, the degree of contrast enhancement (defined as the median absolute density in Hounsfield units) was significantly less in dogs with metastasis compared with dogs without metastasis in their SLNs at both 1 minute and 5 minutes (but better at 1 minute). The size and shape of metastatic and nonmetastatic SLNs were also significantly different with metastatic SLNs having larger minimum and maximum diameters.[59] A similar indirect lymphography technique was reported in 13 dogs with AGASAC[60] and 18 dogs with tumors of oral cavity and head.[61] In the former study, the lymphatic pathway and SLN were identified in 12 dogs (92%) with the SLN being ipsilateral to the local AGASAC in 8 dogs and contralateral in 4 dogs. The SLNs included sacral, internal iliac, and medial iliac lymph nodes.[60] In the latter study, the SLN was identified within 3 minutes of the contrast injection in 16 dogs (89%).[61] The SLN was the superficial cervical lymph node in 1 dog with a pinna tumor and the mandibular lymph node in the remaining dogs; the SLN was ipsilateral in 14 dogs (88%), contralateral in one dog, and bilateral in one dog.[61] In another study, indirect lymphography using a lipid-soluble contrast agent, Lipiodol, was investigated in 29 dogs with 30 tumors.[62] The indirect lymphography technique included 4-quadrant peritumoral injection of up to 2.5 mL Lipiodol (480 mg/mL) under sedation 24 hours before surgery (**Fig. 8**A). On the day of surgery, regional radiographs were performed to identify the SLN preoperatively (**Fig. 8**B). The preoperative SLN mapping was combined with intraoperative 4-quadrant peritumoral injection of 1 to 2 mL of methylene blue (see **Fig. 7**). The SLN was then excised (**Fig. 8**C). The SLN was identified in 97% of dogs with preoperative Lipiodol injection and there was agreement with intraoperative methylene blue in 85% of dogs.[62] This is an attractive alternative to other direct and indirect techniques because it uses facilities readily available in most hospitals (ie, radiology) and is less costly than other SLN mapping techniques. The only

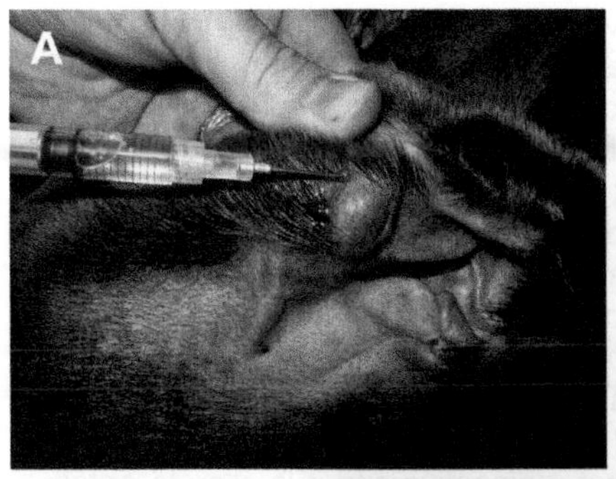

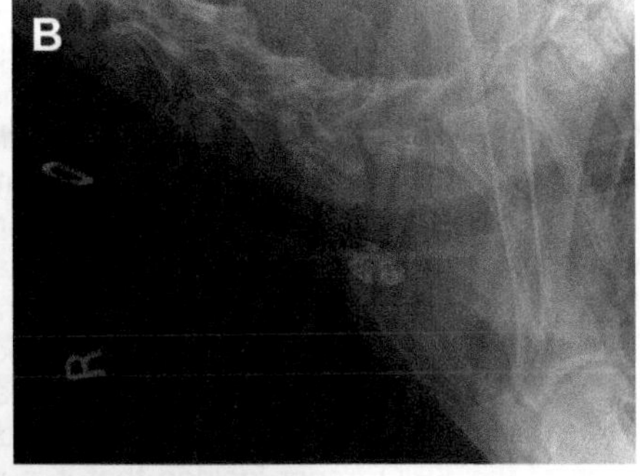

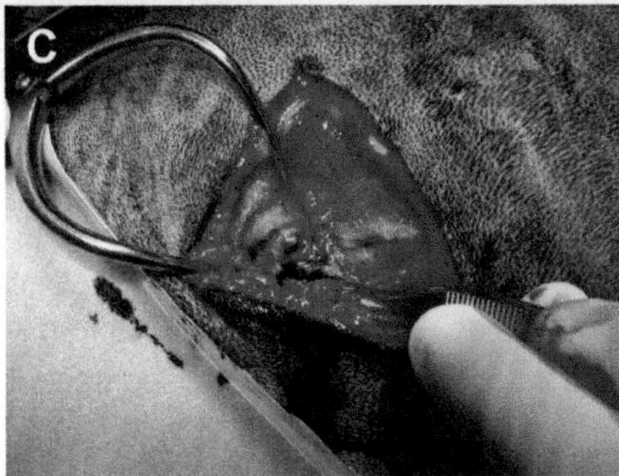

Fig. 8. Indirect lymphography technique using preoperative Lipiodol and intraoperative methylene blue. (*A*) Four-quadrant peritumoral injection of Lipiodol is performed under sedation in a dog with a pinna mast cell tumor. (*B*) Regional radiographs are performed 24 hours after Lipiodol injection. In this case, the SLN is the superficial cervical lymph node. (*C*) Following intraoperative 4-quadrant peritumoral injection of methylene blue (see **Fig. 7**), a directed approach is made over the SLN identified on preoperative radiographs and the blue discolored SLN is extirpated and submitted for histopathology.

disadvantage is that this technique is a two-stage process separated by 24 hours because of the slower uptake of Lipiodol into the peritumoral lymphatics.

The future of SLN mapping and biopsy is exciting with several techniques being developed and investigated. The use of contrast-enhanced ultrasound has shown promise in both people[63,64] and dogs.[12,65,66] First- and second-generation contrast agents have been investigated with the newer products (eg, SonoVue, Sonazoid) stabilizing the microbubbles using an inert gas rather than air.[63] Following intradermal peritumoral injection of the contrast agent, the area is massaged to encourage uptake of the microbubbles into the lymphatic system. Using contrast pulse sequencing, microbubbles are identified within the lymphatics and followed in real time to the presumptive SLN.[63] This SLN is then either aspirated or biopsied. In one meta-analysis, ultrasound-guided biopsies had a 54% sensitivity and 100% specificity for the diagnosis of metastatic SLNs in people.[67]

Alternative intraoperative techniques to radiocolloids and blue dyes include near-infrared image-guided and superparamagnetic iron oxide (SPIO)-guided SLN biopsy.[45] For fluorescent optical intraoperative image-guided SLN biopsies, an optical imaging camera system and a near-infrared fluorescent tracer with an affinity for lymph nodes are required. SLNs are identified by fluorescence emitted from dyes that accumulate in the SLNs. Indocyanine green is the most commonly used tracer for SLN mapping because it fluoresces in the near-infrared spectrum (absorption

765 nm, emission 840 nm), thus providing a very high signal-to-background ratio. In 23 studies reported to date, the SLN identification rate was 93% or greater.[45] Furthermore, identification rates were greater for indocyanine green than blue dyes and comparable to radiocolloids in most of the studies.[45]

SPIO has been used as a contrast agent for MRI for more than 20 years and can respond to an external magnetic field but does not have magnetic properties in the absence of magnetic fields.[45] After subcutaneous injection, SPIO can accumulate in the lymph nodes and then a handheld magnetometer is used to magnetize the SPIO.[45,68] SLN identification is guided by both the magnetometer and brown to black discoloration of the SLN.[68] In one meta-analysis, the SLN identification rate was 97.1% compared with 96.8% for standard radioisotope and/or blue dye.[68] Advantages of the SPIO tracer include that it is not radioactive and it is easy to obtain,[45] which make it a suitable alternative to some of the other techniques commonly used in human surgical oncology and which have limited applicability to veterinary medicine because of either costs, availability, or legislative restrictions.

REFERENCES

1. Szczubiał M, Łopuszynski W. Prognostic value of regional lymph node status in canine mammary carcinomas. Vet Comp Oncol 2011;9:296–303.
2. Hillers KR, Dernell WS, Lafferty MH, et al. Incidence and prognostic importance of lymph node metastases in dogs with appendicular osteosarcoma: 228 cases (1986-2003). J Am Vet Med Assoc 2005;226:1364–7.
3. Tuohy JL, Worley DR. Pulmonary lymph node charting in normal dogs with blue dye and scintigraphic lymphatic mapping. Res Vet Sci 2014;97:148–55.
4. Warland J, Amores-Fuster I, Newbury W, et al. The utility of staging in canine mast cell tumours. Vet Comp Oncol 2014;12:287–98.
5. Williams LE, Gliatto JM, Dodge RK, et al. Carcinoma of the apocrine glands of the anal sac in dogs: 113 cases (1985-1995). J Am Vet Med Assoc 2003;223:825–31.
6. Polton GA, Brearley MJ. Clinical stage, therapy, and prognosis in canine anal sac gland carcinoma. J Vet Intern Med 2007;21:274–80.
7. Hume CT, Kiupel M, Rigatti L, et al. Outcomes of dogs with grade 3 mast cell tumors: 43 cases (1997-2007). J Am Anim Hosp Assoc 2011;47:37–44.
8. Lejeune A, Skorupski K, Frazier S, et al. Aggressive local therapy combined with systemic chemotherapy provides long-term control in grade II stage 2 canine mast cell tumour: 21 cases (1999-2012). Vet Comp Oncol 2015;13:267–80.
9. Williams LE, Packer RA. Association between lymph node size and metastasis in dogs with oral malignant melanoma: 100 cases (1987-2001). J Am Vet Med Assoc 2003;222:1234–6.
10. Paoloni MC, Adams WM, Dubielzig RR, et al. Comparison of results of computed tomography and radiography with histopathologic findings in tracheobronchial lymph nodes in dogs with primary lung tumors: 14 cases (1999-2002). J Am Vet Med Assoc 2006;228:1718–22.
11. Ballegeer EA, Adams WM, Dubielzig RR, et al. Computed tomography characteristics of canine tracheobronchial lymph node metastasis. Vet Radiol Ultrasound 2010;51:397–403.
12. Gelb HR, Freeman LJ, Rohleder JJ, et al. Feasibility of contrast-enhanced ultrasound guided biopsy of sentinel lymph nodes in dogs. Vet Radiol Ultrasound 2010;51:628–33.

13. Boston SE, Lu X, Culp WT, et al. Efficacy of systemic adjuvant therapies administered to dogs after excision of oral malignant melanomas: 151 cases (2001-2012). J Am Vet Med Assoc 2014;245:401–7.
14. Skinner OT, Boston SE, Souza CHM. Patterns of lymph node metastasis identified following bilateral mandibular and medial retropharyngeal lymphadenectomy in 31dogs with malignancies of the head. Vet Comp Oncol 2017;15:881–9.
15. Skinner OT, Boston SE, Giglio RF, et al. Diagnostic accuracy of contrast-enhanced computed tomography for assessment of mandibular and medial retropharyngeal lymph node metastasis in dogs with oral and nasal cancer. Vet Comp Oncol 2018;16:562–70.
16. Fournier Q, Cazzini P, Bavcar S, et al. Investigation of the utility of lymph node fine-needle aspiration cytology for the staging of malignant solid tumors in dogs. Vet Clin Pathol 2018;47:489–500.
17. Grimes JA, Matz BM, Christopherson PW, et al. Agreement between cytology and histopathology for regional lymph node metastasis in dogs with melanocytic neoplasms. Vet Pathol 2017;54:579–87.
18. Palladino S, Keyerleber MA, King RG, et al. Utility of computed tomography versus abdominal ultrasound examination to identify iliosacral lymphadenomegaly in dogs with apocrine gland adenocarcinoma of the anal sac. J Vet Intern Med 2016;30:1858–63.
19. Pollard RE, Fuller MC, Steffey MA. Ultrasound and computed tomography of the iliosacral lymphatic centre in dogs with anal sac gland carcinoma. Vet Comp Oncol 2017;15:299–306.
20. Barnes DC, Demetriou JL. Surgical management of primary, metastatic and recurrent anal sac adenocarcinoma in the dog: 52 cases. J Small Anim Pract 2017;58:263–8.
21. Smith MM. Surgical approach for lymph node staging of oral and maxillofacial neoplasms in dogs. J Vet Dent 2002;19:170–4.
22. Green K, Boston SE. Bilateral removal of the mandibular and medial retropharyngeal lymph nodes through a single ventral midline incision for staging of head and neck cancers in dogs: a description of surgical technique. Vet Comp Oncol 2017;15:208–14.
23. Wainberg SH, Oblak ML, Giuffrida MA. Ventral cervical versus bilateral lateral approach for extirpation of mandibular and medial retropharyngeal lymph nodes in dogs. Vet Surg 2018;47:629–33.
24. Belz GT, Heath TJ. Lymph pathways of the medial retropharyngeal lymph node in dogs. J Anat 1995;186:517–26.
25. Wright T, Oblak ML. An overview of surgical anatomy and removal of peripheral lymph nodes. Today's Vet Pract 2016;6:20–8.
26. McNiel EA, Ogilvie GK, Powers BE, et al. Evaluation of prognostic factors for dogs with primary lung tumors: 67 cases (1985-1992). J Am Vet Med Assoc 1997;211:1422–7.
27. Pfannschmidt J, Klode J, Muley T, et al. Nodal involvement at the time of pulmonary metastasectomy: experiences in 245 patients. Ann Thorac Surg 2006;81: 448–54.
28. Renaud S, Falcoz PE, Alifano M, et al. Systematic lymph node dissection in lung metastasectomy of renal cell carcinoma: an 18 years of experience. J Surg Oncol 2014;109:823–9.
29. Steffey MA, Daniel L, Mayhew PD, et al. Video-assisted thoracoscopic extirpation of the tracheobronchial lymph nodes in dogs. Vet Surg 2015;44(Suppl 1):50–8.

30. Bennett PF, DeNicola DB, Bonney P, et al. Canine anal sac adenocarcinomas: clinical presentation and response to therapy. J Vet Intern Med 2002;16:100–4.
31. Steffey MA, Daniel L, Mayhew PD, et al. Laparoscopic extirpation of the medial iliac lymph nodes in normal dogs. Vet Surg 2015;44(Suppl 1):59–65.
32. Ball CG, Sutherland F, Kirkpatrick AW, et al. Dramatic innovations in modern surgical subspecialties. Can J Surg 2010;53:335–41.
33. Beek MA, Verheuvel NC, Luiten EJ, et al. Two decades of axillary management of breast cancer. Br J Surg 2015;102:1658–64.
34. Abass MO, Gismalla MD, Alsheikh AA, et al. Axillary lymph node dissection for breast cancer: efficacy and complication in developing countries. J Glob Oncol 2018;4:1–8.
35. Thompson JF, Uren RF, Shaw HM, et al. Location of sentinel lymph nodes in patients with cutaneous melanoma: new insights into lymphatic anatomy. J Am Coll Surg 1999;189:195–206.
36. Pereira CT, Luiz Navarro Marques F, Williams J, et al. 99mTc-labeled dextran for mammary lymphoscintigraphy in dog. Vet Radiol Ultrasound 2008;49:487–91.
37. Worley DR. Incorporation of sentinel lymph node mapping in dogs with mast cell tumours: 20 consecutive procedures. Vet Comp Oncol 2014;12:215–26.
38. Herring ES, Smith MM, Roberston JL. Lymph node staging of oral and maxillofacial neoplasms in 31 dogs and cats. J Vet Dent 2002;19:122–6.
39. Gervasoni JJE, Taneja C, Chung MA, et al. Biologic and clinical significance of lymphadenectomy. Surg Clinic North Am 2000;80:1631–73.
40. Newman LA. Lymph node biopsy in breast cancer patients: a comprehensive review of variations in performance and technique. J Am Coll Surg 2004;199:804–16.
41. Somasundaram SK, Chicken DW, Keshtgar MRS. Detection of sentinel lymph node in breast cancer. Br Med Bull 2007;84:117–31.
42. Salem A. Sentinel lymph node biopsy in breast cancer: a comprehensive literature review. J Surg Educ 2009;66:267–75.
43. Wang Z, Wu LC, Chen JQ. Sentinel lymph node biopsy compared with axillary lymph node dissection in early breast cancer: a meta-analysis. Breast Cancer Res Treat 2011;129:675–89.
44. Van Oostrum NHM, Makar APH, Van Den Broeke R. Sentinel node procedures in gynecologic cancers: an overview. Acta Obstet Gynecol Scand 2012;91:174–81.
45. Qiu SQ, Zhang GJ, Jansen L, et al. Evolution of sentinel lymph node biopsy in breast cancer. Crit Rev Oncol Hematol 2018;123:83–94.
46. Balasubramanian SP, Harrison BJ. Systematic review and meta-analysis of sentinel node biopsy in thyroid cancer. Br J Surg 2011;98:344–444.
47. Turner RR, Ollila DW, Krasne DL, et al. Histopathologic validation of the sentinel lymph node hypothesis for breast carcinoma. Ann Surg 1997;226:271–6.
48. Filippakis GM, Zografos G. Contraindications of sentinel lymph node biopsy: are there any really? World J Surg Oncol 2007;5:10.
49. Sullivan SA, Rossi EC. Sentinel lymph node biopsy in endometrial cancer: a standard of care? Curr Treat Options Oncol 2017;18:62.
50. Yang Y, Zhou J, Wu H. Diagnostic value of sentinel lymph node biopsy for cT1/T2N0 tongue squamous cell carcinoma: a meta-analysis. Eur Arch Otorhinolaryngol 2017;274:3843–52.
51. Wang Z, Dong ZY, Chen JQ, et al. Diagnostic value of sentinel lymph node biopsy in gastric cancer: a meta-analysis. Ann Surg Oncol 2012;19:1541–50.

52. Lips DJ, Schutte HW, van der Linden RLA, et al. Sentinel lymph node biopsy to direct treatment in gastric cancer. A systematic review of the literature. Eur J Surg Oncol 2011;37:655–61.
53. Layfield DM, Agrawal A, Roche H, et al. Intraoperative assessment of sentinel lymph nodes in breast cancer. Br J Surg 2011;98:4–17.
54. Van der Noordaa MEM, Peeters MTFDV, Rutgers EJT. The intraoperative assessment of sentinel lymph nodes – standards and controversies. Breast 2017;34: S64–9.
55. Masannat Y, Shenoy H, Speirs V, et al. Properties and characteristics of the dyes injected to assist axillary sentinel node localization in breast surgery. Eur J Surg Oncol 2006;32:381–4.
56. Balogh L, Thuroczy J, Andocs G, et al. Sentinel lymph node detection in canine oncological patients. Nucl Med Rev Cent East Eur 2002;5:139–44.
57. Nwogu CE, Kanter PM, Anderson TM. Pulmonary lymphatic mapping in dogs: use of technetium sulfur colloid and isosulfan blue for pulmonary sentinel lymph node mapping in dogs. Cancer Invest 2002;20:944–7.
58. Cabanas RM. The concept of the sentinel lymph node. Recent Results Cancer Res 2000;157:109–20.
59. Soultani C, Patsikas MN, Karayannopoulou M, et al. Assessment of sentinel lymph node metastasis in canine mammary gland tumors using computed tomographic indirect lymphography. Vet Radiol Ultrasound 2017;58:186–96.
60. Majeski SA, Steffey MA, Fuller M, et al. Indirect computed tomographic lymphography for iliosacral lymphatic mapping in a cohort of dogs with anal sac gland adenocarcinoma: technique description. Vet Radiol Ultrasound 2017;58: 295–303.
61. Grimes JA, Secrest SA, Northrup NC, et al. Indirect computed tomography lymphangiography with aqueous contrast for evaluation of sentinel lymph nodes in dogs with tumors of the head. Vet Radiol Ultrasound 2017;58:559–64.
62. Brissot HN, Edery EG. Use of indirect lymphography to identify the sentinel lymph node in dogs: a pilot study in 30 tumors. Vet Comp Oncol 2017;15:740–53.
63. Sharma N, Cox K. Axillary nodal staging with contrast-enhanced ultrasound. Curr Breast Cancer Rep 2017;9:259–63.
64. Lowes S, Leaver A, Cox K, et al. Evolving imaging techniques for staging axillary lymph nodes in breast cancer. Clin Radiol 2018;73:396–409.
65. Lurie DM, Seguin B, Schneider PD, et al. Contrast-assisted ultrasound for sentinel lymph node detection in spontaneously arising canine head and neck tumors. Invest Radiol 2006;41:415–21.
66. Wang Y, Cheng Z, Li J, et al. Gray-scale contrast-enhanced ultra- sonography in detecting sentinel lymph nodes: an animal study. Eur J Radiol 2010;74:e55–9.
67. Moody AN, Bull J, Culpan AM, et al. Preoperative sentinel lymph node identification, biopsy and localisation using contrast enhanced ultrasound (CEUS) in patients with breast cancer: a systematic review and meta-analysis. Clin Radiol 2017;72:959–71.
68. Zada A, Peek MCL, Ahmed M, et al. Meta-analysis of sentinel lymph node biopsy in breast cancer using the magnetic technique. Br J Surg 2016;103:1409–19.

Towards the Delivery of Precision Veterinary Cancer Medicine

Anna Katogiritis, DVM[a,b], Chand Khanna, DVM, PhD[a,b,*]

KEYWORDS

- Precision medicine • Personalized medicine • (Pmed) • Genomics • Oncology
- Next generation sequencing (NGS)

KEY POINTS

- Genomics in medicine is here. In both human and veterinary medicine the opportunity to integrate the fields of genomics and medicine is now a reality, as part of precision/personalized medicine (Pmed).
- Why now? The use of genomic information in medicine is now feasible through the development of innovations in genomic technology and computing power. Collectively, these advancements provide cost-effective technologies that are suitable for use in human and veterinary clinical medicine.
- Genomic characterization of disease: The advent of new genomic technology, specifically next-generation sequencing (NGS), now allows for the characterization of disease at the genomic level. This new characterization in tissues and/or biofluids can supplement current conventional methods of disease characterization (ie, histology, serology).
- Genomic prediction of disease risks: A distinct application of genomic technology to medicine is the analysis of germline risk factors for disease (so-called disease prediction). This approach most often focuses on the analysis of normal cell DNA, rather than that of diseased cells or genes. Although feasible and readily available, significant work is now needed to determine if and how such resulting early diagnoses will improve outcomes for patients.

Continued

Disclosure: C. Khanna is currently employed by Ethos Veterinary Health and Ethos Discovery. A. Katogiritis has nothing to disclose.

[a] EthosVeterinaryHealth LLC, 20 Cabot Road, Woburn, MA 01801, USA; [b] EthosDiscovery(501c3), Washington, DC, USA
* Corresponding author. EthosVeterinaryHealth LLC, 20 Cabot Road, Woburn, MA 01801.
E-mail address: ckhanna@ethosvet.com
; @DoctorAnnaK (A.K.)

Vet Clin Small Anim 49 (2019) 809–818
https://doi.org/10.1016/j.cvsm.2019.04.011

Continued

- Cancer: It is increasingly recognized that cancer is a disease of mutated genes and dysregulated gene expression, and that conventional cancer care often fails to sufficiently consider this critical aspect of cancer biology. This results in high numbers of patients being left with unmet needs after receiving conventional cancer care. Consequently, oncology has been most explored and may deliver the best opportunities for current and future Pmed offerings. Furthermore, the opportunity to identify a tumor's mutated/diseased genes within the tumor itself or in blood and other biofluids (referred to as a liquid biopsy) using certain Pmed platforms provides an additional rationale for the early study of Pmed in oncology.

A RECENT INTERSECTION OF MEDICINE AND GENOMICS (IE, MOLECULAR MEDICINE) HAS DELIVERED PRECISION/PERSONALIZED MEDICINE

Precision/personalized medicine (Pmed) offers an opportunity to characterize disease states across species through the optics of genomics (ie, molecular medicine), and is now a reality for human and veterinary medicine.[1,2] Innovations in genomic technology, so-called "next generation sequencing" (NGS) has fueled this opportunity.[3,4] In simple terms, this technological advancement is analogous to automobile manufacturing, advancing from the "one mechanic per engine" model to that of one based on the assembly line. In the setting of genomics, this advance in production line technology is referred to as "massively parallel sequencing."[5]

In association with these innovations in genomic technology, advances in computing power now allow the management of large genomic datasets associated with NGS.[6–8] This has created the opportunity for relatively inexpensive genomic and molecular characterization of disease states.[6–8] This novel characterization of disease should be complementary, but could ultimately replace some historical approaches to disease characterization based on serology, serum biochemistry, and even microscopy/histology. Alternatively, these historical approaches may be successfully integrated into a new characterization of disease that is a combination of these conventional methods with genomics and advanced imaging.

In many disease conditions, it is well understood that conventional methods of disease characterization are insufficient to fully inform clinicians of an individual patient's needs.[9] For the most part, the genomic characterization of many disease states can better account for these needs and lead to better selection of initial approaches to therapy, rapid alterations in treatment approach, and individualized planning of disease monitoring.[10,11] From the perspective of need and opportunity, oncology seems most ripe for this evolution in medicine.

FACTORS THAT MAKE CANCER SUCH A CHALLENGE TODAY

In oncology, patient responses to conventional cancer therapies is associated with a diversity in outcomes.[12–14] One potential cause for this limitation can be found in the manner in which these treatments have been developed. More specifically, current treatments have been developed for the "average" patient based on population-based trial findings and not for the individual patient.[11] Furthermore, most conventional treatments have focused on combating neoplasia using cytotoxic mechanisms that overlook the fact that cancer is largely a disease of dysregulated genes that are not all related to the cell cycle.

These shortcomings derive from the heterogeneity of cancer, meaning that even though 2 patients may be diagnosed with the same cancer type, those patients may have different mutations that may respond differently to treatment protocols,[15] and further that the types of mutations within a single tumor are distinct. Two tumors may have the same histologic diagnosis, but their underlying genetic mutations may not be the same and may suggest distinct treatment approaches as optimal for the 2 distinct patients.[15] Currently this molecular and targeted approach to cancer is used in canine mast cell tumors. Mutations in the c-kit gene can be readily analyzed from a mast cell tumor sample, and mutational data can be used to select targeted therapy for that patient.

CANCER GENOMICS AND PERSONALIZED MEDICINE

As described above, a significant challenge facing oncology is the inherent inadequacy of the conventional approaches to disease characterization and therapy selection. However, with the advances made through genomic characterization of disease, potential solutions to these challenges may be delivered by Pmed. Using genomic characterization of cancer, clinicians inherently recognize that cancer is a disease of genes, and may have a more specific understanding of the disease pathogenesis.[11] This may lead to more appropriate diagnosis and treatment selection that will better target the consequences of the dysregulated genes that drive cancer.[11]

THE NEED AND PROMISE OF PRECISION/PERSONALIZED MEDICINE IN ONCOLOGY

In the setting of molecularly guided cancer therapy, efforts will focus on identifying the specific genetic alterations that drive the biology of an individual cancer.[12] These factors will subsequently be prioritized based on a detailed understanding of the biological functions of the affected genes in a given disease.[11] This would allow clinicians to match the most important genetic mutations to specific drugs that most effectively alter those observed aberrant genes. In so doing, delivery of a very precise and individualized approach to cancer therapy can be achieved. This potential of Pmed has begun to receive widespread recognition in humans.[16]

In general, cancer medicine ultimately aims to recommend the most effective treatment for an individual patient based on supporting scientific evidence. The use of a Pmed approach to cancer diagnosis and therapy may deliver a variety of outcomes related to this goal. For example, Pmed could improve therapeutic outcomes for patients with specific types of cancer, including those with cancers that are not effectively managed with conventional treatment approaches.[17] In addition, Pmed technologies may generate new data that might (1) support the grouping of patients in clinical trials (ie, Master protocols or "basket" trials) that are agnostic to histology, and (2) accelerate alternatives to conventional drug development of a specific therapy in a specific cancer (ie, "accelerated reverse directional drug development").[18,19] This accelerated reverse directional drug development begins with the patient rather than beginning in cells or mouse models.

Because cancer is a disease of disordered genes, it is intuitive that a more detailed understanding of the molecular and genomic factors associated with cancer development would improve treatment outcomes. However, the evidence in support of the above-described promise of Pmed in human patients is not widely available in the form of conventional, randomized, controlled prospective studies. Nonetheless, several Pmed studies have been launched to deliver these data. One of the first pilot studies incorporating molecular profiling to guide therapy in advanced cancers was published in 2010.[20] In this study, results showed that 18 out of 68 (27%) human patients with cancer experienced a prolonged response duration following a molecularly derived (ie, Pmed) approach to therapy compared with previous conventional therapy (selected by physician choice). If one assumes that all relapses of a cancer will be associated with a shorter response duration then the initial response to therapy, then the 27% of patients who enjoyed longer response durations following Pmed is supportive of the benefits of Pmed. However, in a diverse population of patients with cancer, it is reasonable that some patients may actually exhibit better outcomes on later rounds of therapy than they do following an initial therapy. In this instance, it is less clear how this 27% supports the potential impact of Pmed on oncology. As more prospective studies are completed, it is likely that this desired evidence will be available.

Even though such definitive evidence remains lacking, a variety of Pmed assays are commercially available for clinical use. For example, a leading product in the human field is the OneTEST, which includes genomic and other analyses of tumors. Moreover, these assays are being requested by patients and physicians at increasing frequencies.

EVIDENCE IN SUPPORT OF THIS PROMISE IN VETERINARY ONCOLOGY

In veterinary oncology we have published the feasibility of delivering a highly detailed genomic analysis of a tumor from a patient with a clinically relevant turnaround time of 10 days.[21] This analysis will provide a list of matched genomically derived therapeutic options. We have not made this published assay commercially available at this time, but continue disease-specific research with Pmed in important canine cancers, including canine hemangiosarcoma (Canine Hemangiosarcoma Molecular Profiling [CHAMP] study, Khanna and colleagues, personal communication, 2018). Indeed, there is no published evidence beyond our feasibility report in precision medicine in veterinary oncology that provides evidence in support of Pmed. Nonetheless, several precision medicine assays have been commercialized by other groups and are available to clinicians and patients.

UNDERSERVED CATS

Despite the fact that cats now outnumber dogs as household pets in the United States, cats remain relatively underserved from the perspective of novel diagnostics and therapeutics.

As a result, the genomic advances described in most of this article largely apply to the dog and are not as advanced in the cat.

On the side of genomics, although progressively advancing, the annotation of the feline genome remains relatively scant and therefore limits some of the applications of genomics described above. One exception is the use of germline risk stratification, which uses a variety of risk factor markers to define the potential risk for disease development.[22]

On the side of therapeutics, significant differences in feline physiology and drug metabolism result in greater gaps in knowledge for drug development in cats compared with dogs. It is nonetheless likely that the need for better care in the setting of complex medical conditions in cats will result in many of these advances migrating to the cat in the near future.

CHOOSING A PLATFORM

A variety of different scientific platforms exist within precision medicine. Two examples are assays that prioritize the identification of mutated genes and those that prioritize detection of RNA expression signatures.[23] Assay platforms that prioritize the identification of mutated genes are likely to be the most valuable in clinical scenarios in which a clinician is interested in finding new options to treat a difficult cancer case. This rationale is based on the concept that mutated genes are most often responsible for the behavior of a cancer. Therefore, targeting mutated genes with novel therapeutics will offer alternative and potentially improved treatments for these uniquely aggressive cancers. This would be true in cases in which uniquely aggressive cancers have failed conventional treatment approaches, or in which the patient presents with advanced, potentially metastatic disease. An additional advantage to a mutation-based platform is the potential use of *blood* samples for genomic analysis (ie, liquid biopsy; for cell-free mutated tumor DNA). Identification of mutated tumor DNA (often circulating and cell free or exosomal) in the blood could provide a faster and easier alternative to traditional tissue biopsy approaches to diagnosis and molecular analysis.[23,24] We have recently completed a prospective, nationwide study of canine hemangiosarcoma including the analysis of circulating mutated cell-free tumor DNA for Pmed analysis (Khanna and colleagues, personal communication, 2018; CHAMP study). Beyond its intent to deliver Pmed to individual patients, this study is most likely to serve a drug development goal by uncovering novel therapeutic approaches for this cancer in patients as part of a reverse accelerated drug development approach. These new data have resulted in the design and imminent launch of more conventional drug development trials for dogs with hemangiosarcoma.

Conversely, assay platforms that prioritize detection of RNA expression signatures would have value in different clinical scenarios. More specifically, these assays would be particularly helpful when determining which conventional therapeutics would be best applied to an individual when there are multiple drugs that could be reasonably considered. In such a case, this type of assay could be used to evaluate drug-resistance profiles of a specific tumor to known drugs. Indeed, Researchers at Colorado State University are currently exploring a Pmed approach for this very scenario in dogs, using a platform developed for similar reasons in human bladder cancer. An RNA-based precision medicine assay is commercially available for dogs through Innogenics (clinical evidence surrounding the use of this assay use has not yet been published).

This type of assay platform is not likely optimal for the identification of new drugs to treat difficult cancers. Furthermore, because RNA is the material analyzed by these approaches, the use of circulating RNA species in the blood is not informative, because it is not possible to discriminate between tumor-associated RNA and normal RNA in the blood (unlike mutated cancer DNA described above).

GERMLINE GENOMICS AND PREDICTION OF DISEASE RISK

The use of Pmed technologies goes beyond the enhancement of disease characterization and treatment matching described above. For example, studies of host or germline genomic variations have revealed immediate opportunities for genomics to influence medicine.[25–28] More specifically, through this technology, we may be able to identify genes that predict risk for future disease development and/or individual variation in a patient's tolerability to a given drug (ie, pharmacogenomics). A current example of this pharmacogenomics approach is the analysis of germline MDR1 mutations; most notably in collie-breed dogs at risk of drug sensitivity (eg, ivermectin or doxorubicin).[29–31]

These innovations applied to germline genomics are also well-established consumer products. For example, products such as 23andMe, Embark, and Wisdom

Panel that may describe ancestral origins in humans and dogs respectively. Similar laboratory-based products also have the capability of identifying well-established, single-gene germline predictors of disease risk (eg, BRCA mutations that predict risk and biology of breast cancer in women).[32] These innovations have also led to laboratory disease prediction panels that may predict an individual's risk for, or susceptibility to, future disease development. Such disease-prediction panels have been developed and commercialized in human and veterinary medicine. Although attractive in many circumstances, it should not be assumed that early diagnosis will lead to improved outcomes for patients in all disease settings. After identifying disease risk genes there is still a need to determine the true value of early detection in a "disease-by-disease" manner.

ARE YOU READY TO INTERPRET A PRECISION/PERSONALIZED MEDICINE ANALYSIS OF DISEASE?

Considering all the factors discussed above, it is important for all veterinary clinicians to consider if they are prepared to offer Pmed services to their veterinary oncology patients. As described above, a variety of Pmed offerings are commercially available, and more clients will request advice on the use of these options. At this time and in the future, clinicians should assess their ability to interpret and act on Pmed data and drug reports. Ideally, practitioners should have access to a multidisciplinary team of veterinary scientists and clinicians to deliver the best value to patients from these types of complex data. These teams should be led by veterinary clinical scientists with experience in molecular biology, drug development, pathology, and medicine. Leveraging this expertise within the veterinary field is important, because professionals in the human field alone will likely have insufficient background and context to deliver effective interpretations of data to veterinary clinicians and patients.

CHALLENGES AND SOLUTIONS FOR PRECISION MEDICINE AND VETERINARY ONCOLOGY

Gene Annotation

Limitations of gene annotation in the dog creates significant challenges for the clinical use of Pmed in veterinary oncology. In brief, gene annotation includes a description of an individual gene (ie, location, structure) and identification of its protein or RNA product.[33] The annotation should ideally include a description of the biological function of the gene.[33] Unfortunately, the annotation of canine genes is incomplete.[33] Furthermore, the determination of gene function and the comparison with human genes can often be complicated.[33] As such, it is unlikely that any current drug-matching algorithm can effectively and consistently match a given canine gene with drugs that are capable of inhibiting its function without additional clinician input and decision-making. Fortunately, through a recent initiative of the Animal Cancer Foundation,[34] progress on the structural annotation of canine genes should be expected in the near future. The more complicated biological characterization of gene function is an inherently slow process, and should be expected from academic research laboratories.

Cancer Geography

As many clinicians who have removed tumors from patients will attest, there is considerable variability in the physical appearance of tissue within a tumor.[35] Therefore, it is reasonable to imagine that a molecular analysis of a tumor may yield varying results depending on which distinct portion of the tumor was sampled. Detailed studies in a variety of cancers are needed to understand the impact of this geographic variability on molecular analysis. Fortunately, the increased availability of blood-based DNA analysis (ie, liquid biopsy) in patients with cancer may prove to effectively circumvent this issue. Because the analysis of blood DNA is expected to identify the most common, persistent, and driving mutations in a patient with cancer,[23,24] the geographic and genomic heterogeneity of a cancer may become less of a concern.

Cancer Evolution

Although the primary tumor in a patient with cancer is typically managed by surgery and/or radiation, it is the recurrence of cancer that often represents the greatest unmet need.[36,37] It is generally understood that molecular alterations in a tumor evolve with the recurrence and metastasis of a tumor.[36] Subsequently, it is reasonable to conclude that the analysis of a metastatic lesion will deliver a distinct Pmed result than that of the primary tumor. Assuming this is true, it is necessary for clinicians to re-biopsy metastatic or recurrent lesions to appropriately match the genomic alterations of the metastatic lesion with therapeutic agents. To complicate the situation further, this process of cancer evolution typically occurs within presumed micrometastatic cells that have left the primary tumor.[38] Therefore, it is these cells that would ideally be assessed through a Pmed approach. In so doing, therapeutics could be identified and delivered to prevent these cells from growing into the recurrent or metastatic lesions that plague most patients with cancer. Similar to the suggestion above, the use of liquid biopsies is expected to address this problem of cancer evolution. The recurrent and metastatic cells in the primary tumor, as well as the cells that become micrometastatic, will shed mutated DNA into the blood at disproportionately high rates.[23,24] As a result, these circulating, mutated DNA species will represent the ideal nucleic acids on which a Pmed platform should be delivered, regardless of the metastatic status of the cancer cells.

The feasibility of this approach is already being demonstrated. For example, CADET *BRAF* from Sentinel Biomedical links the presence of certain mutated DNA species in the urine (and potentially blood) of dogs with bladder cancer. Although this is just a single example specifically within the setting of bladder cancer, more efforts are underway to expand the use of liquid biopsies for other cancer types. As suggested above, our CHAMP study will include the development of a liquid biopsy approach for diagnosis and disease monitoring in canine hemangiosarcoma (Khanna and colleagues, personal communication, 2018).

Context

The concept of tumor context refers to the fact that the biological consequences of a mutated gene are dependent on the microenvironment in which that mutation is found. For example, a mutation in the gene BRAF has been identified in human melanoma and is believed to be a driving event in that cancer. Indeed, administration of BRAF-specific inhibitors results in highly favorable therapeutic benefits to patients with melanoma.[39] However, these inhibitors have not been associated with the same therapeutic benefit in cases of human thyroid cancer, even when the identical BRAF mutation is present.[40]

The above example highlights that the context (or specific cancer) in which a mutation is found should be expected to influence the therapeutic benefit of specific inhibitors. This new understanding of cancer mutations and their influence on cancer biology has profound significance to the underpinnings of Pmed. Although this is certainly true in humans, it may prove to be an even more important factor in the application of Pmed to veterinary patients that will require consideration of species in the development and interpretation of drug-matching reports. In other words, the context of tumor in a canine could be distinct from that of the same cancer in a human. Consequently, veterinary clinicians must be aware that algorithms based on data from human medicine should not be expected to deliver the same benefits in dogs, and the interpretation of these data by veterinary clinicians and clinician scientists is needed.

A remedy to this important problem will be the publication of clinical trials in dogs with specific diseases in which precision medicine approaches are offered, and further biological annotation of canine cancer genomes.

Comparative Oncology

The concept of comparative oncology allows questions in the development of novel diagnostics and therapeutics to be asked in pet animals with naturally occurring disease (most commonly dogs, see above) that cannot be asked or answered in conventional preclinical models in human clinical trials.[21,41] The opportunity for more efficient cancer drug development pipelines to be built from this comparative oncology perspective has been increasingly used.[21,41,42] The rationale for this approach is very likely to accelerate the delivery of evidence on the concept of precision medicine, compared with a challenging quagmire of preclinical and clinical development of precision medicine in humans and conventional preclinical models alone. Efficiencies created by the comparative oncology model are largely based on the heterogeneity of naturally occurring cancers within a population of individuals with the same cancer diagnosis, and the natural emergence of resistance and metastasis associated with this cell-to-cell heterogeneity within a given tumor. It is likely that the challenges around randomization of patients to precision medicine prescribed therapy versus physicians' best choice will be more rapidly accepted in comparative oncology trials and, as a result, of the compressed interval of disease in canine versus human patients with cancer. The benefits of such an approach will be more rapidly realized in the pet animal with cancer than in humans. Nonetheless, the above-described advances in our understanding of normal genomes and cancer genomes in dogs with naturally occurring cancer will be necessary for these comparative Pmed trials to be conducted and translated.

ACKNOWLEDGMENTS

The authors recognize the critical review and creative input of Dr Sam Stewart (Ethos Veterinary Health) in the completion of this article.

REFERENCES

1. Friedman AA, Letai A, Fisher DE, et al. Precision medicine for cancer with next-generation functional diagnostics. Nat Rev Cancer 2015;15(12):747–56.
2. Lloyd KC, Khanna C, Hendricks W, et al. Precision medicine: an opportunity for a paradigm shift in veterinary medicine. J Am Vet Med Assoc 2016;248(1):45–8.
3. Mardis ER. The impact of next-generation sequencing technology on genetics. Trends Genet 2008;24(3):133–41.
4. Schuster SC. Next-generation sequencing transforms today's biology. Nat Methods 2008;5(1):16–8.
5. Tucker T, Marra M, Friedman JM. Massively parallel sequencing: the next big thing in genetic medicine. Am J Hum Genet 2009;85(2):142–54.
6. Berger B, Peng J, Singh M. Computational solutions for omics data. Nat Rev Genet 2013;14(5):333–46.

7. He KY, Ge D, He MM. Big data analytics for genomic medicine. Int J Mol Sci 2017;18(2). https://doi.org/10.3390/ijms18020412.
8. Muir P, Li S, Lou S, et al. The real cost of sequencing: scaling computation to keep pace with data generation. Genome Biol 2016;17:53.
9. Chakraborty S, Rahman T. The difficulties in cancer treatment. Ecancermedicalscience 2012;6:ed16.
10. Kensler TW, Spira A, Garber JE, et al. Transforming cancer prevention through precision medicine and immune-oncology. Cancer Prev Res (Phila) 2016; 9(1):2–10.
11. Stricker T, Catenacci DV, Seiwert TY. Molecular profiling of cancer–the future of personalized cancer medicine: a primer on cancer biology and the tools necessary to bring molecular testing to the clinic. Semin Oncol 2011;38(2):173–85.
12. Burki TK. Variations in breast cancer treatment and outcomes. Lancet Oncol 2018;19(7):e342.
13. Herman KJ, Komorowski AL, Wysocki WM, et al. Variation in treatment modalities, costs and outcomes of rectal cancer patients in Poland. Contemp Oncol (Pozn) 2015;19(5):400–9.
14. Maitland ML, DiRienzo A, Ratain MJ. Interpreting disparate responses to cancer therapy: the role of human population genetics. J Clin Oncol 2006;24(14):2151–7.
15. Kim YA, Cho DY, Przytycka TM. Understanding genotype-phenotype effects in cancer via network approaches. PLoS Comput Biol 2016;12(3):e1004747.
16. Hamburg MA, Collins FS. The path to personalized medicine. N Engl J Med 2010; 363(4):301–4.
17. Verma M. Personalized medicine and cancer. J Pers Med 2012;2(1):1–14.
18. Biankin AV, Piantadosi S, Hollingsworth SJ. Patient-centric trials for therapeutic development in precision oncology. Nature 2015;526(7573):361–70.
19. Chen R, Snyder M. Promise of personalized omics to precision medicine. Wiley Interdiscip Rev Syst Biol Med 2013;5(1):73–82.
20. Von Hoff DD, Stephenson JJ Jr, Rosen P, et al. Pilot study using molecular profiling of patients' tumors to find potential targets and select treatments for their refractory cancers. J Clin Oncol 2010;28(33):4877–83.
21. Paoloni M, Khanna C. Translation of new cancer treatments from pet dogs to humans. Nat Rev Cancer 2008;8(2):147–56.
22. Cannon CM. Cats, cancer and comparative oncology. Vet Sci 2015;2(3):111–26.
23. Nalejska E, Maczynska E, Lewandowska MA. Prognostic and predictive biomarkers: tools in personalized oncology. Mol Diagn Ther 2014;18(3):273–84.
24. Haber DA, Velculescu VE. Blood-based analyses of cancer: circulating tumor cells and circulating tumor DNA. Cancer Discov 2014;4(6):650–61.
25. Phillips JC, Lembcke L, Chamberlin T. A novel locus for canine osteosarcoma (OSA1) maps to CFA34, the canine orthologue of human 3q26. Genomics 2010;96(4):220–7.
26. Rivera P, Melin M, Biagi T, et al. Mammary tumor development in dogs is associated with BRCA1 and BRCA2. Cancer Res 2009;69(22):8770–4.
27. Shearin AL, Hedan B, Cadieu E, et al. The MTAP-CDKN2A locus confers susceptibility to a naturally occurring canine cancer. Cancer Epidemiol Biomarkers Prev 2012;21(7):1019–27.
28. Wang G, Wu M, Maloneyhuss MA, et al. Actionable mutations in canine hemangiosarcoma. PLoS One 2017;12(11):e0188667.
29. Dekel Y, Machluf Y, Stoler A, et al. Frequency of canine nt230(del4) MDR1 mutation in prone pure breeds, their crosses and mongrels in Israel - insights from a worldwide comparative perspective. BMC Vet Res 2017;13(1):333.

30. Mealey KL, Bentjen SA, Gay JM, et al. Ivermectin sensitivity in collies is associated with a deletion mutation of the mdr1 gene. Pharmacogenetics 2001;11(8): 727–33.
31. Mealey KL, Northrup NC, Bentjen SA. Increased toxicity of P-glycoprotein-substrate chemotherapeutic agents in a dog with the MDR1 deletion mutation associated with ivermectin sensitivity. J Am Vet Med Assoc 2003;223(10):1453–5, 34.
32. Pruthi S, Gostout BS, Lindor NM. Identification and management of women with BRCA mutations or hereditary predisposition for breast and ovarian cancer. Mayo Clin Proc 2010;85(12):1111–20.
33. Derrien T, Vaysse A, Andre C, et al. Annotation of the domestic dog genome sequence: finding the missing genes. Mamm Genome 2012;23(1–2):124–31.
34. Global News Wire. Animal Cancer Foundation announces $1 Million gift to inaugurate canine cancer genome project. Secondary Animal Cancer Foundation announces $1 Million gift to inaugurate canine cancer genome project 2017. Available at: https://globenewswire.com/news-release/2017/10/24/1152566/0/en/Animal-Cancer-Foundation-Announces-1-Million-Gift-to-Inaugurate-Canine-Cancer-Genome-Project.html. Accessed October 24, 2017.
35. Meacham CE, Morrison SJ. Tumour heterogeneity and cancer cell plasticity. Nature 2013;501(7467):328–37.
36. McGranahan N, Swanton C. Clonal heterogeneity and tumor evolution: past, present, and the future. Cell 2017;168(4):613–28.
37. Seyfried TN, Huysentruyt LC. On the origin of cancer metastasis. Crit Rev Oncog 2013;18(1–2):43–73.
38. Gangnus R, Langer S, Breit E, et al. Genomic profiling of viable and proliferative micrometastatic cells from early-stage breast cancer patients. Clin Cancer Res 2004;10(10):3457–64.
39. Sullivan RJ, Flaherty KT. BRAF in melanoma: pathogenesis, diagnosis, inhibition, and resistance. J Skin Cancer 2011;2011:423239.
40. Cabanillas ME, Patel A, Danysh BP, et al. BRAF inhibitors: experience in thyroid cancer and general review of toxicity. Horm Cancer 2015;6(1):21–36.
41. Khanna C, Lindblad-Toh K, Vail D, et al. The dog as a cancer model. Nat Biotechnol 2006;24(9):1065–6.
42. Schiffman JD, Breen M. Comparative oncology: what dogs and other species can teach us about humans with cancer. Philos Trans R Soc Lond B Biol Sci 2015;370: 1673.

Diagnosis and Prognosis of Canine Cutaneous Mast Cell Tumors

Dr. med. vet. Dr. habil. Matti Kiupel, BS, MS, PhD[a,b,*],
Melinda Camus, DVM[c]

KEYWORDS

• Canine • Mast cell tumor • Grading • c-Kit

KEY POINTS

- The majority of canine cutaneous mast cell tumors (MCTs) can be diagnosed with fine-needle aspirates, but differentiating cutaneous from subcutaneous MCTs requires a biopsy.
- Cytologic grading helps with initial clinical decisions, whereas histologic grading using the 2-tier system provides the best approach for identifying high-grade MCTs.
- Combining histologic grading with analysis of argyrophilic nucleolus organizer regions (AgNORs), Ki67, KIT expression, and detection of mutations in exons 8 and 11 provides the most detailed prognostic assessment.
- Cross-sectioning (half and radial sections) combined with tangential sectioning of tumor margins is the preferred method to determine surgical excision of canine MCTs.
- Low-grade MCTs with a low AgNORxKi67 index have a low risk of local recurrence regardless of the cleanliness of the surgical margins.

INTRODUCTION

Canine cutaneous mast cell tumors (MCTs) account for approximately 20% of all canine skin tumors.[1] They develop most commonly as solitary nodules in the skin or less commonly in the subcutis, and their gross appearance may range from hairless, raised, erythematous masses to nodular rashes or diffuse swellings. There is no known age or gender predisposition, although several canine breeds have a high

Disclosure Statement: The Authors have nothing to disclose.
[a] Michigan State University Veterinary Diagnostic Laboratory, College of Veterinary Medicine, Michigan State University, 4125 Beaumont Road, Room 152A, Lansing, MI 48910, USA; [b] Department of Pathobiology and Diagnostic Investigation, College of Veterinary Medicine, Michigan State University, 4125 Beaumont Road, Room 152A, Lansing, MI 48910, USA; [c] Department of Pathology, College of Veterinary Medicine, University of Georgia, 501 D.W. Brooks Drive, Athens, GA 30602, USA
* Corresponding author.
E-mail address: kiupel@dcpah.msu.edu

Vet Clin Small Anim 49 (2019) 819–836
https://doi.org/10.1016/j.cvsm.2019.04.002

incidence of developing MCTs.[1] Although the diagnosis rarely represents a diagnostic challenge, except for some poorly differentiated cases, MCTs can have highly variable biologic behavior, and most efforts of the pathologists are focused on accurately identifying more aggressive cases.[2]

DIAGNOSIS

Most neoplastic mast cells in the dog resemble their non-neoplastic counterparts, and both cutaneous and subcutaneous MCTs are identified most readily by fine-needle aspirates. Cytologically, MCTs are characterized by a predominance of individualized, monomorphic round cells, with a central to slightly eccentric round nucleus and typically large numbers of magenta granules. These granules are often termed, *metachromatic*, because they exhibit tinctorial properties different from those exhibited by the stain components themselves. When using aqueous-based manual quick stains, for example, Diff-Quik (Siemens Healthcare, Malvern, PA, USA), occasionally mast cell granules demonstrate only minimal stain uptake, making a diagnosis of an MCT challenging (**Fig. 1**A). The poor stain uptake most likely is the result of dissolution of the granule contents in water due to inadequate fixation. This can be avoided by either leaving the stain in the fixative component (blue) for at least 5 minutes prior to staining or using a methanol-based differentiating stain, for example, Wright (see **Fig. 1**B).[1] It is important to recognize, however, that mast cells may lack typical staining characteristics not associated with artifacts. In poorly differentiated MCTs, neoplastic mast cells may be highly anaplastic, resulting in altered staining characteristics, including an absence of granules in both the cytoplasm of neoplastic cells and in the background (**Fig. 2**A). Alternatively, neoplastic mast cells may degranulate, whether associated with trauma or the tumor microenvironment, resulting in the absence of heavily stained granules within the cytoplasm and an abundance of detectable granules in the background (see **Fig. 2**B). Such MCTs may represent a diagnostic challenge in surgical biopsy specimens, including ancillary diagnostic techniques, such as special stains and immunohistochemistry (IHC). Use of these techniques may fail to differentiate these MCTs accurately from other poorly differentiated round cell neoplasms. For such poorly differentiated MCTs, cytology is the preferred method of accurate diagnosis, because some granules usually can be identified cytologically.

Mast cell granules contain interleukin 5, a cytokine that induces eosinophil migration.[1] Therefore, in most canine MCTs, the neoplastic mast cells are admixed with large numbers of eosinophils. In addition to eosinophils, MCTs often contain abundant fibroblasts (**Fig. 3**A). Tryptase-containing mast cells have been demonstrated to both express and secrete growth factors in the fibroblast growth factor family that stimulate neovascularization and fibroblast proliferation. Therefore, the presence of these plump mesenchymal cells can complicate the cytologic interpretation of such MCTs, because they may be misdiagnosed as mesenchymal neoplasms with secondary mast cell infiltration. Another feature commonly associated with MCTs is the presence of collagen, which appears as brightly eosinophilic bands coursing among neoplastic cells (see **Fig. 3**B). The presence of collagen is attributed to the induction of collagen synthesis by tryptase-containing and chymase-containing mast cells.[1]

A surgical biopsy is necessary to differentiate between cutaneous and subcutaneous MCTs. Cutaneous MCTs can be localized anywhere in the dermis and commonly extend to the epidermis, causing severe ulceration. They also may extend into the subcutis. Only those MCTs that are localized entirely within the subcutis and are

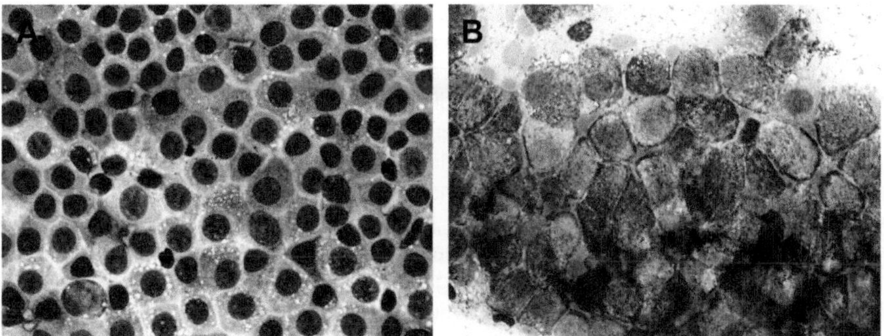

Fig. 1. Aspirate of a canine cutaneous MCT. (*A*) Water-based rapid hematology stain may fail to highlight mast cell granules. (*B*) Methanol-based Romanowsky stain (modified Wright) allows easy recognition of mast cell granules.

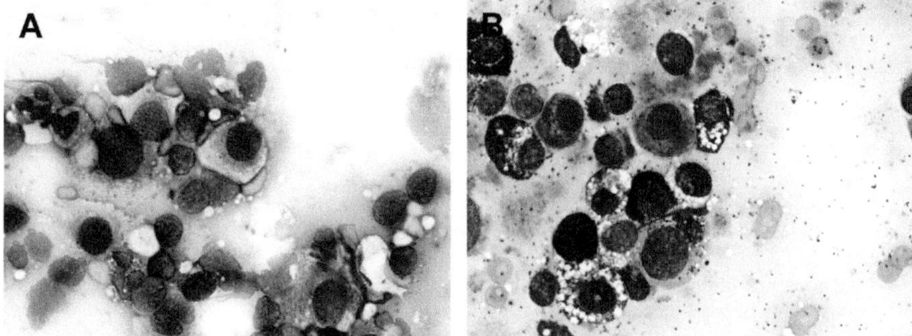

Fig. 2. Aspirate of canine cutaneous MCT. Modified Wright stain. (*A*) Virtual absence of granules in both cytoplasm of neoplastic cells and background in a poorly differentiated MCT. (*B*) Degranulated mast cells with vacuoles within the cytoplasm that indicate the initial granule location. Note the large number of magenta-colored granules in the background.

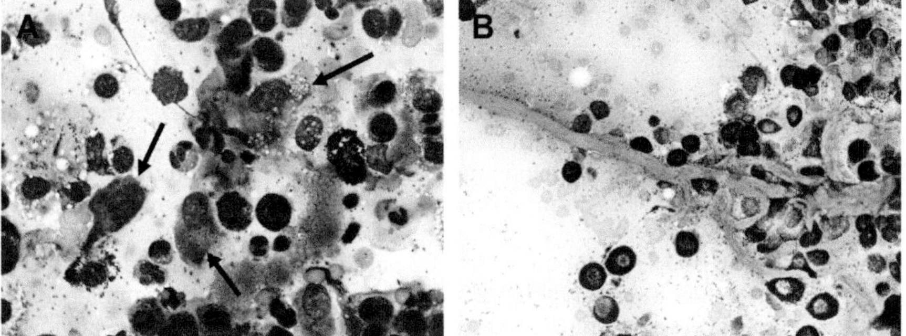

Fig. 3. Aspirate of a canine cutaneous MCT. Modified Wright stain. (*A*) Plump fibroblasts (*arrows*) often are noted in MCTs. (*B*) Abundant brightly eosinophilic, fibrillar collagen strands surrounded by neoplastic mast cells.

surrounded by adipose tissue are identified as subcutaneous MCTs.[3] Although the differentiation into cutaneous or subcutaneous MCTs is of little diagnostic relevance, it bears some important aspects for prognostication, as discussed later.[2] Regardless, in surgical biopsies the neoplastic mast cells appear microscopically similar to what has been described previously for aspirates. In hematoxylin-eosin (H&E)-stained sections, neoplastic mast cells have moderate amounts of pale pink cytoplasm that usually contains abundant light gray/blue granules. These granules are purple with metachromatic stains, for example, toluidine blue.[1] Neoplastic mast cells can be packed into dense sheets or appear individualized, commonly forming rows that infiltrate between collagen bundles (**Fig. 4**A). Most MCTs contain large numbers of eosinophils and occasionally neoplastic cells may be masked by the dense eosinophilic infiltrates (see **Fig. 4**B).[1] Eosinophils also play a role in collagenolysis. Secondary inflammation is common and often associated with severe ulceration and necrosis; these changes may make an accurate diagnosis and the evaluation of surgical margins difficult. In cases of chronic inflammation, sclerosis may be a prominent feature. Commonly, MCTs are surrounded by a clear halo composed of edema admixed with inflammatory cells, reactive stromal cells, and mast cells.[2] This halo may have a thickness of multiple centimeters and can have a negative impact on the ability to identify the margins of the MCT when attempting surgical excision.

Diagnosis of canine cutaneous mast cell tumors

- Fine-needle aspirates identify the majority of MCTs.
- Non-neoplastic mast cells may be found in other cutaneous neoplasms and inflammatory lesions.
- MCTs are difficult to diagnose with Diff Quik.
- Use methanol-based differentiation stain, for example, Romanowsky, to detect granules.
- Even poorly differentiated (high-grade) MCTs are diagnosed easily with cytology but pose a challenge as surgical biopsies.
- Differentiating cutaneous from subcutaneous MCTs requires a biopsy.

PROGNOSIS

Grading

Histologic

Historically, histologic grading has been the method used most commonly to predict the biological behavior of canine cutaneous MCTs. In the past, 2 systems classifying MCTs into 1 of 3 histologic grades, well-differentiated tumors, intermediately differentiated tumors, and poorly differentiated tumors, have been used routinely for surgical biopsies.[4,5] Although the grading system by Patnaik and colleagues[5] has been referenced most widely by pathologists when providing a histologic grade, there has been a high degree of inconsistency among pathologists in accurately applying the criteria of this grading system, and the reproducibility of assigned grades has been poor among pathologists.[6–8] In different studies, there was marked interobserver variation that reached 63% when pathologists adhered strictly to the grading criteria established by Patnaik and colleagues[6,7] There was only 50% agreement among pathologists grading MCTs in a routine setting.[8] Even more concerning was the large number of cases assigned an intermediate grade (72%) that provides little guidance regarding the biological behavior of the tumor.[6,7] Furthermore, 1 parameter that represents a major deciding factor for assigning an intermediate grade instead of a low grade to an MCT is

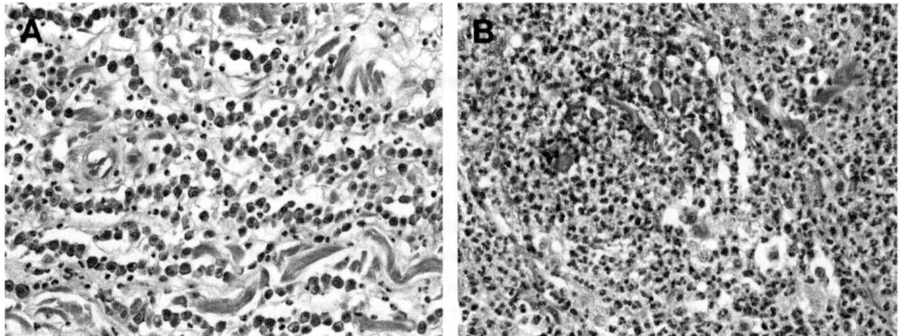

Fig. 4. Low-grade canine cutaneous MCT. H&E stain. (*A*) Well-differentiated, round, monomorphic neoplastic mast cells commonly are arranged in rows that separate collagen bundles and are surrounded by edematous stroma. (*B*) Large numbers of eosinophils commonly are observed and may aggregate around foci of collagenolysis.

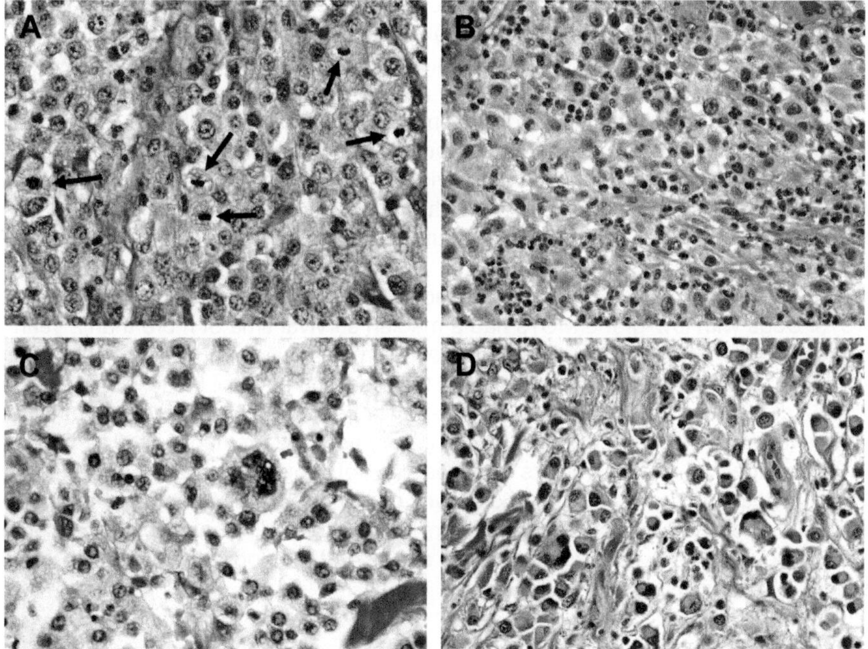

Fig. 5. Features to classify a high-grade canine cutaneous MCT. H&E stain. (*A*) An MC of at least 7 mitotic figures in 10 HPFs, an area of 2.37 mm^2). There are 5 mitoses (*arrows*) in a single field of vision. (*B*) Marked variation in nuclear size with at least 10% of neoplastic cells having a nuclear diameter that varies by 2-fold. There are numerous neoplastic cells with karyomegaly. (*C*) At least 3 bizarre nuclei per 10 HPFs. In the center is a neoplastic mast cell with a giant, abnormally shaped nucleus. (*D*) At least 3 multinucleated giant cells with 3 or more nuclei in 10 HPFs. There are numerous multinucleated neoplastic mast cells.

the depth of the MCT within the dermis. A study investigating tumor depth of canine cutaneous MCTs as an independent parameter found no prognostic significance of this parameter, further challenging the accuracy of the 3-tier grading system.[9] Including the location of the MCT within the dermis as a deciding factor in the histologic grading system also prevented utilization of this grading system for aspirates. Lastly, all 3-tier grading systems determined the grade of a canine cutaneous MCT in order to predict survival times rather than biological behavior.

A 2-tier histologic grading system was established not only to increase interobserver consistency but also, more importantly, to identify more accurately those MCTs that have a high risk of aggressive biological behavior, for example, metastatic disease.[6] In the initial study, the 2-tier grading system was applied first to 95 dogs with cutaneous MCT and was shown statistically significant in predicting survival time. High-grade MCTs were significantly associated with shorter time to metastasis or new tumor development.[6] Using multivariate analysis with Cox proportional hazard models for the Patnaik grading system and the 2-tier system fitted in different orders, the Patnaik grading system provided no statistically significant information over of the 2-tier system, whereas the 2-tier system proved a better statistical predictor of survival than the Patnaik system.[6] Several independent studies confirmed the high interobserver consistency as well as the prognostic significance of the 2-tier system.[10–13] Furthermore, these studies consistently documented that the 2-tier system was superior to the Patnaik system in predicting MCT-associated mortality and metastasis. The 2-tier system, thereby, also is superior in identifying those dogs that require additional therapy beyond surgical excision. Currently, the 2-tier grading system has been applied only in large-scale studies to cutaneous, but not subcutaneous MCTs, partly due to the low incidence of aggressive subcutaneous MCTs. Individual parameters, however, for example, mitotic count (MC), KIT pattern, and the combined AgNORxKi67 index, have been shown to predict behavior of subcutaneous MCTs in a similar manner as of cutaneous MCTs.[3,14]

The 2-tier system divides canine cutaneous MCTs into low-grade and high-grade MCTs. Dogs with low-grade MCTs had a median survival time of more than 2 years, whereas dogs with high-grade MCTs had a median survival time of less than 4 months.[6] High-grade MCTs are identified by observing any 1 of the following criteria (**Fig. 5**): at least 7 mitotic figures in 10 high-power fields (HPFs); (2) at least 3 multinucleated (3 or more nuclei) cells in 10 HPFs; (3) at least 3 bizarre nuclei in 10 HPFs; and (4) karyomegaly (nuclear diameters of at least 10% of neoplastic cells vary by at least 2 times). Fields with the highest mitotic activity or with the highest degree of anisokaryosis were selected to assess the different parameters. HPFs are being measured with an ocular with a field number of 22 and a 40-times objective, resulting in an area of 2.37 mm^2 assessed.[1,2]

Cytologic

Another advantage of the 2-tier grading system is that all the criteria utilized in the histologic grading of MCTs can be appreciated on cytologic specimens. There have been attempts at creating a standardized cytologic grading scheme for canine cutaneous MCTs, although none pervades the veterinary pathology community. Some have attempted to apply the histologic criteria for the 2-tier system directly to cytologic specimens, whereas others have utilized the histologic criteria to develop a predictive algorithm for cytologic grading of cutaneous MCTs in dogs based on outcome assessment.[15–17] Uniformly the cytologic grading schemes correlate reasonably well with histologic grading. However, even those 2 studies which directly applied histologic criteria to cytologic specimens, varied in the way in which they were conducted, the number of fields evaluated, and the type of stains utilized, making the studies difficult to compare and the criteria challenging to utilize on cytologic specimens. The first of these 2 studies applied the histologic grading system to a relatively small series of cases and assessed the criteria in 1000 cells on slides stained with May-Grünwald-Giemsa.[17] The sensitivity of this study was 84% and the specificity was 97%, with an agreement of 94% to the histologic grading system. The second study applied the histologic grading system to 141 cases by evaluating 10 HPFs on both H&E-stained and Giemsa-stained specimens.[16] The reported sensitivity and specificity were 86% and 97%, respectively, with an agreement of 94% to the histologic grading system.[16] Although these numbers are promising, in a 2-tier decision with high-grade MCTs, accounting for 30% or less of the cases, the overall percentages of agreement tend to be high. It is more important, however, to determine how many high-grade MCTs were identified correctly. The second study graded 5 (12%) of 41 histologically high-grade MCTs as low-grade MCTs on cytology and reviewed the limitations of cytologic grading when using the 2-tier system. Even highly cellular cytologic samples contain significantly lower number of neoplastic mast cells per HPF than histologic sections. This disparity is due in part to the way that tissues are collected and processed for histology, allowing entire tissues to be kept intact and, more importantly, because the terminology varies between the 2 modalities, because an HPF in cytology is based on a 100-times objective rather than a 40-times objective in histology. Therefore, the established histologic criteria would have to be validated for future use of the 2-tier system in cytologic preparations. When comparing the individual criteria for malignancy in histologically high-grade MCTs, in cytologic samples, karyomegaly, multinucleated cells, and bizarre nuclei were present in only 82.9%, 47.3%, and 31.6% of cytologically classified high-grade MCTs, respectively.[16] Mitotic figures were identified in approximately 50% of the high-grade MCTs, but the concordance between histology and cytology was poor, with far fewer mitotic figures seen in aspirates than in histologic sections.[16] Furthermore, this study required that cytology slides were first destained and then restained with H&E to properly assess nuclear morphology, which is easily obscured by strongly staining granules in Romanowsky-type stains. H&E staining is not used commonly in cytology because it requires incubation of slides in alcohol or fixation in acetone for 24 hours prior to H&E staining, thereby eliminating the fast turnaround advantage of cytologic preparations.

The third study established cytologic grading criteria based on cytologic findings that correlated with the histologic grade and could easily be assessed with modified Wright stain.[15] MCTs were classified as high grade if they were poorly granulated or had at least 2 of 4 findings: mitotic figures, binucleated or multinucleated cells, nuclear pleomorphism, and greater than 50% anisokaryosis.[15] This cytologic grading scheme had a sensitivity of 88% and a specificity of 94% relative to histologic grading. It tended to overestimate high-grade MCTs, however. Two (11%) of 17 histologic high-grade MCTs were graded as low-grade MCTs on cytology, but 7 (5%) of 135 histologically low-grade MCTs were graded as high-grade MCTs, thereby representing 32% false-positive high-grade MCTs in this study.[15] Although the consequences of a false-positive result for a high-grade tumor could include more aggressive surgery or staging than necessary or, worst case scenario, euthanasia, cytology typically is considered a screening test. Although it may be argued that over-diagnosing high-grade MCTs will ensure that more aggressive staging and potentially more aggressive treatment are not overlooked, it is essential to use caution when basing therapeutic decisions on a single cytologic grading system.[15]

In summary, based on current data, the cytologic feature reported most predictive of the biological behavior is granularity, with poorly granular MCTs exhibiting a greater tendency to metastasize than well granulated mast cell neoplasms (**Fig. 6**).[15] Caution must be used when using aqueous quick stains to ensure that the microscopic absence of granules is reflective of the aspirated cells and not a result of staining artifact. Additionally, manipulation of the mass should be avoided prior to aspiration to minimize degranulation effects, which can compound interpretation. Importantly, the assumption that highly granular MCTs are benign should be avoided, because highly granular tumors may exhibit other criteria correlated with aggressive biological behavior (**Fig. 7**), including the presence of mitotic figures, anisokaryosis, binucleation, multinucleation, and bizarre (nonround) nuclei.[15,18] These features are less predictive of metastatic potential than granularity and should be used together, with the presence of at least 2 of these criteria suggesting aggressive biological behavior.[15] Because cytologic specimens vary in cellularity, quantitative criteria for mitotic figures and other atypical morphologic features should not be used with these specimens. This is a substantial variation that limits direct application of the 2-tier histologic grading system to cytologic specimens, because the 2-tier scheme utilizes the number of criteria per HPF to determine a histologic grade. In heavily granulated specimens where nuclear details are obscured, the use of H&E rather than Romanowsky stains may decrease granular staining and accentuate nuclear and cytoplasmic features (**Fig. 8**). The fact that H&E staining, which is routinely used for histologic sections, minimally stains granules may account for the fact that granularity is not a key component of histologic grading schemes.

Molecular Markers

KIT expression and c-Kit mutations

The tyrosine kinase receptor KIT plays a central role in the survival, proliferation, differentiation, and migration of mast cells. Aberrant expression of KIT protein as detected with IHC has been shown a negative prognostic indicator for canine cutaneous MCTs.[19] Three different KIT expression patterns have been described. Perimembranous labeling (pattern I) is found in non-neoplastic mast cells as well as in well differentiated MCTs (**Fig. 9**A) and has not been associated with aggressive biological behavior.[19] Loss of perimembranous labeling along with focal or stippled cytoplasmic labeling is characteristic of pattern II (see **Fig. 9**B), and diffuse cytoplasmic labeling in at least 10% of neoplastic cells is consistent with pattern III (see **Fig. 9**C). Both patterns II and III have been associated with a decreased overall survival time and an increased incidence of local recurrence. In addition to the IHC pattern, activating mutations in exons 11, 8, and 9 of *c-Kit* have been commonly reported in canine cutaneous MCTs.[20,21] Activating duplication mutations in exon 11 occur in approximately 20% of canine cutaneous MCTs and occur much more commonly in high-grade MCTs.[21,22] They have been associated with a high risk of local recurrence and metastases as well as decreased survival and disease-free times.[21,22] Mutations in exon 8 and 9 occur in less than 5% of canine cutaneous MCTs and mutations in exon 8 have not been associated with a poor prognosis.[23]

Proliferation markers

Uncontrolled cellular proliferation is considered a hallmark of cancer. Several studies have evaluated cellular proliferation in canine MCTs and have shown

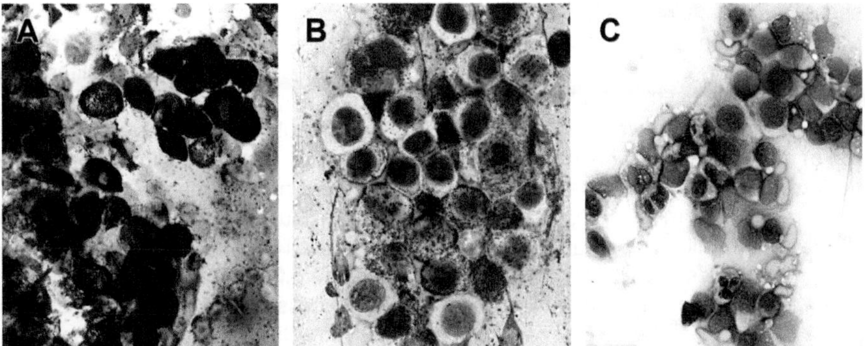

Fig. 6. Variation of granularity in cytologic samples of canine cutaneous MCTs. Modified Wright stain. (*A*) Heavily granulated mast cells with nuclei almost completely obscured by granules. (*B*) Mixed granularity mast cells with a few heavily granulated and more poorly granulated mast cells. (*C*) Poorly granulated mast cells. The absence of granules makes it difficult to accurately diagnose this neoplasm as an MCT.

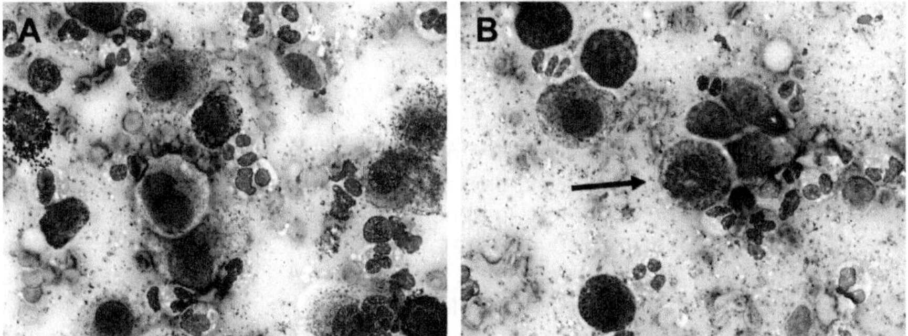

Fig. 7. Aspirate of a high-grade canine cutaneous MCT. Modified Wright stain. (*A*) Neoplastic cells are markedly pleomorphic, including binucleation, anisocytosis, and anisokaryosis. (*B*) Neoplastic cells exhibit variable granularity as well as anisocytosis and anisokaryosis. Mitotic figures (*arrow*) are commonly noticed.

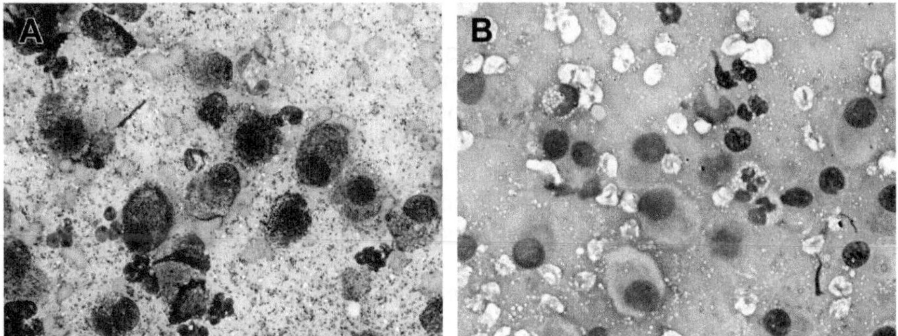

Fig. 8. Assessing nuclear morphology in cytologic samples of canine cutaneous MCTs. (*A*) Modified Wright staining may obscure nuclear morphology in heavily granulated mast cells. (*B*) H&E staining of the same tumor allows for easier examination of nuclear morphology because granules are poorly stained.

assessment of cellular proliferation being a strong prognostic parameter. To evaluate proliferation markers, it is important to understand a few key concepts of tumor growth. Tumor growth is the result of a disturbed balance between cell proliferation and cell death (growth = proliferation × 1/cell death). Any disturbance that results in an increased ratio of proliferation to cell death can result in tumor growth. The degree of cellular proliferation is determined by the number of cells within the cell cycle (growth fraction) and the rate (speed) of cells progressing through the cycle (proliferation rate). The most common proliferation markers used in veterinary medicine include argyrophilic nucleolus organizer regions (AgNORs) (**Fig. 10**), Ki67 (**Fig. 11**), and the MC. These proliferation markers characterize different aspects of proliferation.[2] Ki67 is a nuclear protein that labels all cycling cells but cannot be detected in resting cells. It is, therefore, a marker of the growth fraction. AgNORs represent nuclear proteins that can be visualized by silver stains, and large numbers and small size of AgNORs correlate with an increased speed of cell cycle progression; therefore, AgNORs represent a proliferation rate marker. The MC is a phase index marker that identifies cells in the M phase of the cell cycle. Combining assessment of the growth fraction (Ki67) with the proliferation rate (AgNORs) provides the most accurate approach to determine proliferation of a neoplastic cell population and has been established as an important prognostic indicator for canine cutaneous MCTs.[2,24] In contrast, using a phase index, such as the MC, as a sole predictor of proliferation, may result in both false-positive or false-negative assessments because the MC may reflect the state of proliferation or could be due to karyologic abnormalities.

A major problem when evaluating proliferation markers in canine cutaneous MCTs is standardization of the evaluation methods and, even more importantly, selection of the area to be evaluated. In general, areas with the highest proliferation activity should be used to accurately determine the MC, the Ki67 index, or the number of AgNORs in any given MCT.[1,2] This is especially problematic when determining the MC in highly granulated MCTs in H&E-stained sections and there can be high interobserver variation. In contrast, when using a red chromogen to label Ki67-positive cells, examination of slides at low magnification allows much easier identification of the areas with the highest index and, therefore, a higher consistency among pathologists. The areas of neoplastic cells with the largest numbers of AgNORs also are more easily identifiable than areas of the highest MC. Furthermore, because the MC represents only a phase index, at least 20% of high grade MCTs have a low MC.[3,6] Although a large MC is a clear indicator of more aggressive biological behavior and, therefore, has been included in the current 2-tier grading system, a low MC is not a sensitive marker of a more benign behavior. There is little value in assessing the MC as a sole prognostic marker because it is less sensitive and less specific compared with the current 2-tier grading system. Regardless, all 3 parameters should be determined consistently with the same method and when reporting these numbers the method used should be provided to the client to allow comparison of the results.[2] A standardized method for determining the Ki67 index has been based on the use of an ocular grid and, in this method, an average of more than 23 Ki-67–positive cells per grid area was associated with shorter survival times and MCT-related mortality.[24] When the Ki-67 index was furthermore combined with the AgNOR counts as a product of the value for each parameter, aggressive MCTs were identified with a higher degree of accuracy. A combined AgNORxKi-67 score larger than 54 was associated with an increased risk of MCT-related mortality and metastasis.[24]

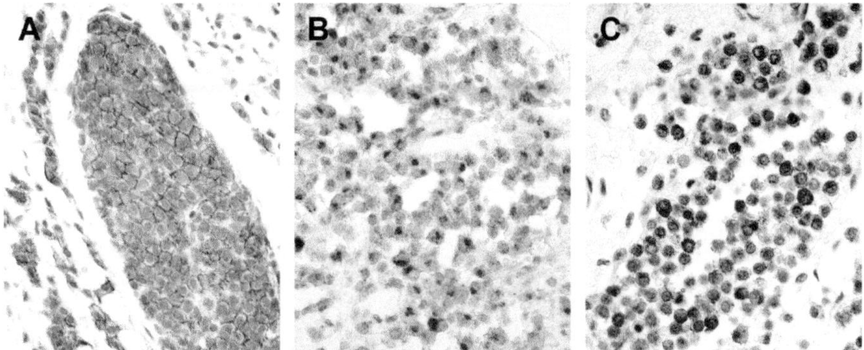

Fig. 9. Evaluating the KIT (CD117) labeling pattern. IHC for KIT (DAB, brown), hematoxylin counterstain. (*A*) Perimembranous labeling characteristic for pattern 1. (*B*) Stippled cytoplasmic labeling and loss of perimembranous labeling characteristic for pattern 2. (*C*) Diffuse cytoplasmic labeling observed in pattern 3.

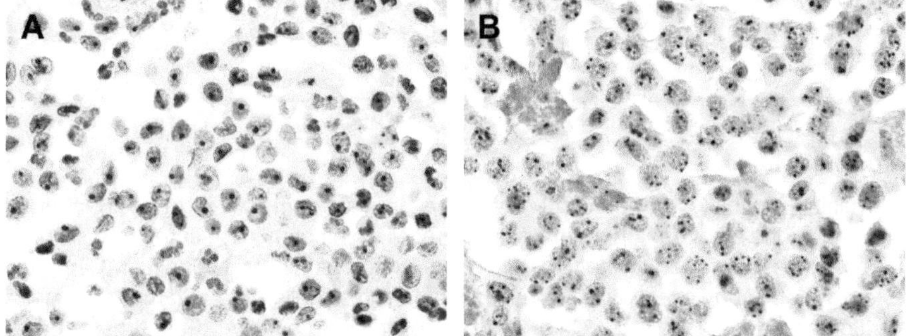

Fig. 10. Evaluating numbers of AgNORs. Silver stain according to Ploton. (*A*) An average of 1 to 3 AgNORs per nucleus is associated with less aggressive biological behavior. (*B*) An average of more than 4 AgNORs per nucleus is associated with poor survival.

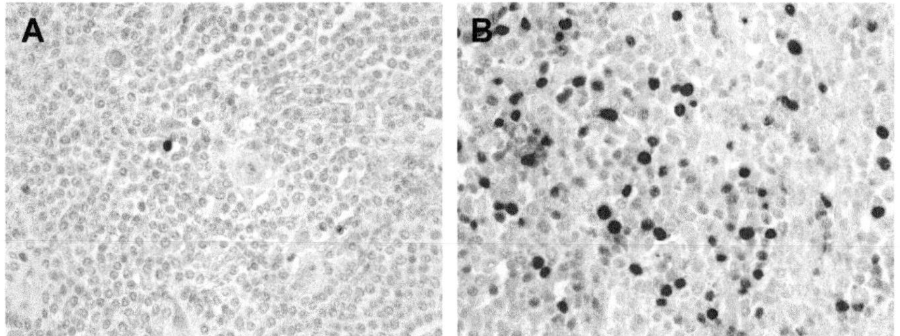

Fig. 11. Evaluating Ki67 index. IHC for Ki67 (Vector red, red), hematoxylin counterstain. (*A*) A low Ki67 index (23 or below per grid) has been associated with longer survival times and unlikely local recurrence. (*B*) A high Ki67 index (>23 per grid) has been associated with shorter survival times and a high risk of metastatic disease.

Prognosis of canine cutaneous mast cell tumors

- No single technique identifies every single aggressive MCT.
- Cytologic grading provides a simple approach for initial clinical decision making.
- The positive predictive value of cytologic grading is low (it falsely detects too many high grade MCTs); a more detailed prognosis has to be based on biopsy.
- Histologic grading using the 2-tier system (Kiupel and colleagues, 2011[6]) provides the best histologic approach for identifying aggressive (high-grade) MCTs with high metastatic risk.
- Between 5% and 15% of low-grade MCTs still exhibit aggressive behavior and additional tools have to be used to detect these neoplasms.
- The mitotic count alone is less sensitive then the 2-tier grading system.
- Other grading systems suffer from low reproducibility and a combination with the 2-tier system has a negative impact on the overall reproducibility and specificity.
- The combined AgNOR and Ki67 values predict aggressive behavior.
- An abnormal expression pattern of KIT predicts aggressive behavior.
- Mutations in exon 11 of *c-Kit* predict aggressive biological behavior.
- Mutations in exon 8 of *c-Kit* are not associated with aggressive behavior.
- Combining the 2-tier histologic grading with analysis of AgNORs, Ki67, KIT expression, and detection of mutations in exons 8 and 11 provides the most detailed prognostic assessment.

Margin Evaluation

Determining cleanliness of surgical margins is an important part in the evaluation of excisional biopsies of canine cutaneous MCTs. Margins should be inked and surgical sutures are used most commonly to help orientate the pathologist. Canine MCTs often are surrounded, however, by edema, reactive stromal cells, and inflammatory cells, including non-neoplastic mast cells, that can form a halo of several-centimeter thickness. This halo poses a challenge to both the veterinary surgeon when grossly determining the surgical margins and the veterinary pathologist when determining cleanliness of the examined margins. Although the distance of neoplastic mast cells to surgical margins has been linked in numerous studies to the likelihood of recurrence, the accuracy of assessing this distance is questionable. Numerous technical factors have an impact on margin distance. After surgical incision, there is marked retraction of the cutaneous margins. Fixation and processing have an impact, especially on the adipose tissue and the halo, causing both shrinkage and distortion. Furthermore, pathologists currently are unable to differentiate neoplastic from non-neoplastic mast cells, and markers used in human medicine, for example, CD25, are not specific for neoplastic mast cells in dogs.[2] Differentiating neoplastic from non-neoplastic mast cells when examining surgical margins most commonly is based on the arbitrary decision that clusters of 3 or more mast cells are considered neoplastic, whereas individual, well-granulated mast cells are considered inflammatory mast cells.[1] Lastly, the method used to trim MCTs for microscopic examination has a major impact on the ability of pathologists to determine cleanliness of margins as well as distance of neoplastic cells to those margins. Routinely, most MCTs are radially sectioned (halves and quarters). This method essentially only examines neoplastic mast cells along the radii of the 4 quarters (**Fig. 12**). For a 1-cm diameter MCT with 2-cm margins, the total excision would have an approximately 5-cm diameter and a circumference of 15.7 cm. A single mast cell measures approximately

10 μm. In order to detect every cluster of 3 or more mast cells extending to the margins, more than 500 radial sections would be required. Examining such large numbers would be technically and economically unfeasible. Therefore, combined radial and tangential sectioning is the preferred method the assess MCT margins and has a more than 20% higher sensitivity in detecting dirty margins.[25] The radial sections are based on palpation of the mass and provide high-quality samples for the diagnosis and future prognostic testing as well as some information about the distance of the tumor to the margins. The tangential sections give the most accurate information about margin cleanliness (see **Fig. 12**).

Considering the technical difficulties in determining clean margins, newer methods, based on molecular pathology, have been more recently applied to determine the need for additional surgery or radiation therapy.[2,24,26–28] High-grade MCTs as well as MCTs with a mutation in exon 11 of *c-Kit* have a high likelihood (up to 40%) of local recurrence despite clean surgical margins.[2,26] Alternatively, low-grade MCTs with a low proliferation activity, as determined by the Ki67 index or the Ki67xAgNOR index, were highly unlikely (less than 10%) to recur regardless of the cleanliness of margins.[27,28] A combination of radial and tangential margin examination with these molecular methods represents currently the most accurate method to determine the likelihood of local recurrence.

Margins of canine cutaneous mast cell tumors

- Individual neoplastic mast cells cannot be differentiated from non-neoplastic mast cells; clusters of 3 or more cells are arbitrarily considered neoplastic.
- Surgical manipulation, fixation, and sectioning of the excised MCT all have an impact on the actual distance of neoplastic mast cells from the surgical margins.
- Cross-sectioning (half and radial sections) based on palpation provides high-quality sections for an accurate diagnosis, prognostic testing, and assessing tumor distance to lateral and deep margins.
- Complete surgical excision is best determined by tangential sectioning.
- Advanced molecular techniques are superior in predicting local recurrence.
- Low-grade MCTs with a low AgNORxKi67 index have a low risk of local recurrence regardless of the cleanliness of the surgical margins.

Lymph Node Assessment

Although there is a lack of consensus among oncologists regarding the steps for MCT staging, evaluation of the draining lymph node represents an essential component in every approach. It is important to remember that the nearest node to the neoplasm may not be the draining node. Review of lymphatic drainage or regional lymphoscintigraphy may be beneficial when determining the node that should be sampled (**Fig. 13**). Approximately 40% of draining nodes would be missed if only the anatomically closest node were sampled.[29] Furthermore, metastatic disease was detected in 50% of nonpalpable/normal-sized regional lymph nodes in 1 study.[30] Such high numbers raise questions about the accuracy and standardization of evaluating lymph node spread of canine cutaneous MCTs. Although both cytologic and histologic classifications for lymph node spread have been proposed, both system suffer from several technical difficulties.[31,32] Regardless, removal of regional nodes with manifestation of metastatic MCTs has been shown to be associated with a better prognostic outcome.[33]

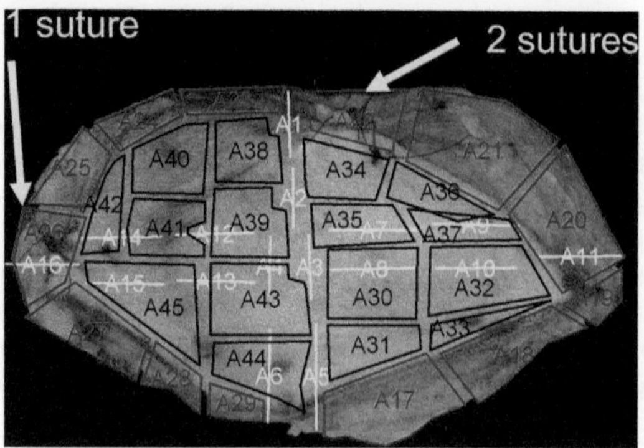

Fig. 12. Margin evaluation of a canine cutaneous MCT. The yellow lines indicate the perpendicular half and quarter sections (radial sectioning) to diagnose the mass accurately and to determine the distance of the closest margin. To determine complete surgical removal, tangential sectioning evaluating the lateral skin margins (*red sections*) and the deep margins (*black sections*) has to be performed. The number of sutures placed within the margins (1 suture = cranial and 2 sutures = medial) determines the orientation of the neoplasm on the body.

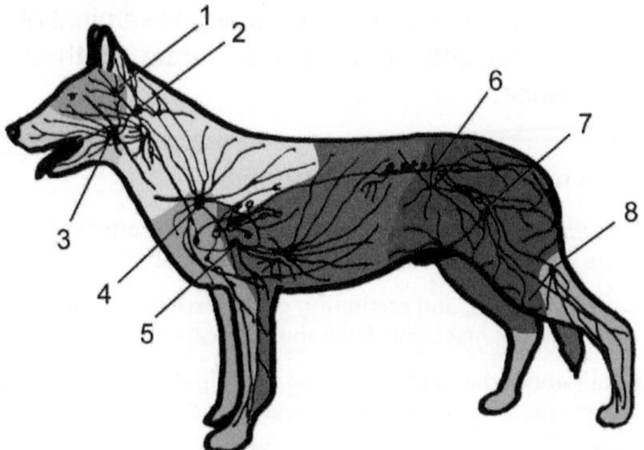

Fig. 13. Diagram of lymphatic drainage. Identification of the tributary lymph node is helpful when determining the appropriate node to aspirate during MCT staging. Major draining lymph nodes: 1 = parotid, 2 = submandibular, 3 = retropharyngeal, 4 = prescapular, 5 = axillary, 6 = iliac, 7 = inguinal, and 8 = popliteal.

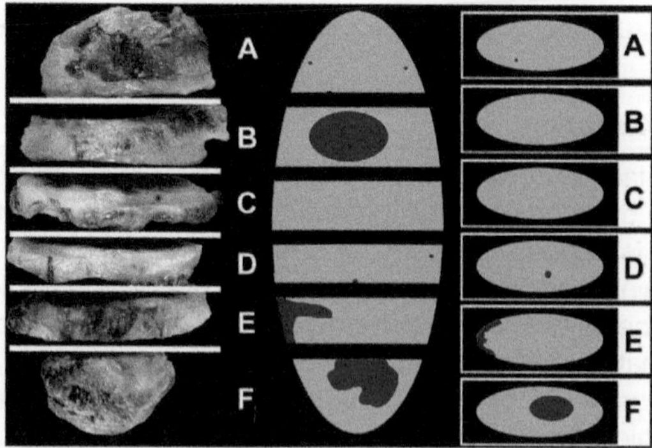

Fig. 14. Sectioning of the lymph node to detect metastatic disease. Sections should be taken at 2-mm intervals to detect manifestation of metastatic disease with at least 2 mm in diameter. Detection of individual mast cells is arbitrary unless sections are cut at 10-μm thickness. Slide A = arbitrary detection of individual cells, slide B = sections missed metastasis smaller than 2 mm in diameter, slide C = no evidence of metastasis, slide D = arbitrary detection of small metastatic focus, slide E = detection of sinusoidal infiltrates of large numbers of neoplastic mast cells, and slide F = detection of a large metastatic mass.

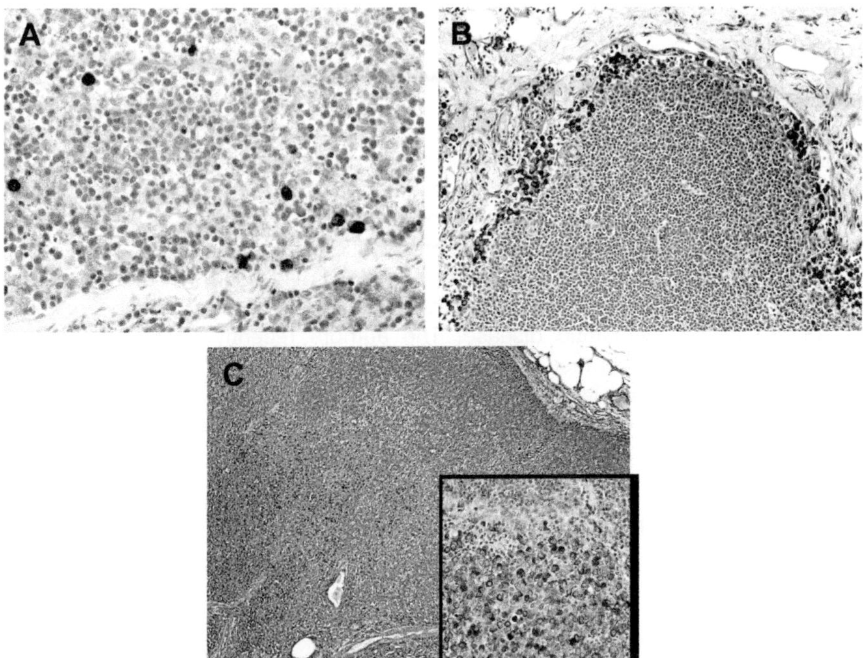

Fig. 15. Microscopic classification of nodal metastasis of canine cutaneous MCTs. Toluidine blue stain. (*A*) Class HN1 = more than 3 individualized mast cells in sinuses in a minimum of 4 HPFs. (*B*) Class HN2 = aggregates of mast cells in sinuses or sinusoidal sheets of mast cells. (*C*) HN3 = effacement of normal nodal architecture by mast cells; (*inset*) large nodule composed of sheets of mast cells.

Cytologic evaluation of lymph node spread of MCTs can be challenging, because lymph nodes normally contain low numbers of mast cells and as neoplastic mast cells can recruit non-neoplastic mast cells via lymphatics. This is particularly problematic when MCTs are manipulated during surgical removal, because physical pressure on the mass and surrounding tissues can induce degranulation and recruitment of non-neoplastic mast cells to the draining lymph nodes.[1] To minimize the effects of manipulation on lymph node evaluation, it is recommended that lymph node aspirates for MCT staging are taken prior to surgical mass removal.

Because it is impossible to definitively distinguish neoplastic from non-neoplastic mast cells, the number and arrangement of mast cells in a lymph node are used as indicators of lymphatic metastasis. Although a standardized system for cytologic lymph node staging has been proposed, it remains largely unutilized, due to the nebulous categories of possible metastasis and probable metastasis that are of little prognostic value to oncologists.[31,34] Although percentages of mast cells in lymph nodes are increased in patients with neoplastic versus allergic disease, distinguishing microscopic metastasis remains difficult and cytopathologists tend to subjectively evaluate the significance of mast cells in lymph nodes based on pleomorphism, arrangement in aggregates, and overall number.[34] Histologic evaluation of the draining lymph node is typically advised in these cases for additional characterization. There is no standard for trimming excised nodes, however, for microscopic examination. To detect individual mast cells of 10-μm diameter, a 1-cm diameter lymph node would have to be sectioned 100 times (**Fig. 14**). Routinely, excised nodes often are simply single sectioned. Sectioning nodes at 0.2-cm intervals, following a recommendation adopted from human medicine to detect overt metastatic disease, is recommended. A 4-tiered histologic classification system (HN0–HN3) has been recommended to more accurate predict the clinical outcomes for dogs with MCT metastasis (**Fig. 15**).[32] Even with nodes sectioned at 0.2-cm intervals, detection of HN1 is purely arbitrary and of little clinical significance. It is also important to recognize that categories HN1 and HN2 do not present a premetastastic or early metastatic disease but rather a different degree of a suspected metastatic disease. Identifying HN3 nodes with overt nodal metastasis represents an important prognostic parameter, but other categories should not be over-interpreted. In a similar manner as discussed with margin evaluation, combing histologic node assessment with molecular markers will improve accuracy of identifying metastatic disease. The authors recently demonstrated that quantitation of RNA of tryptase and carboxypeptidase A3 in lymph node aspirates and biopsies dramatically improved the accuracy of detecting lymph node spread (Matti Kiupel, unpublished data, 2019). Establishing such techniques in routine surgical pathology will advance the ability to predict metastatic spread.

Lymph node spread of canine mast cell tumors

- Sentinel nodes always should be examined for metastatic spread regardless of their clinical presentation.
- In addition, clinically abnormal lymph nodes (eg, enlarged) should be examined for metastatic spread.
- Individual neoplastic mast cells cannot be differentiated from non-neoplastic mast cells.
- Detection of individual or even small clusters of mast cells with cytology or histology is arbitrary and should not be over-interpreted as metastasis.
- Aspirates of a tributary lymph node with a diagnosis of certain or probable metastasis (Krick and colleagues, 2009[31]) are consistent with or highly suggestive of metastatic spread, respectively.
- Microscopic evaluation of the tributary node requires sectioning of the node at 2-mm intervals to detect overt metastatic disease (HN3 [Weishaar and colleagues, 2014[32]]).
- A negative result on either cytology or histology does not confirm absence of neoplastic mast cells or even early metastasis.
- Novel molecular techniques, for example, quantitation of RNA of tryptase and carboxypeptidase A3, will improve accuracy of detecting lymph node spread.

REFERENCES

1. Kiupel M. Mast cell tumors. In: Meuten DJ, editor. Tumors in domestic animals. 5th edition. Ames (IA): Wiley-Blackwell; 2017. p. 176–202.
2. Sledge DG, Webster J, Kiupel M. Canine cutaneous mast cell tumors: a combined clinical and pathologic approach to diagnosis, prognosis, and treatment selection. Vet J 2016;215:43–54.
3. Thompson JJ, Pearl DL, Yager JA, et al. Canine subcutaneous mast cell tumor: characterization and prognostic indices. Vet Pathol 2011;48:156–68.
4. Bostock DE. The prognosis following surgical removal of mastocytomas in dogs. J Small Anim Pract 1973;14:27–41.

5. Patnaik AK, Ehler WJ, MacEwen EG. Canine cutaneous mast cell tumor: morphologic grading and survival time in 83 dogs. Vet Pathol 1984;21:469–74.
6. Kiupel M, Webster JD, Bailey KL, et al. Proposal of a 2-tier histologic grading system for canine cutaneous mast cell tumors to more accurately predict biological behavior. Vet Pathol 2011;48:147–55.
7. Northrup NC, Howerth EW, Harmon BG, et al. Variation among pathologists in the histologic grading of canine cutaneous mast cell tumors with uniform use of a single grading reference. J Vet Diagn Invest 2005;17:561–4.
8. Northrup NC, Harmon BG, Gieger TL, et al. Variation among pathologists in histologic grading of canine cutaneous mast cell tumors. J Vet Diagn Invest 2005;17: 245–8.
9. Kiupel M, Webster JD, Miller RA, et al. Impact of tumour depth, tumour location and multiple synchronous masses on the prognosis of canine cutaneous mast cell tumours. J Vet Med A Physiol Pathol Clin Med 2005;52:280–6.
10. Sabattini S, Scarpa F, Berlato D, et al. Histologic grading of canine mast cell tumor: is 2 better than 3? Vet Pathol 2015;52:70–3.
11. Stefanello D, Buracco P, Sabattini S, et al. Comparison of 2- and 3-category histologic grading systems for predicting the presence of metastasis at the time of initial evaluation in dogs with cutaneous mast cell tumors: 386 cases (2009-2014). J Am Vet Med Assoc 2015;246:765–9.
12. Takeuchi Y, Fujino Y, Watanabe M, et al. Validation of the prognostic value of histopathological grading or c-kit mutation in canine cutaneous mast cell tumours: a retrospective cohort study. Vet J 2013;196:492–8.
13. Vascellari M, Giantin M, Capello K, et al. Expression of Ki67, BCL-2, and COX-2 in canine cutaneous mast cell tumors: association with grading and prognosis. Vet Pathol 2013;50:110–21.
14. Thompson JJ, Yager JA, Best SJ, et al. Canine subcutaneous mast cell tumors: cellular proliferation and KIT expression as prognostic indices. Vet Pathol 2011; 48:169–81.
15. Camus MS, Priest HL, Koehler JW, et al. Development of cytologic criteria for mast cell tumor grading with clinical outcome evaluation. Vet Pathol 2016;53(6): 1117–23.
16. Hergt F, von Bomhard W, Kent MS, et al. Use of a 2-tier histologic grading system for canine cutaneous mast cell tumors on cytology specimens. Vet Clin Pathol 2016;45(3):477–83.
17. Scarpa F, Sabattini S, Bettini G. Cytological grading of canine cutaneous mast cell tumours. Vet Comp Oncol 2014;14(3):245–51.
18. Ressel L, Finotello R. Cytological grading of canine cutaneous mast cell tumours: is haematoxylin and eosin staining better than May-Grünwald-Giemsa? Vet Comp Oncol 2016;15(3):667–8.
19. Kiupel M, Webster JD, Kaneene JB, et al. The use of KIT and tryptase expression patterns as prognostic tools for canine cutaneous mast cell tumors. Vet Pathol 2004;41:371–7.
20. Letard S, Yang Y, Hanssens K, et al. Gain-of-function mutations in the extracellular domain of KIT are common in canine mast cell tumors. Mol Cancer Res 2008;6:1137–45.
21. Webster JD, Yuzbasiyan-Gurkan V, Kaneene JB, et al. The role of c-KIT in tumorigenesis: evaluation in canine cutaneous mast cell tumors. Neoplasia 2006;8: 104–11.

22. Webster JD, Yuzbasiyan-Gurkan V, Thamm DH, et al. Evaluation of prognostic markers for canine mast cell tumors treated with vinblastine and prednisone. BMC Vet Res 2008;4:32.
23. Kiupel M, Catlin C, Collins-Webb A, et al. Prognostic Significance of activating mutations in exons 8 and 11 of c-Kit in canine cutaneous mast cell tumors. Cartagena (Columbia): WSAVA; 2016.
24. Webster JD, Yuzbasiyan-Gurkan V, Miller RA, et al. Cellular proliferation in canine cutaneous mast cell tumors: associations with c-KIT and its role in prognostication. Vet Pathol 2007;44:298–308.
25. Dores CB, Milovancev M, Russell DS. Comparison of histologic margin status in low-grade cutaneous and subcutaneous canine mast cell tumours examined by radial and tangential sections. Vet Comp Oncol 2018;16:125–30.
26. Donnelly L, Mullin C, Balko J, et al. Evaluation of histological grade and histologically tumour-free margins as predictors of local recurrence in completely excised canine mast cell tumours. Vet Comp Oncol 2015;13:70–6.
27. Séguin B, Besancon MF, McCallan JL, et al. Recurrence rate, clinical outcome, and cellular proliferation indices as prognostic indicators after incomplete surgical excision of cutaneous grade II mast cell tumors: 28 dogs (1994-2002). J Vet Intern Med 2006;20:933–40.
28. Smith J, Kiupel M, Farrelly J, et al. Recurrence rates and clinical outcome for dogs with grade II mast cell tumours with a low AgNOR count and Ki67 index treated with surgery alone. Vet Comp Oncol 2017;15:36–45.
29. Worley DR. Incorporation of sentinel lymph node mapping in dogs with mast cell tumours: 20 consecutive procedures. Vet Comp Oncol 2014;12:215–26.
30. Ferrari R, Marconato L, Buracco P, et al. The impact of extirpation of non-palpable/normal-sized regional lymph nodes on staging of canine cutaneous mast cell tumours: a multicentric retrospective study. Vet Comp Oncol 2018; 16(4):505–10.
31. Krick EL, Billings AP, Shofer FS, et al. Cytological lymph node evaluation in dogs with mast cell tumours: association with grade and survival. Vet Comp Oncol 2009;7:130–8.
32. Weishaar KM, Thamm DH, Worley DR, et al. Correlation of nodal mast cells with clinical outcome in dogs with mast cell tumour and a proposed classification system for the evaluation of node metastasis. J Comp Pathol 2014;151:329–38.
33. Marconato L, Polton G, Stefanello D, et al. Therapeutic impact of regional lymphadenectomy in canine stage II cutaneous mast cell tumours. Vet Comp Oncol 2018;16(4):580–9.
34. Mutz ML, Boudreaux BB, Royal A, et al. Cytologic comparison of the percentage of mast cells in lymph node aspirate samples from clinically normal dogs versus dogs with allergic dermatologic disease and dogs with cutaneous mast cell tumors. J Am Vet Med Assoc 2017;251(4):421–8.

Anorexia and the Cancer Patient

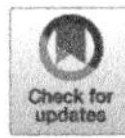

Chad M. Johannes, DVM*, Margaret L. Musser, DVM

KEYWORDS

• Anorexia • Inappetence • Cachexia • Cancer • Ghrelin • Capromorelin
• Mirtazapine

KEY POINTS

- Inappetence occurs commonly and is a key factor in perceived quality of life and clinical management for cats and dogs with cancer.
- Prolonged inappetence can have a negative impact on patient nutritional status, potentially leading to cachexia, which may have a significant effect on overall outcome.
- Understanding the importance of early recognition and intervention for the inappetent dog or cat with cancer is critical.
- Being familiar with the mechanisms of action, safety and efficacy data, and potential clinical utility of the recently approved pharmacologic appetite stimulants (capromorelin [dogs] and mirtazapine [cats]) will pay dividends in practices, with learning how to best integrate these therapeutics.

DEFINING THE CLINICAL CHALLENGE OF INAPPETENCE IN CANCER PATIENTS

Incidence...More Common than One May Think

Presence of a good appetite is a critical element when pet owners consider the overall quality of life of their dog or cat.[1] Lack of appetite often is the first recognizable sign by pet owners that their companion is not feeling well and typically triggers inquiry to their veterinarian's office. Market studies indicate that 14% of canine patients are presented to veterinary clinics in the United States due to the clinical symptom of inappetence.[2] A clinical survey, the aim of which was to determine the most frequently reported clinical presentations in the small animal primary care setting, identified inappetence as the third most common clinical sign reported (3.9%) and the most common

Disclosure Statement: Within the past 3 years, Dr C.M. Johannes has been on the advisory board, has been a paid consultant, and has done clinical trials with Aratana Therapeutics. Dr C.M. Johannes is on the advisory board and receives research grant from Zoetis. Dr M.L. Musser has nothing to disclose.
Department of Veterinary Clinical Sciences, Iowa State University College of Veterinary Medicine, Ames, IA, USA
* Corresponding author.
E-mail address: cmj15@iastate.edu

Vet Clin Small Anim 49 (2019) 837–854
https://doi.org/10.1016/j.cvsm.2019.04.008 vetsmall.theclinics.com

presenting problem overall (8.5%).[3] This survey found that inappetence was more commonly a presenting clinical sign in cats (5.8%) than dogs (2.2%).[3] Similarly, a survey of US veterinarians indicated that the number of cats presenting with weight loss/inappetence due to underlying conditions may approach 9 million annually, with 2 million of those cats receiving medical therapy for their inappetence.[4]

Specifically, in dogs and cats diagnosed with cancer, it also has been found that appetite frequently is a key determinant in pet owners' perceived quality of life.[5] A survey of clients whose cats were treated with a cyclophosphamide, doxorubicin, vincristine, and prednisone (CHOP)-based protocol for lymphoma revealed that appetite, vomiting, and diarrhea were important parameters in assessing the perceived quality of life for their cats. Although overall 75% of responding clients indicated that they were happy that they treated their cats with chemotherapy, these results indicate that a cat's appetite during chemotherapy is an important consideration for clients.[6]

Semantics

Decreased appetite is a nonspecific clinical sign with gradations in severity and many underlying causes, both acute and chronic (**Table 1**). Inappetence is an umbrella term used to describe decreased appetite throughout this article and encompasses the more specifically defined terms associated with decreased appetite outlined[1,2]:

- Anorexia: complete loss of appetite/lack of food intake
- Hyporexia: decreased appetite; not taking in full caloric needs
- Dysrexia: altered eating patterns; eating but not the desired diet(s) (chicken, hamburger, rice, etc., rather than prescribed commercial diet).

Recognizing the Problem

Clinical signs of inappetence (listed later) may be subtle, subjective, patient specific (based on typical routine and patterns at home), and incredibly dependent on client observations. Detailed questioning of clients by veterinarians and their staff is crucial to accurately assessing the severity and duration of inappetence experienced by a patient.

- Taking longer time to eat meals
- Needing to offer more palatable diets to encourage appetite
- Overall decreased food/caloric intake
- Lack of interest or robustness in eating (varying levels)
- May be commonly associated with other clinical signs, including nausea (drooling or lip-smacking), vomiting, diarrhea, and/or weight loss

Table 1
Common causes of inappetence in dogs and cats

Chronic	Acute
Cancer	Gastroenteritis (nonspecific)
Gastrointestinal/inflammatory bowel disease	Pancreatitis
Heart failure	Postoperative
CKD	Pain
Pancreatitis	Infectious (eg, parvovirus)
Secondary to other drugs/therapies	Secondary to other drugs/therapies
Palliative/end of life	

Inappetence in pets with cancer often is multifactorial, with potential contributing factors including the tumor or disease process itself (eg, dysphagia, pain, or ascites), increased systemic inflammatory cytokines, the anticancer treatments (chemotherapy, immunotherapy, and radiation therapy) administered, and/or effects of concomitant, palliative medications (anesthesia and pain relief medications). Although inappetence is a commonly described side effect of many chemotherapeutic agents in dogs and cats, the true incidence is not well defined. Published studies (**Table 2**) reporting the incidence of inappetence in dogs and cats receiving various chemotherapeutics are limited. Another challenge lies in that the methods of evaluating inappetence are variable and inconsistent between studies,[7] despite establishment of Veterinary Cooperative Oncology Group–Common Terminology Criteria for Adverse Events (VCOG-CTCAE) guidelines for anorexia (**Table 3**).[8]

Clinical Impact May Be Profound

If not addressed proactively, severe and/or prolonged inappetence can lead to weight loss and potentially cachexia (a metabolic syndrome leading to loss of lean body mass, described later). Weight loss and the development of cachexia may have a negative impact on a pet's survival and quality of life, as is well documented in human cancer patients.[9] There are many causes of weight loss in cancer patients, key among them inappetence, along with numerous catabolic drivers, including direct tumor metabolism, systemic inflammation, and insulin resistance.[10] This phenomenon is referred to as cancer-related anorexia/cachexia syndrome, a metabolic, paraneoplastic syndrome characterized by decreased food intake, involuntary weight loss, and altered body composition (loss of fat and muscle).[10] Diagnosis of human cancer cachexia is based on a weight loss of greater than 5% over the previous 6 months, any degree of weight loss greater than 2% in patients with concurrent evidence of loss of appendicular skeletal muscle (sarcopenia), or decreasing body mass index.[10] Cachexia is reported in 15% to 40% of human cancer patients, rising to 80% in those

Table 2
Reported incidence of inappetence in dogs & cats receiving chemotherapy (listed in ascending order of reported inappetence incidence)

Chemotherapeutic	Species	Inappetence Incidence	Reference
Vinorelbine	Dogs	17% (4/24)	Grant et al,[84] 2008
Epirubicin	Dogs	19% (27/139)	Marrington et al,[85] 2012
Carboplatin	Dogs and cats	25% (7/28)	Bowles et al,[86] 2010
Doxorubicin	Dogs	35%–51% (n = 49)[a,b]	Rau et al,[69] 2010
Rabacfosadine + doxorubicin	Dogs	35% (18/51)	Thamm et al,[87] 2017
Cyclophosphamide	Dogs	36% (15/42)[a]	Mason et al,[68] 2014
Toceranib phosphate	Dogs	39% (34/87)	London et al,[88] 2009
Vincristine	Dogs	43% (25/57)[a]	Mason et al,[68] 2014
Epirubicin	Dogs	44% (8/18)	Kim et al,[89] 2007
Lomustine	Dogs	48% (39/81)	Vail et al,[90] 2012
Rabacfosadine	Dogs	55% (21/38)	Vail et al,[91] 2009
Paclitaxel	Dogs	76% (128/168)	Vail et al,[90] 2012

[a] Subset of dogs treated with maropitant after chemotherapy administration.
[b] Crossover study.
Data from Refs.[68,69,84–91]

Table 3
Veterinary Cooperative Oncology Group scoring for anorexia

Veterinary Cooperative Oncology Group Grade	Clinical Description
Grade 1	Coaxing or dietary change required to maintain appetite
Grade 2	Oral intake altered (≤3 d) without significant weight loss; oral nutritional supplements/appetite stimulants may be indicated
Grade 3	Of >3 d duration; associated with significant weight loss (≥10%) or malnutrition; intravenous fluids, tube feeding, or force feeding indicated
Grade 4	Life-threatening consequences; total parenteral nutrition indicated; >5 d duration
Grade 5	Death

Data from Veterinary cooperative oncology group – common terminology criteria for adverse events (VCOG-CTCAE) following chemotherapy or biological antineoplastic therapy in dogs and cats. Vet Comp Oncol 2011;14(4):417–46.

with advanced disease. It is estimated that cachexia is the major cause of death in greater than 20% of human cancer patients.[9,11]

The extent to which veterinary cancer patients may develop cachexia-related changes has been only minimally examined. This may be attributed in part to veterinarians not recognizing the syndrome due to lack of awareness and/or absence of established diagnostic criteria or the fact that some veterinary patients may be humanely euthanized before the syndrome becomes clinically evident. Although there is limited information on the incidence of cachexia in pets, it is clear that the impact of inappetence on dogs and cats with cancer, along with their caregivers, can be profound.

It has been proved that in 1 population of dogs, anorexia at time of admission to a veterinary hospital was associated with a higher risk of death (not limited to dogs with cancer).[12] In addition, it was found that inappetence is a key factor in a client's decision-making process when it comes to end-of-life considerations. A recent survey of clients in a primary care setting found that inappetence and nonspecific decline were the 2 most common clinical signs listed by clients for consideration of humane euthanasia in their dog or cat.[13]

Anorexia and weight loss clearly have an impact on outcomes in dogs with cancer. Dogs diagnosed with gastrointestinal lymphoma presenting with clinical signs of anorexia had significantly decreased median survival time compared with dogs without anorexia (50 vs 81 days, respectively; $P = .047$).[14] Similarly, dogs underweight at the time of lymphoma diagnosis have been shown to experience significantly shorter survival times.[15] In addition, a majority (98%) of veterinary oncologists surveyed indicate that inappetence is one of the key clinical signs they use to categorize canine patients with lymphoma as substage b, which is associated with a less favorable clinical prognosis (the median decrease in appetite needed to classify the patient as substage b in this survey was approximately 40%).[16] One study indicated that the mean body condition score (BCS) for dogs diagnosed with cancer was 5.4 ± 1.2 (9-point scale). In this study, there was a significantly lower prevalence of overweight and obese dogs with cancer compared with control dogs without cancer. In addition, dogs with round cell tumors were found to have a significantly higher prevalence of underweight patients compared with healthy, noncancer control dogs.[17] A study by Michel and colleagues[18] reported that although only 4% of 100 evaluated dogs with cancer demonstrated cachexia based on a BCS less than or equal to 3, 15% experienced moderate to severe muscle wasting (muscle score ≤1). Additionally, 37% of the 64 dogs with body weights available from a time prior to the diagnosis of cancer had lost greater than 5% of their body weight at diagnosis. This amount (>5%) of weight loss within a 6-month time period from diagnosis would be defined as cachexia based on established criteria in humans, as outlined previously.[10]

Development of cachexia also is a concern in cats with cancer. In a study by Baez and colleagues,[19] the mean BCS for 57 feline cancer patients was 4.4 ± 2.1 (9-point scale). Although 60% of the cats experienced decreased fat mass, a vast majority (91%) experienced reduced muscle mass. Findings also were prognostic: cats with BCS less than 5 had a median survival time of 3.3 months compared with 16.7 months for cats with BCS greater than or equal to 5 ($P = .008$).

Although limited in number and scope, these studies in dogs and cats illustrate the importance of looking at more than body weight loss and BCS changes to identify veterinary patients experiencing cachexia. Total weight loss is an insensitive measure of muscle loss because lean body mass loss occurs prior to the detection of substantial weight loss.[20] Clinical awareness and consistent quantitative muscle assessment and/or scoring[1,20–23] are critically important for veterinary cancer patients, in addition to trends of percentage change in body weight.

Several studies in veterinary medicine have indicated dogs with cancer experience metabolic alterations similar to those observed in human patients with cachexia: increased resting energy expenditure and decreased rates of protein synthesis in dogs with osteosarcoma[24]; alterations in carbohydrate metabolism in dogs with lymphoma[25] and solid tumors[26]; and differences in serum cytokine profiles in dogs with lymphoma compared with healthy controls.[27]

Beyond cancer, other chronic conditions in dogs and cats associated with inappetence and related weight loss/cachexia include chronic kidney disease (CKD),[28–31] congestive heart failure,[32] and inflammatory bowel disease.[33] Dogs and cats are living longer lives, receiving more advanced medical care, and, not uncommonly, are diagnosed with more than 1 of these chronic conditions concurrently with their cancer diagnosis. In such patients, the importance of early intervention to prevent weight loss/cachexia likely is even more important.

EVOLVING THE CLINICAL MANAGEMENT OF INAPPETENCE

If weight loss/cachexia has an impact on canine and feline survival as it does in humans with cancer and other chronic illnesses, management of this syndrome may improve survival times and quality of life for pets diagnosed with similar conditions. Although most mild (grade 1) to moderate (grade 2) adverse events defined by the VCOG-CTCAE are managed with observation or minimal clinical intervention, anorexia may require a more aggressive approach. Grade 3 anorexia is defined as that greater than 3 days in duration and associated with significant (≥10%) weight loss (see **Table 3**).[8] From both a quality-of-life consideration as well as an enteral nutrition and cachexia prevention standpoint, earlier intervention (in the grade 1–2 timeframe) likely is warranted and important clinically. The challenge for veterinarians lies in having effective, proved therapies available for clinical use. Although identifying and treating the underlying cause(s) of inappetence remain important, the reality is that therapeutic intervention often is clinically necessary to stimulate appetite.

Physiology of Appetite Regulation

Initiation of feeding and appetite control is complicated and multifactorial. If it were simple and straightforward, pharmaceutical companies would have conquered it long ago because there are literally billions of dollars to be had in this field. Most of the focus has been on ways to decrease appetite and reduce obesity. An appetite suppressant, dirlotapide (Slentrol, Zoetis, Parsippany, NJ, USA), previously was approved by the Food and Drug Administration (FDA) in 2007 for management of obesity in dogs[34] but is no longer commercially available. Clinically it was successful but decreased the positive feeding interactions with their dogs most pet owners come to expect and enjoy and thus was not particularly popular.

The primary regulatory center for appetite is located in the hypothalamus. Signals from the periphery (gastrointestinal tract, pancreas, and adipose tissue) (**Fig. 1**) result in changes in activity of 2 neuronal subpopulations[35]:

1. Anorexigenic (appetite-suppressing) neurons
   a. Activate satiety center in ventromedial hypothalamus
   b. Signal the eat-less–metabolize-more effects on muscle, adipose tissue, liver, and so forth
   c. Positively influenced by circulating leptin and insulin
   d. Cross-communication occurs between the anorexigenic and orexigenic neurons
2. Orexigenic (appetite stimulating) neurons
   a. Activate hunger center in lateral hypothalamus
   b. Signal the eat-more–, metabolize-less effects on muscle, adipose tissue, liver, and so forth

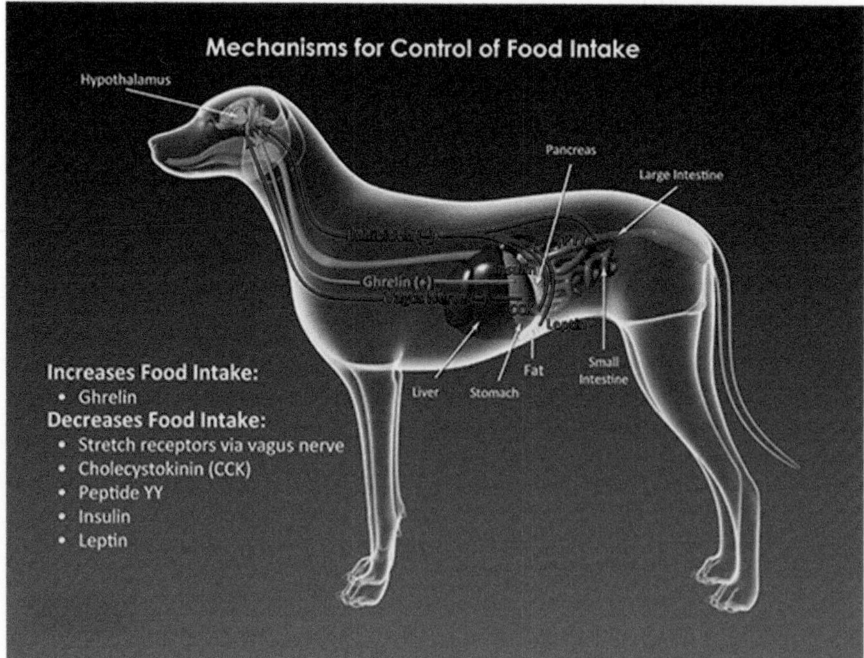

Fig. 1. Summary of appetite regulation signals. (*Courtesy of* Aratana Therapeutics, Inc., Leawood, KS; with permission.)

c. Positively influenced by circulating ghrelin (produced primarily in the oxyntic glands of the gastric fundus)[36,37]
d. Negatively influenced by circulating peptide YY, leptin, and insulin
e. Cross-communication occurs between the anorexigenic and orexigenic neurons

As noted previously, many of the peripheral signals exert a negative effect on appetite whereas ghrelin is the only known mediator with a stimulatory effect on orexigenic neurons. As such, ghrelin is believed the key driver for initiation of feeding behavior, appetite stimulation, and subsequent food intake.[37]

Therapeutic Options—Challenges and Opportunities

The list of therapies (most not approved for this indication) utilized historically in an attempt to stimulate appetite in dogs and cats is extensive (**Box 1**), with common choices including mirtazapine, cyproheptadine, corticosteroids, and antiemetics (**Table 4**). The challenge with these drugs is none of them has stimulation of appetite as a primary mechanism. The appetite stimulation component is a secondary or side effect of these drugs, explaining the lack of reliability from patient to patient. Except for mirtazapine in cats, additional challenges arise from limited data on dosing and pharmacokinetics and sparse to nonexistent data on efficacy for appetite stimulation in dogs and cats. New FDA-approved options are now available and outlined later.

Although the importance of proactive enteral nutritional support has been well recognized in veterinary medicine for some time, active treatment has been somewhat limited due to the lack of reliable pharmacologic clinical interventions. The availability of recent FDA approvals for appetite stimulation in dogs and cats has renewed interest and discussion around this topic. The availability of approved therapeutics for appetite stimulation has the potential to significantly alter the course of case management for many dogs and cats with cancer, similar to that experienced in the realm of emesis control when maropitant citrate (Cerenia [Zoetis, Parsippany, NJ, USA]) was approved in 2007. The remainder of this article focuses on updates on the key pharmacologic

Box 1
Medical treatments for inappetence in dogs and cats (not approved for this indication)

Anabolic steroids (stanozolol/Winstrol)

Benzodiazepines (diazepam)

CBD oil

Cobalamin (vitamin B_{12})

Cyproheptadine

Fish oil

Glucocorticoids (prednisone)

Hemp (Canna-Pet, LLC, Seattle, WA, USA)

Maropitant (Cerenia)

Medical marijuana

Megestrol acetate (Ovaban)

Propofol

Table 4
Appetite stimulant utilization by specialists for chemotherapy-induced signs in dogs (2016)

Appetite Stimulant	Very Likely to Use (%)	Somewhat Likely to Use (%)
Cerenia (maropitant)	57.7	28.2
Mirtazapine	52.9	34.1
Metoclopramide	15.3	45.9
Cyproheptadine	11.8	31.8
Corticosteroid	8.2	18.9
Canna-Pet	5.9	1.1
Acupuncture	4.7	3.5

Data from Punt NP, Johannes CM, Hackbarth LR, Fox LE. Clinical survey of veterinary specialists evaluating management of chemotherapy induced vomiting and inappetence in dogs. In: ACVIM Forum Proceedings. 2017; 45. Available at: https://onlinelibrary.wiley.com/doi/epdf/10.1111/jvim.14778. Accessed December 19, 2018.

appetite stimulant therapeutics currently available in veterinary practice and how they may have an impact on cancer patients.

Ghrelin receptor agonists

Mechanism of action Ghrelin receptor agonists (GRAs)were first identified in the late 1980s when a small peptide (growth hormone-releasing peptide 6 [GHRP-6]) was found to stimulate growth hormone (GH) release from the pituitary through a novel receptor (GH secretagogue receptor 1a [GHS-R1a]). This receptor has been identified to be expressed in the hypothalamus, pituitary gland, bone, heart, lung, liver, kidney, pancreas, and immune cells. These findings ultimately led to development of a class of orally administered small molecules called GH secretagogues (GHS) or GRAs that caused GH release by the pituitary. Endogenous ghrelin was later identified to be the natural ligand of GHS-R1a.[36]

The primary physiologic actions of GRAs have been identified to include appetite stimulation, GH release from the pituitary gland with subsequent increase in insulin-like growth factor 1 (IGF-1) via the liver, muscle mass increase, bone formation stimulation, gastrointestinal motility enhancement, and anti-inflammatory activity. Although endogenous ghrelin has a short serum half-life, the GRAs have been designed for therapeutic use with improved oral bioavailability and extended half-lives. Given the numerous systemic effects of ghrelin, which are still being fully defined, the potential therapeutic roles of GRAs are widespread.[36]

Defining clinical use Based on the demonstrated physiologic functions of endogenous ghrelin and actions of GRAs, pharmaceutical investigation of these molecules has included evaluation for treatment of gastroparesis associated with diabetes mellitus, GH deficiency, cancer anorexia–cachexia syndrome, frailty in elderly humans, and nutrition disorders.[36]

Given the significant clinical challenge presented by inappetence in dogs and cats and the important role played by ghrelin in the appetite control process, the interest in utilization of GRAs for appetite stimulation was a natural fit. GHS-R1a is expressed in key areas of the hypothalamus (arcuate and ventromedial nuclei) associated with feeding behavior.[36,38] Studies in multiple species have helped define the role of ghrelin in the control of preprandial hunger and initiation of meal intake.[39] Administration of exogenous ghrelin has been shown to stimulate eating when administered at times of minimal spontaneous food intake.[39] Studies in dogs[40,41] and cats[42] have shown that ghrelin levels are increased in the fasting state and suppressed with food intake, and exogenous administration of ghrelin increased daily food intake of healthy beagle dogs.[40]

The potential for appetite stimulation combined with the increase in IGF-1 noted with GRAs and the role of IGF-1 in muscle mass maintenance/hypertrophy in dogs,[43] makes the investigation of GRAs in cancer anorexia-cachexia syndrome highly desirable. Anamorelin, a GRA, has been studied in treatment of cancer-related cachexia in human non–small cell lung cancer (NSCLC). Two studies (ROMANA 1 and 2) together enrolled 979 patients with unresectable, advanced (stage III or stage IV) NSCLC in randomized, placebo-controlled manner utilizing anamorelin. Results showed that anamorelin significantly increased lean body mass and provided a significant, meaningful improvement of anorexia and cachexia symptoms. Findings indicated that anamorelin may be a valid treatment option for human patients experiencing cancer anorexia and cachexia.[44,45] The key advantage of GRAs, such as anamorelin, in the treatment of cachexia lies in their unique ability to stimulate appetite and potentially food intake as well as promote anabolism and increase muscle mass, without the deleterious side effects of other anabolic drugs.[45]

IGF-1 has been implicated with a potential role in cellular proliferation and increased metastatic ability in some human cancers.[46,47] Promotion of tumor growth was not demonstrated in the 2 large anamorelin human clinical trials in patients with NSCLC, described previously.[44] It is unclear what role, if any, the increased IGF-1 levels produced by GRAs could have in the clinical progression of various canine cancers.

Capromorelin oral solution Capromorelin is an orally active small molecule GRA that mimics the action of ghrelin, resulting in GH secretion and appetite stimulation. Approved by the FDA (May 2016) for appetite stimulation in dogs, capromorelin oral solution (Entyce [Aratana Therapeutics, Leawood, KS, USA]) became available to veterinarians in the fall of 2017. Capromorelin is the first GRA to be approved by the FDA.[36]

Capromorelin oral solution dosed at 3 mg/kg, orally, every 24 hours, has been shown to cause increased food intake and weight gain in both healthy laboratory and inappetent client-owned dogs.[48–50] In the pivotal field safety and effectiveness study, dogs with a reduced appetite or no appetite for a minimum of 2 days prior to presentation were eligible for enrollment. A total of 177 evaluable dogs (121 treated with capromorelin and 56 placebo) were enrolled. Dogs were treated with capromorelin at label dose (3 mg/kg, orally, every 24 hours) for 4 consecutive days. Owners completed an evaluation of their dog's appetite at days 0 and 3 $\pm$ 1. Improvement in appetite at day 3 was defined as treatment success. Capromorelin treatment resulted in significantly improved appetite compared with placebo (68.6% vs 44.6%, respectively; $P = .008$). Capromorelin treatment also produced a significant increase in mean body weight compared with placebo (1.8% vs 0.1%, respectively; $P<.001$).[49]

Capromorelin oral solution also has demonstrated a wide margin of safety, being well-tolerated at daily doses up to 17.5 times the label dose once daily for 12 consecutive months.[51] It is due to this robust safety data that capromorelin has no treatment duration, age, or weight restrictions on the label. Although the efficacy of capromorelin has not been clinically tested in client-owned dogs for longer than 4 days, at this time there is no restriction on treatment duration. This means that capromorelin can be used for chronic, long-term administration in dogs as clinically indicated.[52] The most common adverse clinical signs reported in capromorelin-treated dogs in the pivotal clinical study were diarrhea (7.0%), vomiting (6.4%), polydipsia (4.1%), and hypersalivation (2.3%).[49,52]

When administered to healthy dogs for 7 days, capromorelin treatment produced increased IGF-1 concentrations on day 1 and this increase was sustained through day 7. Mean serum IGF-1 levels 8 hours post–capromorelin dosing on days 4 and 7 were approximately 60% to 70% higher in dogs dosed at 3 mg/kg, orally, every 24 hours, compared with dogs in the placebo group. These sustained IGF-1 serum concentrations may increase lean muscle mass when capromorelin is administered to dogs over extended periods.[48]

Although capromorelin currently is not FDA approved for use in cats, some data are available in healthy cats. In 1 short-term study, cats were dosed at up to 60 mg/kg, orally, every 24 hours, for 14 days; another longer-term study treated cats at up to 6 mg/kg, orally, every 24 hours, for 91 consecutive days. Capromorelin administration in the 91-day study produced increases in IGF-1 (which were sustained, similar to what is seen in dogs) and increased food intake and body weight in cats. Individual serum fructosamine levels did not exceed the upper end of reference range for any capromorelin-treated cat.[53] Aratana also is developing a cat-specific formulation and has initiated a pivotal field effectiveness study for weight management in cats with CKD (dosing at 2 mg/kg, orally, every 24 hours,).

It is exciting to have an approved GRA in veterinary medicine even before this category of therapeutic is available in human medicine. That also means, however, fewer comparative data are available to help inform clinical use of capromorelin in dogs. Although further studies are needed to more fully define the best use of capromorelin in veterinary practice, this therapeutic has significant potential to have a positive impact on the clinical management of inappetence and cachexia related to chemotherapy/cancer and other chronic medical conditions in dogs and cats (off-label use in cats).

Mirtazapine

Mechanism of action Mirtazapine as a human noradrenergic and specific serotonergic antidepressant has ancillary properties, including anxiolytic, sedative, antiemetic, and appetite stimulant effects. Although the exact mechanism of appetite stimulation is not clearly defined, mirtazapine has been shown to antagonize (block): presynaptic α_2-receptors, postsynaptic serotonin (serotonin 2A, serotonin 2C, and serotonin 3) receptors, and histamine (H_1) receptors. Antagonism of the serotonin 2 and serotonin 3 receptors increases serotonergic stimulation via serotonin 1 receptors.[4,54]

Appetite stimulation is believed to occur through interaction with nuclei within the hypothalamus and enhanced release of norepinepherine.[4,55] Other studies have indicated that anti-H_1 activity is the strongest predictor of weight gain in humans treated with antidepressants.[56] The bodyweight gain noted in humans on mirtazapine has been associated with increases in body fat mass, rather than lean body mass.[57]

Defining clinical use Mirtazapine therapeutic dosing in healthy young cats has been established at 1.88 mg, orally, every 24 hours.[58] Additional studies have shown that dosing of 1.88 mg, orally, every 48 hours, is more appropriate in cats with CKD.[59] A double-masked, placebo-controlled crossover clinical trial in cats with CKD demonstrated that mirtazapine administration at 1.88 mg, orally, every 48 hours, for 3 weeks resulted in a significant increase in appetite and activity and a significant decrease in vomiting compared with placebo. Mirtazapine-treated cats also experienced a significant gain in bodyweight (median gain 0.18 kg) compared with placebo.[60] Decreased vomiting (likely via serotonin 3 antagonism) may contribute to appetite stimulation if vomiting or nausea is contributing to decreased appetite in a particular patient. The antiemetic effect noted in cats with CKD is interesting as mirtazapine sometimes is used for refractory chemotherapy-induced nausea and vomiting in humans.[61]

Clinical experience would indicate that mirtazapine is a less reliable/predictable appetite stimulant in dogs. A small pilot study evaluating the pharmacokinetics in healthy Beagle dogs has been described. Dogs in this study (weighing between 15 kg and 17 kg) were dosed at 20 mg of mirtazapine per dog orally, once. Results indicated that mirtazapine is metabolized more quickly in dogs (compared with cats) with mean half-life of 6.17 hours.[62] The ideal dose and frequency of mirtazapine in dogs need to be more fully defined with additional studies. Based on the limited information currently available, twice-daily dosing may be more appropriate in this species. Given the wide variation of dosing used in dogs in practice at this time, it is not surprising that its clinical effect is variable and rather unpredictable.

Mirtazapine transdermal ointment Indicated for the management of weight loss in cats, mirtazapine transdermal ointment (Mirataz [Kindred Biosciences, Burlingame, CA, USA]) received FDA approval in May 2018.[63] It is applied topically (inner pinna) as a transdermal ointment at 2 mg/cat (1.5-in ribbon) once daily for 14 days.[64]

The pivotal field safety and effectiveness study included 177 cats with a documented loss (≥5%) in body weight, 83 treated with Mirataz and 94 with vehicle control. The primary efficacy endpoint was percent change in body weight at 14 days. At study end, the mean percent increase in body weight from day 1 was 3.94% in the mirtazapine group compared with 0.41% in the vehicle control group. The difference between the 2 groups was significant (P<.0001). The most common side effects reported in cats (>10%) treated with Mirataz included vocalization (11.3%), vomiting (11.3%), and erythema at the application site (10.4%).[64,65] The finding of vomiting in approximately 11% of mirtazapine-treated cats is interesting because it is believed to have antiemetic properties due to serotonin 3 inhibition. Vomiting in the control group was similar, at 13%.

Further clinical studies need to be performed to more fully define the use of Mirataz in clinically inappetent cats with various underlying conditions, including cancer. Of particular interest will be the effect beyond the 14-day time constraint of the current study and the metabolic changes that might occur in relation to this weight gain (fat vs lean body mass).

Maropitant citrate

Mechanism of action Maropitant is a neurokinin (NK1) receptor antagonist that blocks the action of substance P in the central nervous system. Maropitant citrate (Cerenia) oral tablets are indicated for the prevention of acute vomiting and vomiting due to motion sickness in dogs. The injectable solution is indicated for the prevention and treatment of acute vomiting in dogs and treatment of vomiting in cats.[66]

Defining clinical use As an antiemetic, the potential for Cerenia to stimulate appetite likely exists only if nausea or vomiting is a primary cause of a dog's or cat's inappetence. Prior to the approval of Entyce, however, it was one of the most commonly used appetite stimulants in dogs by veterinary specialists (see **Table 4**).

A prospective, blinded, placebo-controlled study evaluating chronic (14 days) maropitant treatment in cats with CKD has been reported. This study found that cats treated with maropitant had statistically decreased vomiting but no difference in appetite scores or body weight was noted. Thus, although maropitant palliated vomiting associated with CKD in this 14-day study, it did not have an impact on appetite or weight.[67]

A few canine chemotherapy studies have prospectively evaluated the clinical signs observed in dogs receiving maropitant in the days immediately after treatment with various cytotoxic chemotherapeutics, including vincristine, cyclophosphamide, and doxorubicin. In these studies, no difference in incidence of inappetence was seen between dogs treated with maropitant and nontreated dogs.[68,69] A separate study evaluated the safety of chronic maropitant administered for 28 consecutive days to dogs with lymphoma and being treated with a CHOP-based chemotherapy protocol. Although appetite status for dogs in the study was not reported, dogs in the study did experience increase in body weight over the 28-day period.[70]

Maropitant often may be a necessary concurrent therapy for inappetent dogs and cats that have nausea and/or vomiting as a component of their clinical picture. It is, however, unlikely to be effective alone in patients where other causes of inappetence are the driving factors.

Cannabidiol oil

Mechanism of action The cannabinoids exert their effects via 1 of 2 receptors or through nonreceptor interactions. Cannabinoid type 1 receptors are expressed on neurons and in the gastrointestinal tract, resulting in release of γ-aminobutyric acid (inhibitory neurotransmitter). This receptor is present in high concentration in the canine cerebellum. Cannabinoid type 2 receptors are expressed on cells of the immune system.[71] In addition to possible appetite stimulation, reported pharmacologic actions of cannabidiol (CBD) include anti-inflammatory, anticonvulsant, analgesia, antioxidant, antiseborrheic, anti–methicillin-resistant *Staphylococcus aureus*, antifungal, antidepressant, anxiolytic, antiemetic, anticancer, immunomodulation, neuroprotection, and neurogenesis.[71–74] The effects of CBD on food intake has been inconclusive in both human and animal studies.[72–74] Some human cancer studies indicate that patients treated with CBD report that food tastes better, their appetite is improved, and the proportion of protein calories was increased compared with placebo groups.[74]

Although the exact mechanism for appetite stimulation is not fully understood and results in human and other animal species has been variable, CBD remains of interest for its potential clinical utility in dogs and cats with cancer. These clinical benefits could be multifactorial and include appetite stimulation, antiemesis, pain modulation, and anticancer effects.

Defining clinical use Pet owners may, not infrequently, inquire about use of CBD oil therapy in their dogs or cats with cancer, often with the goal of appetite stimulation or antiemesis. One of the many limitations in this drug category is that data regarding pharmacokinetics, safety, and clinical efficacy of CBD in dogs are limited but recently expanding. One study has evaluated 3 formulations of CBD products (oral microencapsulated oil beads, oral CBD-infused oil, and CBD-infused transdermal cream) in healthy dogs. In this evaluation, the oral CBD-infused oil formulation provided the most favorable pharmacokinetics profile for further evaluation.[75] Another study evaluated Bedrocan (20% delta-9-tetrahydrocannabinol [THC] and 0.5% CBD) in fasting and fed healthy dogs. The oral bioavailability in fed dogs was reported to be 48%.[76]

CBD oil has been evaluated in treatment of osteoarthritis in dogs. A randomized placebo-controlled, double-blinded, cross-over study evaluated CBD oil (administered at a dose of 2 mg/kg, orally, every12 hours) in dogs with osteoarthritis. Findings revealed significant decrease in pain and increase in activity via standardized owner-based evaluation in dogs treated with CBD oil. Decreased pain was also noted on veterinarian assessments of dogs in the CBD treatment group.[77]

Another significant barrier to clinical use of CBD products in dogs and cats at this time is that most CBD products, and all those marketed for pets, remain a Schedule 1 controlled substance in the United States (January 2019). A recent decision by the US Drug Enforcement Administration, however, has lowered a very small sector of human CBD products to Schedule 5. Drugs, including CBD with THC content below 0.1%, that have been approved by the FDA are now classified as Schedule 5.[78] Despite that all pet-related CBD products are Schedule 1, many different formulations of CBD (oil, capsules, and treats) are readily available to pet owners online and in stores. These products are not FDA approved and have no regulatory quality/manufacturing oversight.[79] Testing of several CBD-containing products by the FDA over the past several years, including those marketed for pets, has indicated that many do not contain the amount of CBD listed on the label. Some products contained no detectable CBD; others also contained unlabeled THC.[79,80]

Given the few data available and legal status of CBD-products, the American Veterinary Medical Association recently has provided guidance for veterinarians as a resource to answer client questions.[71] Although it is possible that CBD-containing products may be approved for clinical use (appetite stimulation or other indications) in dogs and/or cats in the future, insufficient data currently are available to warrant use.

Diet and Feeding Tubes

One of the most common questions veterinarians receive after diagnosing a pet with cancer is, Should I change my pet's diet? A recent survey of 75 clients visiting a referral oncology service with their dog after a diagnosis of cancer indicated that 25% changed their dog's primary diet within 6 months of diagnosis. This change in diet often included exclusion of a conventional diet and/or inclusion of a homemade diet; 90% of the clients instituting a diet change for their dog indicated that the change was made due to the diagnosis of cancer.[81] The next question from pet owners often is, What is the best diet for my pet with cancer? The answer to this question is not well defined in dogs and cats, or in humans, with cancer. Wide-ranging recommendations on the best diet and supplements for dogs and cats with cancer can be found online, making it challenging for pet owners to know whom to believe in this aspect of their pet's care. At this time, the best recommendation for pet owners is to emphasize the importance of ensuring that their pet's caloric and essential nutrients are met, whether it is via a commercial or veterinarian-designed homemade diet.[82]

When pharmacologic appetite stimulation is not successful or when patients are in need of rapid correction of their nutritional state, enteral feeding support with tubes is critically important. When to intervene, which diet(s) are best for dogs and cats with high potential for cachexia, and so forth are beyond the scope of this article and are well described elsewhere.[1,20,83]

SUMMARY

Although a nonspecific clinical finding, inappetence is a key factor in perceived quality of life and case management in cats and dogs with cancer. Prolonged inappetence can have a negative impact on patient nutritional status, potentially leading to cachexia, which may have a significant effect on overall outcome. Understanding the importance of early recognition and intervention for the inappetent dog or cat with cancer is critical. Being familiar with the mechanisms of action, safety and efficacy data, and potential clinical utility of the more recently available pharmacologic appetite stimulants will support a practice when learning how to best utilize these therapeutics. The potential end benefits include improved quality of life for canine and feline cancer patients, improved patient outcomes, less hospitalization time, and happier pet owners.

REFERENCES

1. Johnson LN, Freeman LM. Recognizing, describing, and managing reduced food intake in dogs and cats. J Am Vet Med Assoc 2017;251:1260–6.
2. Entyce® Inappetence Overview. Available at: https://entyce.aratana.com. Accessed December 18, 2018.
3. Robinson NJ, Dean RS, Cobb M, et al. Investigating common clinical presentations in first opinion small animal consultations using direct observations. Vet Rec 2015;176(18):463.
4. MIRATAZ® product detailer, US-MAZ-1800011. Burlingame (CA): Kindred Biosciences, Inc.; 2018.
5. Williams J, Phillips C, Byrd HM. Factors which influence owners when deciding to use chemotherapy in terminally ill pets. Animals 2017;7(3):E18.
6. Thornton LA, Cave N, Bridges JP, et al. Owners perception of their cat's quality of life when treated with a modified University of Wisconsin-Madison protocol for lymphoma. J Feline Med Surg 2018;20(4):356–61.
7. Malone EK, Rassnick KM, Bailey DB, et al. Comparison of two questionnaires to assess gastrointestinal toxicity in dogs and cats treated with chemotherapy. Vet Comp Oncol 2011;9(3):225–31.
8. Veterinary cooperative oncology group – common terminology criteria for adverse events (VCOG-CTCAE) following chemotherapy or biological antineoplastic therapy in dogs and cats. Vet Comp Oncol 2011;14(4):417–46.
9. Mondello P, Lacquaniti A, Mondello S, et al. Emerging markers of cachexia predict survival in cancer patients. BMC Cancer 2014;14:828.
10. Fearon K, Strasser F, Anker SD, et al. Definition and classification of cancer cachexia: an international consensus. Lancet Oncol 2011;12:489–95.
11. Bennani-Baiti N, Walsh D. What is cancer anorexia-cachexia syndrome? A historical perspective. J R Coll Physicians Edinb 2009;39:257–62.
12. Molina J, Hervera M, Manzanilla EG, et al. Evaluation of the prevalence and risk factors for undernutrition in hospitalized dogs. Front Vet Sci 2018;5:205.
13. Gates MC, Hinds HJ, Dale A. Preliminary description of aging cats and dogs presented to a New Zealand first-opinion veterinary clinic at end-of-life. N Z Vet J 2017;65(6):313–7.
14. Sogame N, Ribson R, Burgess KE. Intestinal lymphoma in dogs: 84 cases (1997-2012). J Am Vet Med Assoc 2018;252:440–7.
15. Romano FR, Heinze CR, Barber LG, et al. Association between body condition score and cancer prognosis in dogs with lymphoma and osteosarcoma. J Vet Intern Med 2016;30:1179–86.
16. Barber LG, Weishaar KM. Criteria for designation of clinical substage in canine lymphoma: a survey of veterinary oncologists. Vet Comp Oncol 2016;14(Suppl 1):32–9.
17. Weeth LP, Fascetti AJ, Kass PH, et al. Prevalence of obese dogs in a population of dogs with cancer. Am J Vet Res 2007;68:389–98.
18. Michel KE, Sorenmo K, Shofer FS. Evaluation of body condition and weight loss in dogs presented to a veterinary oncology service. J Vet Intern Med 2004;18:692–5.
19. Baez JL, Michel KE, Sorenmo K, et al. A prospective investigation of the prevalence and prognostic significance of weight loss and changes in body condition in feline cancer patients. J Feline Med Surg 2007;9(5):411–7.
20. Freeman LM. Cachexia and sarcopenia: emerging syndromes of importance in dogs and cats. J Vet Intern Med 2012;26:3–17.

21. Freeman LM, Sutherland-Smith J, Prantil LR, et al. Quantitative assessment of muscle in dogs using a vertebral epaxial score. Can J Vet Res 2017;81(4):255–60.
22. Muscle condition score, feline. WSAVA Global Nutrition Committee, 2014. Available at: https://www.wsava.org/WSAVA/media/Documents/Committee%20Resources/Global%20Nutrition%20Committee/Muscle-condition-score-chart-Cats-1.pdf. Accessed December 18, 2018.
23. Muscle condition score, canine. WSAVA Global Nutrition Committee, 2013. Available at: https://www.wsava.org/WSAVA/media/Documents/Committee%20Resources/Global%20Nutrition%20Committee/Muscle-condition-score-chart-2013-1.pdf. Accessed December 18, 2018.
24. Mazzaferro EM, Hackett TB, Stein TP, et al. Metabolic alterations in dogs with osteosarcoma. Am J Vet Res 2001;62(8):1234–9.
25. Vail DM, Ogilvie GK, Wheeler SL, et al. Alterations in carbohydrate metabolism in canine lymphoma. J Vet Intern Med 1990;4(1):8–11.
26. Ogilvie GK, Walters L, Salman MD, et al. Alterations in carbohydrate metabolism in dogs with nonhematopoietic malignancies. Am J Vet Res 1997;58(3):277–81.
27. Calvalido J, Wood GA, Mutsaers AJ, et al. Comparison of serum cytokine levels between dogs with multicentric lymphoma and healthy dogs. Vet Immunol Immunopathol 2016;182:106–14.
28. O'Neill DG, Elliott J, Church DB, et al. Chronic kidney disease in dogs in UK veterinary practices: prevalence, risk factors and survival. J Vet Intern Med 2013;27:814–21.
29. Greene JP, Lefebvre SL, Wang M, et al. Risk factors associated with the development of chronic kidney disease in cats evaluated at primary care veterinary hospitals. J Am Vet Med Assoc 2014;244(3):320–7.
30. Markovich JE, Freeman LM, Labato MA, et al. Survey of dietary and medication practices of owners of cats with chronic kidney disease. J Feline Med Surg 2015;17(12):979–83.
31. Freeman LM, Lachaud MP, Matthews S, et al. Evaluation of weight loss over time in cats with chronic kidney disease. J Vet Intern Med 2016;30:1661–6.
32. Freeman LM, Rush JE, Kehayias JJ, et al. Nutritional alterations and the effect of fish oil supplementation in dogs with heart failure. J Vet Intern Med 1998;12:440–8.
33. Craven M, Simpson JW, Ridyard AE, et al. Canine inflammatory bowel disease: retrospective analysis of diagnosis and outcome in 80 cases (1995-2002). J Small Anim Pract 2004;45:336–42.
34. Wren JA, Ramudo AA, Campbell SL, et al. Efficacy and safety of dirlotapide in the management of obese dogs evaluated in two placebo-controlled, masked clinical studies in North America. J Vet Pharmacol Ther 2007;30(Suppl 1):81–9.
35. Hormonal control. Available at: https://image.slidesharecdn.com/5appetiteregulation-150512035442-lva1-app6892/95/appetite-regulation-18-638.jpg?cb=1431402972. Accessed December 29, 2018.
36. Rhodes L, Zollers B, Wofford JA, et al. Capromorelin: a ghrelin receptor agonist and novel therapy for stimulation of appetite. Vet Med Sci 2017;4(1):3–16.
37. Howick K, Griffin BT, Cryan JF, et al. From belly to brain: targeting the ghrelin receptor in appetite and food intake regulation. Int J Mol Sci 2017;18(2):E273.
38. Kojima M, Kangawa K. Ghrelin: structure and function. Physiol Rev 2005;85(2):495–522.
39. Cummings DE, Frayo RS, Marmonier C, et al. Plasma ghrelin levels and hunger scores in humans initiating meals voluntarily without time- and food-related cues. Am J Physiol Endocrinol Metab 2004;287(2):E297–304.

40. Yokoyama M, Nakahara K, Kojima M, et al. Influencing the between-feeding and edocrine responses of plasma ghrelin in healthy dogs. Eur J Endocrinol 2005; 152(1):155–60.
41. Bhatti SF, Hofland LJ, van Koetsveld PM, et al. Effects of food intake and food withholding on plasma ghrelin concentrations in healthy dogs. Am J Vet Res 2006;67(9):1557–63.
42. Ida T, Miyazato M, Naganobu K, et al. Purification and characterization of feline ghrelin and its possible role. Domest Anim Endocrinol 2007;32(2):93–105.
43. Molon-Noblot A, Laroque P, Prahalada S, et al. Effect of chronic growth hormone administration on skeletal muscle in dogs. Toxicol Pathol 1998;26(2):207–12.
44. Temel JS, Abernethy AP, Currow DC, et al. Anamorelin in patients with non-small-cell lung cancer and cachexia (ROMANA1 and ROMANA 2): results from two randomized, double-blind, phase 3 trials. Lancet Oncol 2016;17(4):519–31.
45. Currow DC, Maddocks M, Cella D, et al. Efficacy of anamorelin, a novel non-peptide ghrelin analogue, in patients with advanced non-small cell lung cancer (NSCLC) and cachexia – review and expert opinion. Int J Mol Sci 2018;19(11): E3471.
46. Burtscher I, Christofori G. The IGF/IGF-1 receptor signaling pathway as a potential target for cancer therapy. Drug Resist Updat 1999;2:3–8.
47. Armakolas N, Armakolas A, Antonopoulos A, et al. The role of the IGF-1 Ec in myoskeletal system and osteosarcoma pathophysiology. Crit Rev Oncol Hematol 2016;108:137–45.
48. Zollers B, Rhodes L, Smith RG. Capromorelin increases food consumption, body weight, growth hormone, and sustained insulin-like growth factor 1 concentrations when administered to healthy adult beagle dogs. J Vet Pharmacol Ther 2017;40(2):140–7.
49. Zollers B, Wofford JA, Heinen E, et al. A prospective, randomized, masked, placebo-controlled clinical study of capromorelin in dogs with reduced appetite. J Vet Intern Med 2016;30(6):1851–7.
50. Zollers B, Rhodes L, Heinen E. Capromorelin oral solution (ENTYCE®) increases food consumption and body weight when administered for 4 consecutive days to healthy adult beagle dogs in a randomized, masked, placebo controlled study. BMC Vet Res 2017;13(1):10.
51. Zollers B, Huebner M, Armintrout G, et al. Evaluation of the safety in dogs of long-term, daily oral administration of capromorelin, a novel drug for stimulation of appetite. J Vet Pharmacol Ther 2017;40(3):248–55.
52. ENTYCE® (capromorelin oral solution) [package insert]. Leawood (KS): Therapeutics, Inc; 2016.
53. Wofford JA, Zollers B, Rhodes L, et al. Evaluation of the safety of daily administration of capromorelin in cats. J Vet Pharmacol Ther 2018;41(2):324–33.
54. Alam A, Voronovich Z, Carley JA. A review of therapeutic uses of mirtazapine in psychiatric and medical conditions. Prim Care Companion CNS Disord 2013; 15(5) [pii:PCC.13r01525].
55. Agnew W, Korman R. Pharmacological appetite stimulation: rational choices in the inappetent cat. J Feline Med Surg 2014;16(9):749–56.
56. Salvi V, Mencacci C, Barone-Adesi F. H1-histamine receptor affinity predicts weight gain with antidepressants. Eur Neuropsychopharmacol 2016;26(10):1673–7.
57. Laimer M, Kramer-Reinstadler K, Rauchenzauner M, et al. Effect of mirtazapine treatment on body composition and metabolism. J Clin Psychiatry 2006;67(3): 421–4.

58. Quimby JM, Gustafson DL, Samber BJ, et al. Studies on the pharmacokinetics and pharmacodynamics of mirtazapine in healthy young cats. J Vet Pharmacol Ther 2011;34(4):388–96.
59. Quimby JM, Gustafson DL, Lunn KF. The pharmacokinetics of mirtazapine in cats with chronic kidney disease and in age-matched control cats. J Vet Intern Med 2011;25:985–9.
60. Quimby JM, Lunn KF. Mirtazapine as an appetite stimulant and anti-emetic in cats with chronic kidney disease: a masked placebo-controlled crossover clinical trial. Vet J 2013;197(3):651–5.
61. Kast RE, Foley KF. Cancer chemotherapy and cachexia: mirtazapine and olanzapine are 5-HT3 antagonists with good antinausea effects. Eur J Cancer Care 2007;16(4):351–4.
62. Giorgi M, Hyoin Y. Pharmacokinetics of mirtazapine and its main metabolites in beagle dogs: a pilot study. Vet J 2012;192(2):239–41.
63. Kindred Biosciences receives FDA approval of Mirataz (mirtazapine transdermal ointment) for the management of weight loss in cats. Available at: https://kindredbio.com/frontpage/kindred-biosciences-receives-fda-approval-of-mirataz-mirtazapine-transdermal-ointment-for-the-management-of-weight-loss-in-cats/. Accessed December 19, 2018.
64. MIRATAZ® (mirtazapine transdermal ointment) [package insert]. Burlingame (CA): Kindred Biosciences, Inc; 2018.
65. Poole M, Quimby JM, Hu T, et al. A double-blind, placebo-controlled, randomized study to evaluate the weight gain drug, mirtazapine transdermal ointment, in cats with unintended weight loss. J Vet Pharmacol Ther 2018. https://doi.org/10.1111/jvp.12738.
66. CERENIA® (maropitant citrate) tablets and injectable solution [package inset]. Kalamazoo (MI): Zoetis, Inc; 2015.
67. Quimby JM, Brock WT, Moses K. Chronic use of maropitant for the management of vomiting and inappetence in cats with chronic kidney disease: a blinded, placebo-controlled clinical trial. J Feline Med Surg 2015;17(8):692–7.
68. Mason SL, Grant IA, Elliott J, et al. Gastrointestinal toxicity after vincristine or cyclophosphamide administered with or without maropitant in dogs: a prospective randomised controlled study. J Small Anim Pract 2014;55:391–8.
69. Rau SE, Barber LG, Burgess KE. Efficacy of maropitant in the prevention of delayed vomiting associated with administration of doxorubicin to dogs. J Vet Intern Med 2010;24:1452–7.
70. Clifford C, Bergman P, Trettien A, et al. Evaluation of safety of maropitant citrate dosed orally at 2 mg/kg once daily for 28 consecutive days in dogs with lymphoma. In: Veterinary Cancer Society Proceedings. Orlando, FL, USA, October 20–22, 2016.
71. AVMA Council on Biologic and Therapeutic Agents. Cannabis: what veterinarians need to know. 2018. Available at: https://www.avma.org/KB/Resources/Reference/Documents/Cannabis-What-Veterinarians-Need-to-Know.pdf. Accessed December 29, 2018.
72. Iffland K, Grotenhermen F. An update on safety and side effects of cannabidiol: a review of clinical data and relevant animal studies. Cannabis Cannabinoid Res 2017;2(1):139–54.
73. Bergamaschi MM, Queiroz RH, Zuardi AW, et al. Safety and side effects of cannabidiol, a cannabis sativa constituent. Curr Drug Saf 2011;6(4):237–49.
74. Abrams DI, Guzman M. Cannabis in cancer care. Clin Pharmacol Ther 2015;97(6):575–86.

75. Bartner LR, McGrath S, Rao S, et al. Pharmacokinetics of cannabidiol administered by 3 delivery methods at 2 different dosages to healthy dogs. Can J Vet Res 2018;82(3):178–83.
76. Lebkowska-Wieruszewska B, Stefanelli F, Chericoni S, et al. Pharmacokinetics of Bedrocan®, a cannabis oil extract, in fasting and fed dogs: an explorative study. Res Vet Sci 2018;123:26–8.
77. Gamble LJ, Boesch JM, Frye CW, et al. Pharmacokinetics, safety, and clinical efficacy of cannabidiol treatment in osteoarthritic dogs. Front Vet Sci 2018;5:165.
78. Marijuana Business Daily. DEA moves some CBD medicines off Schedule 1, a limited expansion of cannabis access. Available at: https://mjbizdaily.com/dea-moves-cbd-medicines-off-schedule-1-a-limited-expansion-of-cannabis-access/. Accessed January 12, 2019.
79. Brutlag A, Hommerding H. Toxicology of marijuana, synthetic cannabinoids, and cannabidiol in dogs and cats. Vet Clin North Am Small Anim Pract 2018;48(6):1087–102.
80. US Food & Drug Administration. Warning letters and test results for cannabidiol-related products. Available at: https://www.fda.gov/NewsEvents/PublicHealthFocus/ucm484109.htm. Accessed December 29, 2018.
81. Rajagopaul S, Parr JM, Woods JP, et al. Owners' attitudes and practices regarding nutrition of dogs diagnosed with cancer presenting at a referral oncology service in Ontario, Canada. J Small Anim Pract 2016;57:484–90.
82. Feeding pets with cancer. Available at: http://vetnutrition.tufts.edu/2017/08/cancer_diet/. Accessed January 2, 2019.
83. Chan D. The inappetent hospitalized cat: clinical approach to maximizing nutritional support. J Feline Med Surg 2009;11:925–33.
84. Grant IA, Rodriguez CO, Kent MS, et al. A phase II clinical trial of vinorelbine in dogs with cutaneous mast cell tumors. J Vet Intern Med 2008;22:388–93.
85. Marrington AM, Killick DR, Grant IA, et al. Toxicity associated with epirubicin treatments in a large case series of dogs. Vet Comp Oncol 2012;10(2):113–23.
86. Bowles DB, Robson MC, Galloway PE, et al. Owners' perception of carboplatin in conjunction with other palliative treatments for cancer. J Small Anim Pract 2010;51:104–12.
87. Thamm DH, Vail DM, Post GS, et al. Alternating rabacfosadine/doxorubicin: efficacy and tolerability in naïve canine multicentric lymphoma. J Vet Intern Med 2017;31:872–8.
88. London CA, Malpas PB, Wood-Follis SL, et al. Multi-center, placebo-controlled, double-blind, randomized study of oral toceranib phosphate (SU11654), a receptor tyrosine kinase inhibitor, for the treatment of dogs with recurrent (either local or distant) mast cell tumor following surgical excision. Clin Cancer Res 2009;15(11):3856–65.
89. Kim SE, Liptak JM, Gall TT, et al. Epirubicin in the adjuvant treatment of splenic hemangiosarcoma in dogs: 59 cases (1997-2004). J Am Vet Med Assoc 2007;231:1550–7.
90. Vail DM, von Euler H, Rusk AW, et al. A randomized trial investigating the efficacy and safety of water soluble micellar paclitaxel (Paccal Vet) for treatment of nonresectable grade 2 or 3 mast cell tumors in dogs. J Vet Intern Med 2012;26(3):598–607.
91. Vail DM, Thamm DH, Reiser H, et al. Assessment of GS-9219 in a pet model of non-Hodgkin's lymphoma. Clin Cancer Res 2009;15(10):3503–10.

Histiocytic Sarcoma and Hemangiosarcoma Update

Christine Mullin, VMD*, Craig A. Clifford, DVM, MS

KEYWORDS

• Hemangiosarcoma • Histiocytic sarcoma • Hepatosplenic neoplasia
• Hemoabdomen • Pericardial effusion

KEY POINTS

- Both tumor types are much more common in dogs than in cats.
- Both tumors are highly aggressive and patient prognosis depends upon tumor type, location, stage of disease, treatment employed, and various prognostic factors.
- Adjuvant chemotherapy improves patient prognosis following surgery.
- Palliative radiation and chemotherapy can improve quality of life and prolong survival for patients who are not surgical candidates.
- Work is underway toward understanding the genetic alterations of each disease with the hope of identifying driver mutations that may aid in the development of more targeted therapies.

HISTIOCYTIC SARCOMA

Histiocytic sarcoma (HS) is an uncommon neoplasm of dendritic cell origin.[1,2] This disease may present as a localized tumor (internally or externally), regional tissue or organ involvement, or disseminated multiorgan involvement.[3] The previously used term "malignant histiocytosis" is now considered antiquated, as distinctive subtypes including localized, disseminated, and hemophagocytic HS have been identified.[1,2] Reported anatomic sites for HS include lung, lymph node, liver, spleen, stomach, intestine, pancreas, mediastinum, skin and subcutaneous tissue, skeletal muscle, central nervous system, bone, joint space, bone marrow, nasal cavity, and eyes.[1–10] HS is the most common periarticular tumor in dogs, and immunohistochemistry (IHC) is generally required to differentiate periarticular HS (PAHS) from synovial cell sarcoma.[5] HS accounts for 5% of primary brain tumors and 4.5% of secondary (ie, metastatic) brain tumors in dogs.[11–13] Hemophagocytic HS (HHS) is a highly aggressive subtype of HS that occurs in dogs and rarely in cats. This form arises from splenic red pulp or bone marrow macrophages and can only be definitively differentiated through confirmation of a specific IHC staining pattern; however, clinical factors and hematologic and biochemical abnormalities may increase clinical suspicion.[6,14]

Hope Veterinary Specialists, 40 Three Tun Road, Malvern, PA 19355, USA
* Corresponding author.
E-mail address: mullinvet@gmail.com

Vet Clin Small Anim 49 (2019) 855–879
https://doi.org/10.1016/j.cvsm.2019.04.009

Incidence

HS represents less than 1% of canine cancers of the lymphoreticular system and is more common in dogs than any other species.[1,2] True incidence in cats is unclear, but HS is thought to be rare in this species.[1]

Cause

Although the definitive cause of HS remains unclear, multiple risk factors have been reported for dogs, including genetic predispositions and chronic inflammation.

Genetics

Although first reported in the Bernese mountain dog (BMD), a predisposition to the development of HS has been identified in several other breeds, including the Flat-Coated Retriever (FCR), Rottweiler, Miniature Schnauzer, and Pembroke Welsh Corgi.[15–20] An inheritance study found that the genetic predisposition of BMD for HS was widespread within the breed.[18] Specific genetic alterations have been identified, including deletions of the tumor suppressor genes *CDKN2A/B*, *RB1*, and *PTEN* in HS samples from BMD and FCR. There were breed-associated differences in the DNA copy number aberrations noted, and these were thought to contribute to differences in tumor location between breeds, where FCR are most likely to develop PAHS. These chromosomal aberrations found in dogs were highly conserved with those reported in human histiocytic diseases.[20]

Inflammation

A correlation between prior joint disease and risk of PAHS in BMD and other breeds has been reported.[21–23] Specifically, dogs with PAHS were 2.5 times more likely to have preexisting orthopedic disease in the tumor-affected joint as compared with control populations.[21] Dogs receiving antiinflammatory medications had a lower risk of developing PAHS.[23]

Signalment

Dogs with HS are commonly middle aged or older; however, HS has been reported in dogs as young as 3 years old. Any breed can develop HS, but BMD, FCR, Miniature Schnauzers, Pembroke Welsh Corgis, and Golden Retrievers are the most commonly affected breeds.[3,4,15–19,22,23]

HISTORY AND CLINICAL PRESENTATION

Historical findings and clinical signs vary depending on the location and extent of disease. Common signs associated with disseminated HS and HHS include lethargy, weakness, inappetence, weight loss, abdominal distension, dyspnea, and coughing. Lameness is the most common sign in dogs with PAHS.[24]

PHYSICAL EXAMINATION FINDINGS

Examination findings vary depending on the location and extent of disease. Common clinical abnormalities associated with disseminated HS and HHS include fever, pale mucous membranes, bruising, palpable mass with the skin/subcutaneous space, peripheral lymphadenopathy, tachypnea, dyspnea, muffled heart and lung sounds, abdominal distension with cranial organomegaly, and/or palpable fluid wave.[1–3,6,7,15–19,23] Patients with PAHS generally display lameness and often a periarticular mass effect; regional lymphadenopathy may also be present.[24]

DIAGNOSIS

A definitive diagnosis of HS can be obtained via cytologic or histologic examination of tumor tissue. In some cases, neoplastic cells are so pleomorphic or undifferentiated that special stains may be necessary for differentiation from other round cell tumors, carcinomas, or other sarcomas. For staging purposes, standard laboratory analysis (complete blood count, chemistry profile, urinalysis), 3-view thoracic radiographs, and abdominal ultrasound are recommended. Bone marrow analysis may be indicated and if applicable and available, computed tomography (CT) or MRI may be used. The results of clinical staging allow accurate determination of whether the disease is localized or disseminated, thus informing expected prognosis and guiding therapy.

Pathologic Evaluation

Cytology

Cytologic samples may be obtained via fine-needle aspiration of a tumor or in some cases, evaluation of malignant effusion, if present. HS cytology samples typically consist of large, discrete, mononuclear cells with marked anisocytosis and anisokaryosis. Nuclei are round, oval, or reniform with prominent nucleoli, and cytoplasm is moderate to abundant, lightly basophilic, and vacuolated. Mitotic activity is generally high and there may be bizarre mitotic figures and multinucleated giant cells present (**Fig. 1**). In addition, tumor cells may display erythrophagocytosis.[1,2,14,25,26] Often, marked pleomorphism and lack of differentiation can preclude definitive confirmation of HS via cytology.[26] In such cases, although, immunocytochemistry (ICC) using antibodies against the class A macrophage scavenger receptor CD204 may be useful.[27] Ultimately, if cytology and ICC are not definitive, histopathology is indicated.

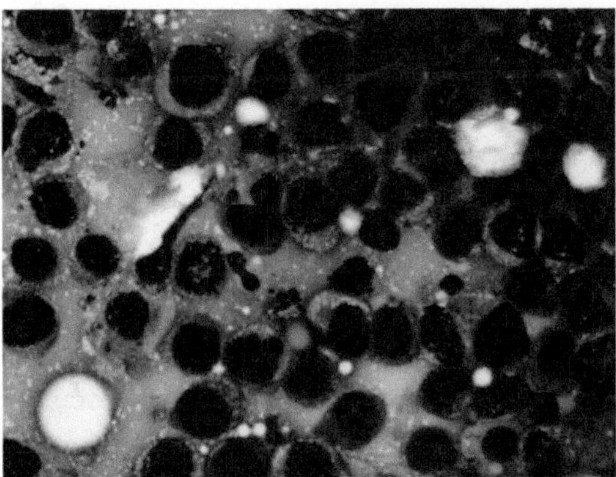

Fig. 1. Impression smear from an extradural spinal mass in a 9-year-old male castrated Japanese Chin that presented for acute-onset paraparesis. Slides contained numerous large, individualized, discrete round cells as shown earlier. These cells had sharply defined margins, moderately abundant blue cytoplasm with punctate clear vacuoles, a high nuclear-to-cytoplasmic ratio, and pleomorphic nuclei 1.5 to 3x the diameter of a neutrophil with fine chromatin and single to multiple dark nucleoli. Anisocytosis and anisokaryosis were moderate. A mitotic figure can be seen toward the middle of the photomicrograph. The histopathologic diagnosis was histiocytic sarcoma based on immunohistochemistry showing strong, diffuse cytoplasmic immunoreactivity to IBA-1 and lack of reactivity to lymphoid antigens (CD3, Pax5). (*Courtesy of* E. Fish, DVM, DACVP, Auburn, AL.)

Histopathology

Diagnosis of HS can be achieved via multiple biopsy methods, including submission of an entire affected organ after removal, local excision of a mass, or a simple diagnostic (ie, incisional, wedge, or tru-cut) biopsy of either internal or external lesions. Histologically, HS is composed of sheets of large, pleomorphic, round mononuclear and multinucleated giant cells, often with frequent bizarre mitotic figures.[1,3,6,26] Alternatively, cells may have a spindyloid appearance similar to other sarcomas, either alone or mixed with the mononuclear and multinucleated giant cells. Immunohistochemistry (IHC) can be performed on formalin-fixed tissue using antibodies to CD18 or CD204 in order to differentiate HS from other round cell tumors, other sarcomas, and carcinomas.[1,2,26,28] In HHS, phagocytosis of red cells and leukocytes is common and is somewhat distinctive for this disease, as the prevalence is low in other forms of HS.[14,26] Antibodies to CD11d can be used to differentiate HHS, particularly when the constellation of clinicopathologic findings supports a suspicion for this subtype.[14,26]

Laboratory Evaluation

Complete blood count

- Anemia is common and usually regenerative especially when the underlying cause is erythrophagocytosis by neoplastic cells.[9,14,24]
- Thrombocytopenia or pancytopenias may be present a result of bone marrow infiltration.[9,29] In one study HS was the second most common cause of pancytopenia in dogs.[3]

Serum biochemistry, urinalysis

- Elevated liver enzymes, hypocholesterolemia, and hypoalbuminemia are common findings, particularly with HHS.[9,14,24]
- Hypercalcemia is a rarely reported finding in dogs with HS.[9]

Diagnostic Imaging

Thoracic radiographs

When present, pulmonary involvement with HS may be characterized by a diffuse interstitial infiltrate, patchy consolidation, or multifocal mass lesions.[30] The right middle lung lobe is the most common location for primary pulmonary HS.[30,31] Sternal and tracheobronchial lymphadenopathy may also be noted.[30]

Abdominal ultrasound

Ultrasonography can be used to identify lesions in visceral organs. Specifically, hepatosplenomegaly, mottling of the liver and spleen, discrete nodules or masses in multiple organs (liver, spleen, kidneys, adrenals), lymphadenopathy, and abdominal effusion may be noted.[32]

Advanced Imaging

CT and MRI: both CT and MRI can be used for evaluation of patients with localized or disseminated HS. These modalities may aid in determining the exact anatomic origin and invasiveness of localized tumors, thereby aiding in the planning of surgical resection and/or radiation therapy. In addition, thoracic CT has been shown to have superior sensitivity to radiography in detecting early pulmonary metastasis for multiple tumor types.[33,34] CT and MRI may also have utility in identifying hepatosplenic metastatic HS lesions.[35,36]

Novel Diagnostics and Biomarkers

CADET histiocytic malignancy

The CADET histiocytic malignancy assay is a commercially available test by which either cytology or biopsy samples are evaluated for copy number aberrations consistent with those found in HS. Sensitivity and specificity of the assay have been estimated to be 78% and 95%, respectively.[37]

Serum ferritin

Hyperferritinemia has been documented in dogs with HS and is thought to be secondary to production by neoplastic cells, erythrocyte destruction, injury to hepatocytes, and release from tissue damage. Serum ferritin was significantly higher in dogs with HS and IMHA as compared with those with inflammatory disease and lymphoma.[38–40] Because of its elevation in other disease processes, its utility as a specific biomarker for HS is limited.

TREATMENT

Because of the highly aggressive nature of HS, effective treatment of this disease often requires both local therapy and systemic therapy, even for localized forms. Disseminated forms are generally treated with systemic therapy only.[1,2,9,24]

Local Therapy

Surgery

In most cases of localized HS, wide margin surgical tumor removal (ie, amputation, splenectomy, lung lobectomy) is the local therapy of choice. There are limited data available on outcomes of dogs undergoing local therapy only. In a series of 18 dogs with periarticular HS, the median survival time for dogs undergoing amputation only was 6 months, with a reported metastatic rate of 91%.[5] A recent study evaluating dogs with primary pulmonary HS showed that dogs undergoing surgery and chemotherapy had significantly prolonged progression-free survival (~9 months) and overall survival (~1 year) as compared with dogs not undergoing surgery.[41]

Radiation therapy

Limited data regarding the true efficacy of radiation therapy against HS exist. In a study of 37 FCR with mostly joint origin HS, dogs undergoing radiation therapy lived longer than those not receiving radiation therapy, with a median survival time of approximately 6 months.[42] Dogs treated with a combined protocol of a palliative radiation and lomustine (CCNU) had a median survival time of approximately 7 months. Further investigation is warranted to determine optimal protocols.

Systemic Therapy

Chemotherapy

- Lomustine (CCNU, CeeNU; 60–90 mg/m^2 by mouth every 3 weeks in dogs, 40–50 mg/m^2 every 3 to 6 weeks in cats) seems to be the most effective chemotherapy agent against HS.[9,40] For dogs with measurable disease, response rate ranges from 29% to 46%, with median response duration of approximately 3 months.[9,43] In one study, responders lived a median of almost 6 months, whereas nonresponders only lived a median of 2 months.[9,40] The use of adjuvant lomustine has been shown to improve survival for dogs with localized HS, resulting in a median survival time of 19 months.[44,45]

- Doxorubicin (30 mg/m^2 for dogs >15 kg or 1 mg/kg for cats and dogs <15 kg, intravenously [IV] over 15–20 minutes every 2–3 weeks) has been given in combination with lomustine in an alternating fashion, every 2 weeks. This regimen yielded a response rate of 58% and a median time to progression of approximately 6 months.[46]
- Dacarbazine (900–1000 mg/m^2 IV every 3 weeks) has been evaluated in the rescue setting and was associated with a response rate of 17.6%, with an event-free survival time in responders of 70 days.[47]
- Epirubicin (30 mg/m^2 IV every 3 weeks) has been evaluated as a single agent in the rescue setting as well as in combination with lomustine as first-line treatment and was associated with an overall response rate of 29% and median time to progression of just greater than 2 months.[48]
- Vinorelbine (15 mg/m^2 IV every 1–2 weeks) was evaluated in a small group of dogs with HS; 2 of 9 dogs had a partial response for 5.4 months and 2.1 years, and 4 of 9 had stable disease for a median of 2 months.[49]
- Metronomic lomustine (2.84 mg/m^2 by mouth daily) and chlorambucil (4 mg/m^2 by mouth daily) have also been used for dogs with HS.[50,51] Efficacy was unable to be determined due to small case numbers.

Novel therapy

- Bisphosphonates: this class of drugs may have utility as agents against HS due to their ability to deplete macrophages as well as their potential to increase effectiveness of cytotoxic chemotherapy.[52]
    - Liposomal clodronate (LC) was effective at inducing apoptosis in HS cell lines. LC was then shown to elicit significant tumor responses in 2 of 5 dogs with HS.[51] Results of larger studies are not yet available.
    - The combination of clodronate and vincristine was found to elicit synergistic killing associated with a significant increase in cell cycle arrest in vitro.[53]
    - Zoledronate significantly increased the uptake of doxorubicin by malignant histiocytic cells and significantly increased cell killing in vitro.[53]

Other medical management

- Corticosteroids: although often prescribed for alleviation of clinical signs associated with advanced HS, corticosteroid use has been associated as a significant negative prognostic factor for survival in 2 studies.[2,24]

FOLLOW-UP

Patients are routinely reevaluated with examinations, blood work, and periodic restaging with thoracoabdominal imaging (radiographs, ultrasound, CT/MRI) as indicated based on form and location of the disease.

PROGNOSIS

As discussed, patients with localized disease treated with adjuvant therapy enjoy longer survival times compared with those with disseminated disease. PAHS is generally associated with a better prognosis than that of other localized forms, with an overall median survival time of 13 months versus 4.2 months for dogs with non-PAHS.[24] This outcome was despite the presence of suspected metastasis at diagnosis in 13 of 19 dogs with PAHS. A recent study evaluating dogs with primary pulmonary HS documented an overall survival of 4.4 months for dogs receiving chemotherapy alone, whereas dogs undergoing both surgery and chemotherapy lived just more than 1 year.[41] HHS is a significantly more aggressive form of HS that commonly involves widespread organ infiltration and severe blood and bone marrow dyscrasias. To date, no effective treatment of HHS has been described with reported survival times ranging from days to 1 to 2 months, regardless of therapy.[2,9,14] Negative prognostic factors for HS include use of corticosteroids (which may be due to selection bias of prednisone administration to sicker patients) as well as anemia, thrombocytopenia, and hypoalbuminemia, all of which may in part be secondary to their association with the HHS form.[2,24]

HEMANGIOSARCOMA

Hemangiosarcoma (HSA) is a highly malignant tumor arising from bone marrow–derived endothelial cell precursors.[54,55] The most common primary anatomic sites for HSA include the spleen, heart, skin/subcutaneous tissues, and liver. Other less commonly reported primary tumor sites include kidney, retroperitoneal space, muscle, bone, eye, oral cavity, nasal cavity, urinary bladder, and lungs.[56–77] The biological behavior of HSA varies depending on primary tumor location, with the skin (dermal) carrying a more favorable prognosis in comparison to visceral locations.[78]

HSA is a rapidly growing and locally invasive tumor with high metastatic potential. Microscopic metastasis typically occurs often early in the course of disease via hematogenous spread to other organs or direct intracavitary tumor seeding following tumor rupture. Metastasis can occur at any site; however, the liver, omentum, and lungs are the most frequently reported metastatic locations.[56–77] HSA is the most common secondary (ie, metastatic) intracranial tumor, and one necropsy study found that 14% of dogs with HSA had metastasis to the brain.[12]

Incidence

HSA is diagnosed more frequently in dogs than in any other domestic species but accounts for only 2% of all canine tumors.[56,60] The spleen is the most commonly affected organ in dogs.

The summary of several studies suggests that approximately two-thirds of ruptured canine splenic tumors are malignant, with approximately two-thirds of that group being HSA.[61,63,64,79–81] This has led to the unofficial adoption of the clinical guideline, the "rule of two-thirds" or "double two-thirds rule." The presence of a nontraumatic hemoabdomen increases the chance that HSA is the underlying cause but does not rule out the possibility for a benign tumor.

The true incidence of HSA in cats is unclear, but it seems to be much less common than in dogs.[62,82–86] A study evaluating spontaneous hemoabdomen in cats reported that 46% of the cats had neoplasia and the remaining 54% had benign conditions. Of the cats with neoplasia, splenic HSA was the most common histology, accounting for ~37% of diagnoses within that group.[87]

Cause

The definitive cause of canine HSA remains unclear; however, several risk factors have been reported including ultraviolet (UV) light exposure, spay/neuter status, and genetic abnormalities.

Ultraviolet light exposure

Chronic UV light exposure is associated with the development of superficial cutaneous HSA along the ventral abdomen and conjunctiva in lightly pigmented, short-haired dog breeds such as Whippets and Italian Greyhounds.[88,89]

Hormonal status

A few studies have suggested a hormonal link with HSA related to neutering status.

- Cardiac HSA was 4x more common in spayed versus intact females,[90] and spayed females had >2x the risk of splenic HSA compared with intact females.[58]
- Late neutering in Golden Retrievers was associated with an increased risk of developing HSA, where females spayed after 1 year of age had 4x the risk compared with intact dogs or dogs neutered at less than 1 year of age.[91]
- Spayed female Vizslas were 9x more likely to develop HSA than intact female Vizslas. Furthermore, male Vizslas castrated after 1 year of age were also 5x more likely to develop HSA compared with intact male Vizslas.[92]

Genetics

The tumor suppressor gene PTEN was shown to be inactivated in more than half of HSA samples in one study,[93] whereas other studies have shown overexpression of the critical cell cycle–regulating proteins pRB, cyclin D1, Bcl2, and survivin.[94,95] Multiple angiogenic factors including VEGF, PDGF, and endothelin-1 are elevated in the blood and effusions of dogs with HSA and their associated receptors are overexpressed in tumor tissue.[96–100] This dysregulation of angiogenic pathways likely plays a role in the pathogenesis of HSA. Recent genome analysis has brought forth evidence of several molecularly distinct subtypes of HSA, although the clinical significance of these findings has yet to be elucidated.[101–103]

Signalment

Older dogs (median age 10 years) are typically affected and several reports suggest a male predominance. German Shepherds, Golden Retrievers, and Labrador Retrievers seem predisposed.[56,58–60,62] HSA most commonly affects older cats, with no sex or breed predisposition identified.[56,60,62,82–86]

HISTORY AND CLINICAL PRESENTATION

Most of the patients with visceral HSA present in an emergent scenario secondary to tumor rupture and internal hemorrhage, with clinical signs related to blood loss anemia and in the case of cardiac HSA, tamponade, and/or right-sided congestive heart failure. Acute weakness, lethargy, and collapse are common signs at presentation. Other historical findings include anorexia, weight loss, abdominal distension, vomiting, and dyspnea.[66,67,79–81]

Cutaneous HSA presentations vary depending on whether the lesion is dermal, subcutaneous, or intramuscular, but most patients present for a visible mass. A history of sunbathing may be reported for patients presenting with dermal HSA.[78,88,89]

PHYSICAL EXAMINATION FINDINGS

Examination findings vary depending on the location and extent of disease. Common findings associated with visceral HSA include pale mucous membranes, tachycardia, heart murmur, cardiac arrhythmia, weak or "snappy" pulses, tachypnea, dyspnea, muffled heart and lung sounds, abdominal distension, cranial organomegaly, and palpable fluid wave.

Patients with dermal HSA typically exhibit small, discrete, often blood blister–like lesions in the skin, most commonly on ventral abdomen, inguinal region, and/or conjunctiva. Subcutaneous and intramuscular HSA are generally larger, deeper, dark masses or mass effects, often having a bruised appearance. Distal limb swelling and lameness are possible when the tumor originates on or near a limb.

DIAGNOSIS

Histopathology is still considered the gold standard for diagnosis of HSA, although cytology may be diagnostic in some cases. A presumptive diagnosis is often made based on the history, signalment, and physical examination findings, and as such, it is common to perform clinical staging before obtaining a definitive histologic diagnosis. Complete staging includes standard laboratory analysis (complete blood count, chemistry profile, urinalysis), 3-view thoracic radiographs, and abdominal ultrasound. If applicable and available, echocardiography, CT, or MRI may be used. The results of clinical staging allow accurate assessment of the patient's stage of disease (**Box 1**), information that helps inform prognosis and guide therapy.

Pathologic Evaluation

Cytology

The diagnostic yield from cytology of HSA masses or effusion is reportedly low, mostly because of the large peripheral blood component.[104,105] In some cases of subcutaneous or intramuscular tumors, cytologic samples obtained from a solid portion of tumor may provide a diagnosis (**Fig. 2**). HSA cells are typically spindyloid to stellate with indistinct cytoplasmic borders and many small clear punctate vacuoles. Cells are generally found individually or in small aggregates. Nuclei are typically large with a coarsely stippled chromatin pattern and 1 to 3 prominent nucleoli. Anisocytosis and anisokaryosis are typically moderate to marked, and bizarre mitotic figures may be present.

Histology

HSA is composed of irregular anastomosing vascular-like structures lined by pleomorphic spindle cells forming large multifocal cavities filled with blood. Areas of necrosis

Box 1
Canine hemangiosarcoma TNM clinical staging system

T = Tumor (Primary Tumor)

T0 = No evidence of tumor

T1 = Tumor confined to primary site and/or dermis and <5 cm in diameter

T2 = Tumor invading SQ tissues and/or ≥5 cm in diameter

T3 = Any T1 or T2 with tumor invading adjacent structures and/or muscle

N = Node (Regional Lymph Nodes)

N0 = No evidence of regional lymph node involvement

N1 = Regional lymph node involvement

N2 = Distant lymph node involvement

M = Metastasis (Distant)

M0 = No evidence of distant metastasis

M1 = Distant metastasis

TNM Stages

I = T0 or T1, N0, M0

II = T1 or T2, N0 or N1

III = T2 or T3, N0 or N1 or N2, M1

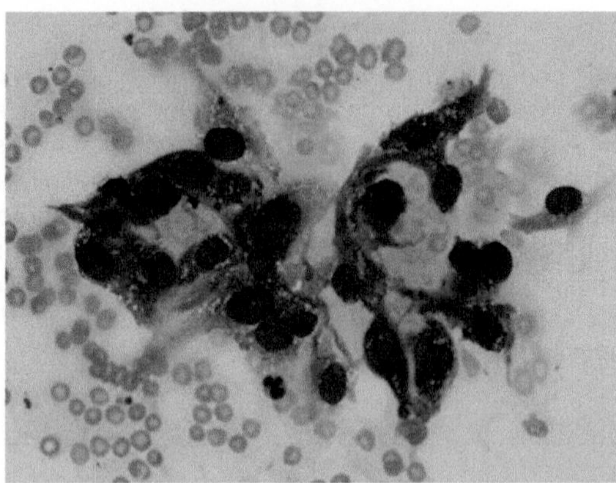

Fig. 2. Fine-needle aspirate of a pulmonary mass in an 11-year-old neutered male Catahoula Leopard Hound that also had multiple masses within the liver. The slides consisted of several spindle to stellate cells, found individually and in small aggregates, with indistinct cytoplasmic borders and many small clear punctate vacuoles. The large oval nuclei exhibited a coarsely stippled chromatin pattern and 1 to 3 prominent nucleoli. Anisokaryosis was mild to moderate. Subsequent histopathology confirmed HSA. (*Courtesy of* by C. LeBlanc, DVM, PhD, DACVP, Bethesda, MD.)

are commonly noted within the tumor. The tumor cells often display marked anisokaryosis and anisocytosis, typically with a high mitotic index. Generally, most of the nondermal tumors are classified histologically as high grade.[57,58]

Laboratory Evaluation

Complete blood count

- Anemia is the most common blood work abnormality in patients with HSA and is usually regenerative, with schistocytes, acanthocytes, and nucleated red blood cells noted, consistent with red blood cell membrane damage secondary to vasculitis, hepatic insufficiency, and a deficient reticuloendothelial system.[56,60,106,107]
- Thrombocytopenia is noted in up to 75% of dogs with HSA.[67,106] This may be a result of consumption and/or sequestration related to tumor hemorrhage, destruction within the tumor vasculature, and secondary consumptive coagulopathies.[108,109]
- Neutrophilic leukocytosis is common with visceral HSA and is likely a result of a paraneoplastic syndrome, secondary to tumor necrosis, or an increase in myeloid-derived suppressor cells, a subset of granulocytes whose role is to suppress innate antitumor immunity.[67,106,110,111]

Serum biochemistry, urinalysis

These tests rarely aid in the diagnosis of HSA, given their lack of specificity. In one study of cats with visceral HSA, 53% of patients had increased aspartate transaminase levels.[87]

Coagulation profile

Up to 50% of dogs with HSA have clinical and biochemical parameters consistent with disseminated intravascular coagulation, including prolongation of prothrombin time and partial thromboplastin time and increases in fibrin degradation product, fibrinogen, and d-dimers.[108,109]

Diagnostic Imaging

Thoracic radiographs

Pulmonary metastasis is most commonly characterized as a multifocal to coalescing miliary to nodular pattern (**Fig. 3**). The reported radiographic sensitivity for detecting pulmonary metastasis is 78%.[33] Dogs with cardiac HSA and pericardial effusion typically have a globoid cardiac silhouette on thoracic radiographs.

Abdominal ultrasound

Ultrasonography can be used to detect effusion and identify lesions in visceral organs and omentum. HSA lesions are most often cavitated but can have a variety of echogenic characteristics ranging from solid to heterogeneous to anechoic (**Fig. 4**).[112]

Echocardiogram

Echocardiography is used to identify cardiac tumors in patients in whom there is pericardial effusion and a suspicion of cardiac HSA.[67,113,114] Its use in routine staging for HSA of noncardiac locations is somewhat controversial, because data suggest the overall detection of splenic and cardiac tumors is low (7.8%).[115] Echocardiography can also be used to evaluate heart function before the initiation of and during chemotherapy, particularly in breeds at risk for dilated cardiomyopathy.[116]

Electrocardiogram

Perioperative ventricular arrhythmias are relatively common, being reported in up to 44% of dogs undergoing splenectomy for HSA.[117–119] In one study, dogs that developed intraoperative arrhythmias had an increased risk of death compared with dogs not experiencing intraoperative arrhythmias.[119]

Advanced Imaging

Computed tomography and magnetic resonance imaging

Both modalities can be used for evaluation of subcutaneous, intramuscular, cardiac, and intraabdominal forms of HSA. CT and MRI may aid in determining the exact anatomic origin and extent and invasiveness of a tumor, thereby aiding in the planning of surgical resection and/or radiation therapy (**Fig. 5**). Thoracic CT has been shown to have superior sensitivity to radiography in detecting early pulmonary metastasis

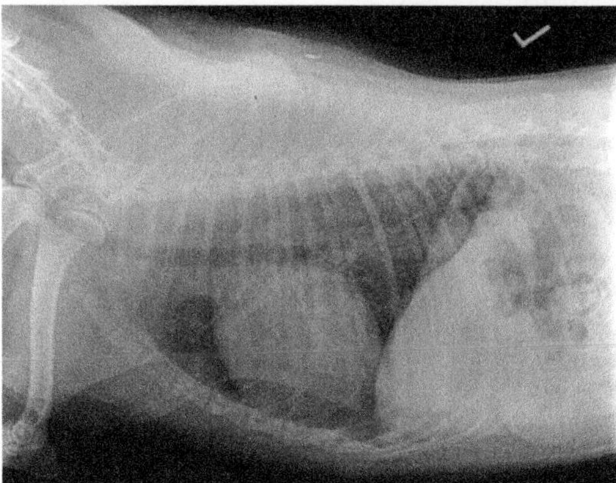

Fig. 3. Lateral thoracic radiograph of a 10-year-old Australian shepherd presenting for a bleeding intramuscular mass, cytologically consistent with hemangiosarcoma. Note the diffuse nodular to miliary pulmonary pattern, consistent with HSA metastasis.

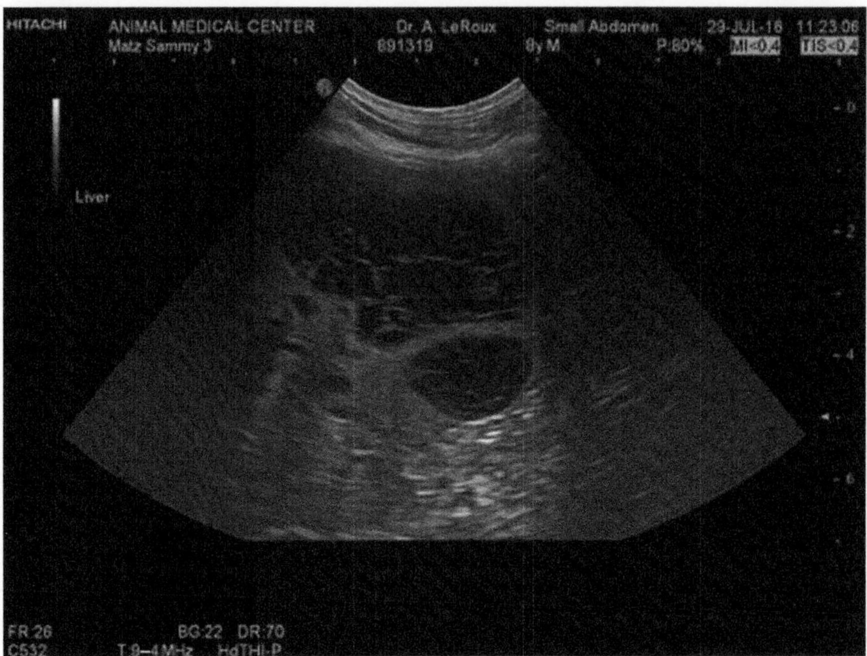

Fig. 4. Ultrasound from a 7-year-old Golden Retriever with hepatic HSA. Note the multicameral cavitary complex splenic mass. The fluid components of the mass exhibit through transmission. The mass bulges the liver's capsule. (*Courtesy of* Anthony Fischetti, DVM, MS, DACVR, New York, NY.)

detection.[34] Both MRI and CT carry a high sensitivity and specificity in discriminating benign from malignant splenic and hepatic lesions[35,36]; however, their routine use is limited due to associated cost and the requirement for anesthesia, which is of particular concern in unstable patients.

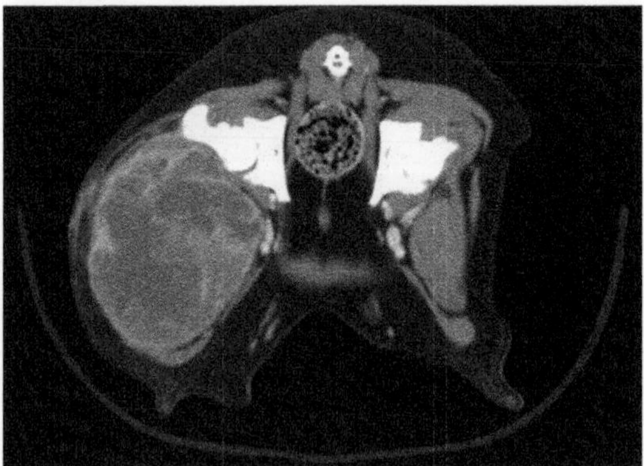

Fig. 5. Computed tomography images from a 10-year-old Minnesota mix breed with a history of lameness and a palpable mass along the right hindlimb. Aspirates were consistent with peripheral blood. Not the large, heterogeneously contrast enhancing soft tissue mass extending cranially from the right femur, intimately associated with the quadriceps muscle. Adjacent bone is normal, without evidence of pressure necrosis or lysis. The mass deforms skin margins. (*Courtesy of* Anthony Fischetti, DVM, MS, DACVR, New York, NY.)

Contrast harmonic ultrasound

Contrast harmonic ultrasound seems to improve diagnostic yield for hepatic and splenic HSA. In one small study, contrast harmonic ultrasound was able to detect hepatic HSA nodules not seen during traditional gray-scale ultrasound examination.[120] Multiple studies evaluating splenic lesions demonstrated that hypoechogenicity of the splenic lesion during the early and late vascular phases was highly associated with malignancy.[121–123] Thus far this modality is not widely available and so clinical application currently remains limited.

Biomarkers

HSA-specific biomarkers might enable early detection of the disease, which in turn could lead to earlier intervention and a potential for improved prognosis. In addition, biomarkers may serve as surrogates of disease status during and after treatment. The development and clinical application of such tests are still in their infancy.

Cardiac troponin I

Cardiac troponin I (cTnI) is a highly specific and sensitive marker for myocardiocyte damage. The median plasma cTnI concentration in dogs with cardiac HSA was shown to be significantly higher than the median concentration in dogs with pericardial effusion of other causes.[124,125]

Serum collagen XXVII peptide

Serum collagen XXVII peptide is a protein breakdown product thought related to invasive and angiogenic processes such as HSA. The concentration of collagen XXVII was found to be significantly higher in dogs with HSA, particularly those with large metastatic burdens, compared with healthy dogs. Reductions in collagen XXVII peptide levels after surgical resection of HSA and subsequent increases with tumor recurrence support the potential of this peptide as a useful HSA biomarker.[126]

Thymidine kinase

Thymidine kinase (TK1) is a cytosolic enzyme that is involved in DNA synthesis and its expression is restricted to proliferating cells. One study demonstrated significantly higher serum TK1 activity in the serum HSA dogs compared with that of healthy dogs.[127] A specific cutoff value to differentiate benign splenic masses versus HSA has not been established; this may limit its diagnostic utility.

TREATMENT

Initial Emergency Therapy

Because most of the patients with HSA present in a critical state secondary to hemorrhagic shock, initial treatment is focused on patient stabilization. Intravenous therapy with crystalloids, colloids, and blood products is indicated to improve endpoints related to anemia and hypovolemic shock.[128] When patients present in shock secondary to pericardial effusion and cardiac tamponade, immediate therapeutic pericardiocentesis is indicated and generally provides rapid relief.[67]

Local Therapy

Surgery

- Cardiac HSA: although a few case reports and series describing surgical excision of cardiac HSA exist, resection of these tumors is rarely feasible and thus not typically attempted.[67] Surgical intervention typically consists of pericardiectomy, which can be performed via an open thoracotomy or minimally invasive thoracoscopy. Removal of the pericardium can prevent recurrence of cardiac tamponade, but is considered palliative only because it does not address the tumor itself.[129]

- Splenic/hepatic/renal HSA: once the patient is stabilized, laparotomy should be performed for exploratory purposes, removal of the affected tissue, and biopsy of other organs (ie, liver).[56–61,63,64] In a recent study evaluating hepatic abnormalities found at the time of splenectomy for splenic HSA, 50% of dogs with grossly abnormal livers had histologic evidence of hepatic metastasis,[130] thus it is imperative that any abnormalities noted at surgery should be biopsied.
- Dermal HSA: wide margin surgical excision is the treatment of choice for dermal HSA and is generally curative for individual lesions.[68,78]
- Subcutaneous/intramuscular HSA: wide margin surgical excision is the treatment of choice for subcutaneous and intramuscular HSA. Some cases may require radical resections such as amputation.[56,60,131,132]

Radiation therapy

Hypofractionated external beam radiation therapy can be used in the palliative setting for nonresectable subcutaneous/intramuscular HSA and is associated with a high response rate but not necessarily a positive impact on survival.[133] Hypofractionated radiation therapy has also been evaluated for cardiac HSA and can reduce the frequency of cardiac tamponade. The use of radiation therapy for cardiac HSA was associated with a median survival time of 2.5 months.[134]

Systemic Therapy

Given the highly metastatic nature of HSA and the expected poor prognosis, adjuvant chemotherapy is indicated for nondermal presentations of the disease.[56,60] Chemotherapy can also be used in the macroscopic setting for nonresectable subcutaneous and intramuscular HSA, cardiac HSA, and advanced stage visceral HSA.

Chemotherapy

- Doxorubicin (30 mg/m^2 for dogs >15 kg or 1 mg/kg for cats and dogs <15 kg, IV over 15–20 minutes every 2–3 weeks) is the most active and widely used chemotherapy agent for HSA. It is most commonly given as an adjuvant following splenectomy and is associated with median survival times of 5 to 8 months.[135–137] It has also been evaluated for dogs with nonresectable cardiac and subcutaneous HSA and yielded a 38% to 41% response rate in these settings.[67,138]
- Vincristine (0.5–0.7 mg/m^2 IV weekly) and cyclophosphamide (200–250 mg/m^2 by mouth or IV weekly) may be given together as a rescue protocol for dogs with HSA or along with doxorubicin (VAC protocol) as part of first-line treatment of HSA.[139]
- Dacarbazine (DTIC; 800–1000 mg/m^2 IV every 3 weeks or 200 mg/m^2 IV daily x 5 days) has been evaluated for dogs with HSA in 2 studies. In one study, DTIC was given along with vincristine and doxorubicin (DAV protocol) to dogs with advanced stage HSA and was associated with a 47% response rate.[140] In another study, when administered with doxorubicin to dogs with various forms, there were significant improvements in both the time to metastasis and median survival time (both >1.5 years) as compared with those of dogs receiving doxorubicin and cyclophosphamide.[141]
- Epirubicin (30 mg/m^2 IV every 3 weeks) can be used as a substitute for doxorubicin in dogs with cardiac disease, as it is noncardiotoxic. It seemed as efficacious as an adjuvant for splenic HSA as doxorubicin in one study.[142]

- Ifosfamide (350–375 mg/m^2 IV every 2–3 weeks, along with saline diuresis and mesna) has been given as a single agent and in combination with doxorubicin in alternating fashion to dogs with various forms HSA.[143]
- Metronomic cyclophosphamide (12.5–15 mg/m^2 by mouth every 24 hours) can be given in combination with a nonsteroidal antiinflammatory drug (NSAID) (eg, piroxicam ,0.3 mg/kg, by mouth every 24 hours; deracoxib, 1–2 mg/kg, by mouth every 24 hours; carprofen, 2.2 mg/kg, by mouth every 12 hours) following, concurrent to, or as an alternative to doxorubicin. A pilot study evaluated an adjuvant metronomic cyclophosphamide/piroxicam protocol in a small group of dogs (n = 9) with stage II HSA and documented a median survival time (~6 months) comparable to the outcome achieved for dogs receiving adjuvant doxorubicin.[144] A more recent study evaluating dogs treated with splenectomy and doxorubicin found no significant improvement in outcome in the group receiving metronomic cyclophosphamide after doxorubicin.[145]
- Thalidomide (2–3 mg/kg by mouth every 24–48 hours or 8.7 mg/kg by mouth every 24 hours) has been evaluated as maintenance therapy for dogs with HSA. One study assessing dogs receiving thalidomide along with metronomic cyclophosphamide after doxorubicin reported significantly longer median time to metastasis and survival time as compared with dogs receiving doxorubicin alone.[146] Another study documented significantly improved outcomes for dogs receiving adjuvant single-agent thalidomide postsplenectomy.[147]
- Metronomic chlorambucil (4 mg/m^2 by mouth every 24 hours) can be given with or without an NSAID. One study reported that low-dose administration of chlorambucil resulted in stable disease in 3 of 5 dogs with macroscopic HSA.[50]

Targeted therapy

- Toceranib phosphate (Palladia; 2.5–3 mg/kg by mouth every 48 hours) was evaluated in dogs with stage I or II HSA following splenectomy and doxorubicin chemotherapy, but there was no significant improvement in median disease-free interval or survival time.[148]
- eBAT, a bispecific epidermal growth factor-urokinase angiotoxin, was evaluated in a small group of dogs before adjuvant doxorubicin and was associated with an improved median survival time of 8.5 months and 6-month survival rate of ~70%. This was superior to those of a historical control group receiving adjuvant doxorubicin only.[149] This product is not yet commercially available.

Immunotherapy

- Liposomal muramyl tripeptide phosphatidylethanolamine, a synthetic macrophage activator derived from mycobacterial cell wall, improved survival times (median 9 months) when given concurrent to a doxorubicin/cyclophosphamide protocol.[150] This agent is not currently commercially available in the United States.

Complementary and alternative therapy

- Yunnan Baiyao is a Chinese herbal medicine that has been anecdotally used to control bleeding in dogs with multiple hemorrhagic conditions, including HSA. An in vitro study documented a dose- and time-dependent cell death via caspase-mediated apoptosis in HSA cell lines[151]; however, 2 laboratory studies demonstrated no modulation of coagulation parameters in normal dogs receiving oral

Yunnan Baiyao.[152,153] A recent retrospective study evaluating a combination of Yunnan Baiyao and epsilon aminocaproic acid in dogs with presumed cardiac HSA suggested no benefit in time to recurrence of pericardial effusion or overall survival time.[154] Dosing of this agent remains anecdotal.

- Polysaccharopeptide (PSP) is the bioactive agent from the mushroom *coriolus versicolor* and main ingredient in the commercial product I'm-Yunity. In a recent double-blind, randomized, multidose pilot study, high-dose (100 mg/kg/d by mouth) PSP delayed the progression of metastases and improved survival times for a small group of postsplenectomy dogs with HSA (n = 5) when compared with historical control data of dogs undergoing splenectomy alone.[155]

FOLLOW-UP

Patients are routinely reevaluated with examinations and blood work, periodic restaging with thoracoabdominal imaging (radiographs, ultrasound, echocardiography, CT/MRI) as indicated based on form and location of the disease.

PREVENTION

Dermal Hemangiosarcoma

Limit sun exposure for lightly pigmented, shorthaired breeds such as Salukis, Whippets, Italian Greyhounds, and Greyhounds.

PROGNOSIS

For dermal HSA, wide margin surgical excision is often curative. Median survival times of greater than 2 years have been reported after excision of dermal HSA.[78] Long-term outcomes for dogs with subcutaneous/intramuscular HSA vary depending on the study referenced, where reported median survival times for dogs underdoing surgery plus adjuvant chemotherapy range from 9 months to more than 3 years.[131,132] For splenic HSA, median survival times with surgery alone range from less than 1 to 2.5 months, whereas the addition of adjuvant doxorubicin-based chemotherapy improves the median survival time to 5 to 8 months.[135–137,139–145] Despite the use of chemotherapy, the 1-year survival rate remains less than 10%. The median survival time for dogs with renal HSA undergoing nephrectomy with or without adjuvant chemotherapy is ~9 months.[70] For cardiac HSA, the median survival time without chemotherapy is ~2 weeks versus 4 months with doxorubicin.[67] A small group of dogs treated with surgical tumor excision and adjuvant doxorubicin chemotherapy had a median survival of nearly 6 months.[156] Limited survival data are available for feline HSA. Cutaneous presentations are typically associated with a superior prognosis (median survival time 9 months to 4 years) compared with that seen with visceral forms (median survival time 2.5 months).[82–87]

SUMMARY

HS and HSA remain 2 of the most aggressive cancers seen in companion animals; however, positive strides have been made on multiple fronts over the last 20 years. Specifically, there is a continually evolving understanding of the genetic abnormalities behind these diseases along with the identification of certain breed predispositions. Improvements in survival related to the use of surgery and adjuvant chemotherapy have changed the perception of HS from an immediately life-threatening cancer to one that can be managed for months or even years. Nondermal forms of HSA remain uniformly terminal. The discovery of driver mutations may lead to the development of more targeted therapies that could further improve the outlook for these difficult diseases.

REFERENCES

1. Moore PF. A review of histiocytic diseases in dogs and cats. Vet Pathol 2014;51: 167–84.
2. Dervisis NG, Kiupel M, Quin Q, et al. Clinical prognostic factors in canine histiocytic sarcoma. Vet Comp Oncol 2017;15:1171–80.
3. Affolter VK, Moore PF. Localized and disseminated histiocytic sarcoma of dendritic cell origin in dogs. Vet Pathol 2002;39:74–83.
4. Dobson J, Hoather T, McKinley TJ, et al. Mortality in a cohort of flat-coated retrievers in the UK. Vet Comp Oncol 2009;7:115–21.
5. Craig LE, Julian ME, Ferracone JD. The diagnosis and prognosis of synovial tumors in dogs: 35 cases. Vet Pathol 2002;39:66–73.
6. Hayden DW, Waters DJ, Burke BA, et al. Disseminated malignant histiocytosis in a golden retriever: clinicopathologic, ultrastructural, and immunohistochemical findings. Vet Pathol 1993;30:256–64.
7. Kohn B, Arnold P, Kaser-Hotz B, et al. Malignant histiocytosis of the dog: 26 cases (1989-1992). Kleintierpraxis 1993;38:409–24.
8. Fant P, Caldin M, Furlanello T, et al. Primary gastric histiocytic sarcoma in a dog—a case report. J Vet Med A Physiol Pathol Clin Med 2004;51:358–62.
9. Skorupski K, Clifford C, Paoloni M, et al. CCNU for the treatment of dogs with histiocytic sarcoma. J Vet Intern Med 2007;21:121–6.
10. Naranjo C, Dubielzig R, Friedrichs K. Canine ocular histiocytic sarcoma. Vet Ophthalmol 2007;10:179–85.
11. Vernau KM, Higgins RJ, Bollen AW, et al. Primary canine and feline nervous system tumors: intraoperative diagnosis using the smear technique. Vet Pathol 2001;38:47–57.
12. Snyder J, Lipitz L, Skorupski K, et al. Secondary intracranial neoplasia in the dog: 177 cases (1986-2003). J Vet Intern Med 2008;22:172–7.
13. Mariani CL, Jennings MK, Olby NJ, et al. Histiocytic sarcoma with central nervous system involvement in dogs: 19 cases (2006–2012). J Vet Intern Med 2015;29:607–13.
14. Moore PF, Affolter VK, Vernau W. Canine hemophagocytic histiocytic sarcoma: a proliferative disorder of CD11d+ macrophages. Vet Pathol 2006;43:632–45.
15. Moore PF. Malignant histiocytosis of Bernese mountain dogs. Vet Pathol 1986; 23:1–10.
16. Rosin A, Moore P, Dubielzig R. Malignant histiocytosis in Bernese Mountain dogs. J Am Vet Med Assoc 1986;188:1041–5.
17. Lenz JA, Furrow E, Craig LE, et al. Histiocytic sarcoma in 14 miniature schnauzers-a new breed predisposition? J Small Anim Pract 2017;58:461–7.
18. Takahashi M, Tomiyasu H, Hotta E, et al. Clinical characteristics and prognostic factors in dogs with histiocytic sarcomas in Japan. J Vet Med Sci 2014;76: 661–6.
19. Voegeli E, Welle M, Hauser B, et al. Histiocytic sarcoma in the Swiss population of Bernese mountain dogs: a retrospective study of its genetic predisposition. Schweiz Arch Tierheilkd 2006;148:281–8.
20. Hedan B, Thomas R, Motsinger-Reif A, et al. Molecular cytogenetic characterization of canine histiocytic sarcoma: a spontaneous model for human histiocytic

cancer identifies deletion of tumor suppressor genes and highlights influence of genetic background on tumor behavior. BMC Cancer 2011;11:201.

21. Manor EK, Craig LE, Sun X, et al. Prior joint disease is associated with increased risk of periarticular histiocytic sarcoma in dogs. Vet Comp Oncol 2017;16(1): E83–8.
22. van Kuijk L, van Ginkel K, de Vos JP, et al. Peri-articular histiocytic sarcoma and previous joint disease in bernese mountain dogs. J Vet Intern Med 2013;27: 293–9.
23. Ruple A, Moreley PS. Risk factors associated with development of histiocytic sarcoma in bernese mountain dogs. J Vet Intern Med 2016;30:1197–203.
24. Klahn SL, Kitchell B, Dervisis N. Evaluation and comparison of outcomes in dogs with periarticular and nonperiarticular histiocytic sarcoma. J Am Vet Med Assoc 2001;239:90–6.
25. Brown DE, Thrall MA, Getzy DM, et al. Cytology of canine malignant histiocytosis. Vet Clin Pathol 1994;23:118–23.
26. Erich SA, Constantino-Casas F, Dobson JM, et al. Morphological distinction of histiocytic sarcoma from other tumor types in bernese mountain dogs and flat-coated retrievers. In Vivo 2018;32(1):7–17.
27. Kato Y, Funato R, Hirata A, et al. Immunocytochemical detection of the class A macrophage scavenger receptor CD204 using air-dried cytologic smears of canine histiocytic sarcoma. Vet Clin Pathol 2014;43:589–93.
28. Kato Y, Murakami M, Hoshino Y, et al. The class a macrophage scavenger receptor CD204 is a useful immunohistochemical marker of canine histiocytic sarcoma. J Comp Pathol 2013;148:188–96.
29. Weiss DJ, Evanson OA, Sykes J. A retrospective study of canine pancytopenia. Vet Clin Pathol 1999;28:83–8.
30. Tsai S, Sutherland-Smith J, Burgess K, et al. Imaging characteristics of intrathoracic Histiocytic sarcoma in dogs. Vet Radiol Ultrasound 2012;53:21–7.
31. Barrett LE, Pollard RE, Zwingenberger A, et al. Radiographic characterization of primary lung tumors in 74 dogs. Vet Radiol Ultrasound 2014;55:480–7.
32. Cruz-Arambulo R, Wrigley R, Powers B. Sonographic features of histiocytic neoplasms in the canine abdomen. Vet Radiol Ultrasound 2004;45:554–8.
33. Holt D, Van Winkle T, Schelling C, et al. Correlation between thoracic radiographs and postmortem findings in dogs with hemangiosarcoma: 77 cases (1984-1989). J Am Vet Med Assoc 1992;200(10):1535–9.
34. Armbrust LJ, Biller DS, Bamford A, et al. Comparison of three-view thoracic radiography and computed tomography for detection of pulmonary nodules in dogs with neoplasia. J Am Vet Med Assoc 2012;240:1088–94.
35. Clifford CA, Pretorius ES, Weisse C, et al. Magnetic resonance imaging of focal splenic and hepatic lesions in the dog. J Vet Intern Med 2004;18(3):330–8.
36. Fife WD, Samii VF, Drost WT, et al. Comparison between malignant and nonmalignant splenic masses in dogs using contrast-enhanced computed tomography. Vet Radiol Ultrasound 2004;45(4):289–97.
37. The CADETSM HM assay. 2018. Available at: https://www.sentinelbiomedical.com/cadet-hm-for-vets/.
38. Newlands CE, Houston DM, Vasconcelos DY. Hyperferritinemia associated with malignant histiocytosis in a dog. J Am Vet Med Assoc 1994;205:849–51.
39. Friedrichs K, Thomas C, Plier M, et al. Evaluation of serum ferritin as a tumor marker for canine histiocytic sarcoma. J Vet Intern Med 2010;24:904–11.

40. Nielsen LN, McEvoy F, Jessen LR, et al. Investigation of a screening programme and the possible identification of biomarkers for early disseminated histiocytic sarcoma in Bernese Mountain dogs. Vet Comp Oncol 2012;10:124–34.
41. Marlowe KW, Robat CS, Clarke DM, et al. Primary pulmonary histiocytic sarcoma in dogs: a retrospective analysis of 37 cases (2000-2015). Vet Comp Oncol 2018;16:658–63.
42. Fidel J, Schiller I, Hauser Y, et al. Histiocytic sarcomas in flat-coated retrievers: a summary of 37 cases (November 1998-March 2005). Vet Comp Oncol 2006;4: 63–74.
43. Rassnick K, Moore A, Russell D, et al. Phase II, open-label trial of single-agent CCNU in dogs with previously untreated histiocytic sarcoma. J Vet Intern Med 2010;24:1528–31.
44. Skorupski K, Rodriguez C, Krick E, et al. Long-term survival in dogs with localized histiocytic sarcoma treated with CCNU as an adjuvant to local therapy. Vet Comp Oncol 2009;7:139–44.
45. Cannon C, Borgatti A, Henson M, et al. Evaluation of a combination chemotherapy protocol including lomustine and doxorubicin in canine histiocytic sarcoma. J Small Anim Pract 2015;56:425–9.
46. Kezer KA, Barber LG, Jennings SH. Efficacy of dacarbazine as a rescue agent for histiocytic sarcoma in dogs. Vet Comp Oncol 2017;1–7.
47. Mason SL, Finotello R, Blackwood L. Epirubicin in the treatment of canine histiocytic sarcoma: sequential, alternating and rescue chemotherapy. Vet Comp Oncol 2018;16(1):77–80.
48. Wouda RM, Miller ME, Chon E, et al. Clinical effects of vinorelbine administration in the management of various malignant tumor types in dogs: 58 cases (1997–2012). J Am Vet Med Assoc 2015;246:1230–7.
49. Tripp CD, Fidel J, Anderson CL, et al. Tolerability of metronomic administration of lomustine in dogs with cancer. J Vet Intern Med 2011;25:278–84.
50. Leach TN, Childress MO, Greene SN, et al. Prospective trial of metronomic chlorambucil chemotherapy in dogs with naturally occurring cancer. Vet Comp Oncol 2011;10(2):102–12.
51. Hafeman S, London C, Elmslie R, et al. Evaluation of liposomal clodronate for treatment of malignant histiocytosis in dogs. Cancer Immunol Immunother 2010;59:441–52.
52. Hafeman SD, Varland D, Dow SW. Bisphosphonates significantly increase the activity of doxorubicin or vincristine against canine malignant histiocytosis cells. Vet Comp Oncol 2012;10:44–56.
53. Elliot J. Lomustine chemotherapy for the treatment of presumptive haemophagocytic histiocytic sarcoma in Flat-coated Retrievers. Aust Vet J 2018;96(12): 502–7.
54. Lamerato-Kozicki AR, Helm KM, Jubala CM, et al. Canine hemangiosarcoma originates from hematopoietic precursors with potential for endothelial differentiation. Exp Hematol 2006;34(7):870–8.
55. Fosmire SP, Dickerson EB, Scott AM, et al. Canine malignant hemangiosarcoma as a model of primitive angiogenic endothelium. Lab Invest 2004;84(5):562–72.
56. Mullin CM, Clifford CS. Hemangiosarcoma. In: Withrow SJ, Vail DM, Thamm DH, et al, editors. Small animal clinical oncology. 6th edition. St Louis (MO): Saunders/Elsevier; 2019.
57. Spangler WL, Culbertson MR. Prevalence, type, and importance of splenic diseases in dogs: 1,480 cases (1985-1989). J Am Vet Med Assoc 1992;200: 829–34.

58. Prymak C, McKee LJ, Goldschmidt MH, et al. Epidemiologic, clinical, pathologic, and prognostic characteristics of splenic hemangiosarcoma and splenic hematoma in dogs: 217 cases (1985). J Am Vet Med Assoc 1988;193:706–12.
59. Brown NO, Patnaik AK, MacEwen EG. Canine hemangiosarcoma: retrospective analysis of 104 cases. J Am Vet Med Assoc 1985;186(1):56–8.
60. Clifford CA, de Lorimier LP. Hemangiosarcoma. In: Ettinger SJ, Feldman EC, Cote E, editors. Textbook of veterinary internal medicine. 8th edition. St Louis (MO): Elsevier; 2017. p. 2093–102.
61. Spangler WL, Kass PH. Pathologic factors affecting postsplenectomy survival in dogs. J Vet Intern Med 1997;11(3):166–71.
62. Schultheiss PC. A retrospective study of visceral and nonvisceral hemangiosarcoma and hemangiomas in domestic animals. J Vet Diagn Invest 2004;16(6): 522–6.
63. Johnson KA, Powers BE, Withrow SJ, et al. Splenomegaly in dogs: predictors of neoplasia and survival after splenectomy. J Vet Intern Med 1989;3:160–6.
64. Eberle N, von Babo V, Nolte I, et al. Splenic masses in dogs. Part 1: epidemiologic, clinical characteristics as well as histopathologic diagnosis in 249 cases (2000-2011). Tierarztl Prax Ausg K Kleintiere Heimtiere 2012;40(4):250–60.
65. Aronsohn M. Cardiac hemangiosarcoma in the dog: a review of 38 cases. J Am Vet Med Assoc 1985;187:922–6.
66. Yamamoto S, Hoshi K, Hirakawa A. Epidemiological, clinical and pathological features of primary cardiac hemangiosarcoma in dogs: a review of 51 cases. J Vet Med Sci 2013;75(11):1433–41.
67. Mullin CM, Arkans MA, Sammarco CD, et al. Doxorubicin chemotherapy for presumptive cardiac hemangiosarcoma in dogs. Vet Comp Oncol 2016;14(4): e171–83.
68. Ward H, Fox LE, Calderwood-Mays MB, et al. Cutaneous hemangiosarcoma in 25 dogs: a retrospective study. J Vet Intern Med 1994;8:345–8.
69. Aupperle H, Marz I, Ellenberger C, et al. Primary and secondary heart tumours in dogs and cats. J Comp Pathol 2007;136:18–26.
70. Locke JE, Barber LG. Comparative aspects and clinical outcomes of canine renal hemangiosarcoma. J Vet Intern Med 2006;20(4):962–7.
71. Liptak JM, Dernell WS, Ehrhart EJ, et al. Retroperitoneal sarcomas in dogs: 14 cases (1992-2002). J Am Vet Med Assoc 2004;224(9):1471–7.
72. Giuffrida MA, Bacon NJ, Kamstock DA. Use of routine histopathology and factor VIII-related antigen/von Willebrand factor immunosthochemistry to differentiate primary hemangiosarcoma of bone from telangiectatic osteosarcoma in 54 dogs. Vet Comp Oncol 2017;15(4):1232–9.
73. Dennis MM, Ehrhart N, Duncan CG, et al. Frequency of and risk factors associated with lingual lesions in dogs: 1,196 cases (1995-2004). J Am Vet Med Assoc 2006;228(10):1533–7.
74. Fujita M, Takaishi Y, Yasuda D, et al. Intranasal hemangiosarcoma in a dog. J Vet Med Sci 2008;70(5):525–8.
75. Pirie CG, Knollinger AM, Thomas CB, et al. Canine conjunctival hemangioma and hemangiosarcoma: a retrospective evaluation of 108 cases (1989-2004). Vet Ophthalmol 2006;9(4):215–26.
76. Liptak JM, Dernell WS, Withrow SJ. Haemangiosarcoma of the urinary bladder in a dog. Aust Vet J 2004;82:215–7.
77. Wobeser BK, Kidney BA, Powers BE, et al. Diagnoses and clinical outcomes associated with surgically amputated canine digits submitted to multiple veterinary diagnostic laboratories. Vet Pathol 2007;44(3):355–61.

78. Szivek A, Burns RE, Gericota B, et al. Clinical outcome in 94 cases of dermal haemangiosarcoma in dogs treated with surgical excision: 1993-2007. Vet Comp Oncol 2012;10(1):65–73.
79. Pintar J, Breitschwerdt EB, Hardie EM, et al. Acute nontraumatic hemoabdomen in the dog: a retrospective analysis of 39 cases (1987-2001). J Am Anim Hosp Assoc 2003;39(6):518–22.
80. Hammond TN, Pesillo-Crosby SA. Prevalence of hemangiosarcoma in anemic dogs with a splenic mass and hemoperitoneum requiring a transfusion: 71 cases (2003-2005). J Am Vet Med Assoc 2008;232(4):553–8.
81. Aronsohn MG, Dubiel B, Roberts B, et al. Prognosis for acute nontraumatic hemoperitoneum in the dog: a retrospective analysis of 60 cases (2003-2006). J Am Anim Hosp Assoc 2009;45(2):72–7.
82. Scavelli TD, Patnaik AK, Mehlhaff CJ, et al. Hemangiosarcoma in the cat: retrospective evaluation of 31 surgical cases. J Am Vet Med Assoc 1985;187(8): 817–9.
83. Miller MA, Ramos JA, Kreeger JM. Cutaneous vascular neoplasia in 15 cats: clinical, morphologic, and immunohistochemical studies. Vet Pathol 1992; 29(4):329–36.
84. Kraje AC, Mears EA, Hahn KA, et al. Unusual metastatic behavior and clinicopathologic findings in eight cats with cutaneous or visceral hemangiosarcoma. J Am Vet Med Assoc 1999;214(5):670–2.
85. McAbee KP, Ludwig LL, Bergman PJ, et al. Feline cutaneous hemangiosarcoma: a retrospective study of 18 cases (1998-2003). J Am Anim Hosp Assoc 2005;41(2):110–6.
86. Culp WT, Drobatz KJ, Glassman MM, et al. Feline visceral hemangiosarcoma. J Vet Intern Med 2008;22(1):148–52.
87. Culp WT, Weisse C, Kellogg ME, et al. Spontaneous hemoperitoneum in cats: 65 cases (1994-2006). J Am Med Assoc 2010;236:978–82.
88. Hargis AM, Ihrke PJ, Spangler QL, et al. A retrospective clinicopathologic study of 212 dogs with cutaneous hemangiomas and hemangiosarcomas. Vet Pathol 1992;29(4):316–28.
89. Nikula KJ, Benjamin SA, Angleton GM, et al. Ultraviolet radiation, solar dermatosis, and cutaneous neoplasia in Beagle dogs. Radiat Res 1992;129(1):11–8.
90. Ware WA, Hopper DL. Cardiac tumors in dogs: 1982- 1995. J Vet Intern Med 1999;13(2):95–103.
91. Torres de la Riva G, Hart BL, Farver TB, et al. Neutering dogs: effects on joint disorders and cancers in golden retrievers. PLoS One 2013;8(2):e55937.
92. Zink MC, Farhoody P, Elser SE, et al. Evaluation of the risk and age of onset of cancer and behavioral disorders in gonadectomized Vizslas. J Am Vet Med Assoc 2014;244(3):309–19.
93. Dickerson EB, Thomas R, Fosmire P, et al. Mutations of phosphatase and tensin homolog deleted from chromosome 10 in canine hemangiosarcoma. Vet Pathol 2005;42:618–32.
94. Yonemaru K, Sakai H, Murakami M, et al. The significance of p53 and retinoblastoma pathways in canine hemangiosarcoma. J Vet Med Sci 2007;69:271–8.
95. Murakami M, Sakai H, Kodama A, et al. Expression of the anti-apoptotic factors Bcl-2 and survivin in canine vascular tumours. J Comp Pathol 2008;139:1–7.
96. Clifford CA, Hughes D, Beal MW, et al. Plasma vascular endothelial growth factor concentrations in healthy dogs and dogs with hemangiosarcoma. J Vet Intern Med 2001;15:131–5.

97. Yonemaru K, Sakai H, Murakami M, et al. Expression of vascular endothelial growth factor, basic fibroblast growth factor, and their receptors (flt-1, flk-1, and flg-1) in canine vascular tumors. Vet Pathol 2006;43(6):971–80.
98. Kodama A, Sakai H, Matsuura S, et al. Establishment of canine hemangiosarcoma xenograft models expressing endothelial growth factors, their receptors, and angiogenesis-associated homeobox genes. BMC Cancer 2009;14(9):363.
99. Göritz M, Müller K, Krastel D, et al. Canine splenic haemangiosarcoma: influence of metastases, chemotherapy and growth pattern on post-splenectomy survival and expression of angiogenic factors. J Comp Pathol 2013;149:30–9.
100. Abou Asa S, Mori T, Maruo K, et al. Analysis of genomic mutation and immunohistochemistry of platelet-derived growth factor receptors in canine vascular tumours. Vet Comp Oncol 2015;13(3):237–45.
101. Gorden BH, Kim JH, Sarber AL, et al. Identification of three molecular and functional subtypes in canine hemangiosarcoma through gene expression profiling and progenitor cell characterization. Am J Path 2014;184(4):985–95.
102. Tamburini BA, Phang TL, Fosmire SP, et al. Gene expression profiling identifies inflammation and angiogenesis as distinguishing features of canine hemangiosarcoma. BMC Cancer 2010;10:619.
103. Thomas R, Borst L, Rotroff D, et al. Genomic profiling reveals extensive heterogeneity in somatic DNA copy number aberrations of canine hemangiosarcoma. Chromosome Res 2014;22:305–19.
104. Bertazzolo W, Dell'Orco M, Bonfanti U, et al. Canine angiosarcoma: cytologic, histologic, and immunohistochemical correlations. Vet Clin Pathol 2005;34(1):28–34.
105. Cagle LA, Epstein SE, Owens SD, et al. Diagnostic yield of cytologic analysis of pericardial effusion in dogs. J Vet Intern Med 2014;28(1):66–71.
106. Childress MO. Hematologic abnormalities in the small animal cancer patient. Vet Clin Small Anim 2012;42:123–55.
107. Hirsch VM, Jacobsen J, Mills JH. A retrospective study of canine hemangiosarcoma and its association with acanthocytosis. Can Vet J 1981;22(5):152–5.
108. Hargis AM, Feldman BF. Evaluation of hemostatic defects secondary to vascular tumors in dogs: 11 cases (1983-1988). J Am Vet Med Assoc 1991;198(5):891–4.
109. Maruyama H, Miura T, Sakai M, et al. The incidence of disseminated intravascular coagulation in dogs with malignant tumor. J Vet Med Sci 2004;66:573–5.
110. Sherger M, Kisseberth W, London C, et al. Identification of myeloid derived suppressor cells in the peripheral blood of tumor bearing dogs. BMC Vet Res 2012;8:209.
111. Goulart MR, Pluhar E, Ohlfest JR. Identification of myeloid derived suppressor cells in dogs with naturally occurring cancer. PLoS One 2012;7(3):e33274.
112. Wrigley RH, Park RD, Konde LJ, et al. Ultrasonographic features of splenic hemangiosarcoma in dogs: 18 cases (1980-1986). J Am Vet Med Assoc 1988;192(8):1113–7.
113. MacDonald KA, Cagney O, Magne ML. Echocardiographic and clinicopathologic characterization of pericardial effusion in dogs: 107 cases (1995-2006). J Am Vet Med Assoc 2009;235:1456–61.
114. Fruchter A, Miller C, O'Grady M. Echocardiographic results and clinical considerations in dogs with right atrial/auricular masses. Can Vet J 1992;33:171–4.
115. Boston SE, Higginson G, Monteith G. Concurrent splenic and right atrial mass at presentation in dogs with HSA: a retrospective study. J Am Anim Hosp Assoc 2011;47:336–41.

116. Ratterree W, Gieger T, Pariaut R, et al. Value of echocardiography and electrocardiography as screening tools prior to doxorubicin administration. J Am Anim Hosp Assoc 2012;48(2):89–96.
117. Keyes M, Rush J. Ventricular arrythmias in dogs with splenic masses. J Vet Emerg Crit Care 1994;3:33–8.
118. Marino DJ, Matthiesen DT, Fox PR, et al. Ventricular arrhythmias in dogs undergoing splenectomy: a prospective study. Vet Surg 1994;23:101–6.
119. Wendelburg KM, O'Toole TE, McCobb E, et al. Risk factors for perioperative death in dogs undergoing splenectomy for splenic masses: 539 cases (2001-2012). J Am Vet Med Assoc 2014;245(12):1382–90.
120. O'Brien RT. Improved detection of metastatic hepatic hemangiosarcoma nodules with contrast ultrasound in three dogs. Vet Radiol Ultrasound 2007;48(2): 146–8.
121. Ohlerth S, Dennler M, Ruefli E, et al. Contrast harmonic imaging characterization of canine splenic lesions. J Vet Intern Med 2008;22(5):1095–102.
122. Rossi F, Leone VF, Vignoli M, et al. Use of contrast-enhanced ultrasound for characterization of focal splenic lesions. Vet Radiol Ultrasound 2008;49(2): 154–64.
123. Nakamura K, Sasaki N, Murakami M, et al. Contrast-enhanced ultrasonography for characterization of focal splenic lesions in dogs. J Vet Intern Med 2010;24(6): 1290–7.
124. Shaw SP, Rozanski EA, Rush JE. Cardiac troponins I and T in dogs with pericardial effusion. J Vet Intern Med 2004;18(3):322–4.
125. Chun R, Kellihan HB, Henik RA, et al. Comparison of plasma cardiac troponin I concentrations among dogs with cardiac hemangiosarcoma, noncardiac hemangiosarcoma, other neoplasms, and pericardial effusion of nonhemangiosarcoma origin. J Am Vet Med Assoc 2010;237:806–11.
126. Kirby GM, Mackay A, Grant A, et al. Concentration of lipocalin region of collagen XXVII alpha I in the serum of dogs with hemangiosarcoma. J Vet Intern Med 2011;25:497–503.
127. Thamm DH, Kamstock DA, Sharp CR, et al. Elevated serum thymidine kinase activity in canine splenic hemangiosarcoma. Vet Comp Oncol 2012;10(4): 292–302.
128. Herold LV, Devey JJ, Kirby R, et al. Clinical evaluation and management of hemoperitoneum in dogs. J Vet Emerg Crit Care 2008;18(1):40–53.
129. Case BL, Maxwell M, Aman A, et al. Outcome evaluation of a thoracoscopic pericardial window procedure or subtotal pericardectomy via thoracotomy for the treatment of pericardial effusion in dogs. J Am Vet Med Assoc 2013;242: 493–8.
130. Clendaniel DC, Sivacolundhu RK, Sorenmo KU, et al. Association between macroscopic appearance of liver lesions and liver histology in dogs with splenic hemangiosarcoma: 70 cases (2004-2009). J Am Anim Hosp Assoc 2014;50(4): e6–10.
131. Bulakowski EJ, Philibert JC, Siegal S, et al. Evaluation of outcome associated with subcutaneous and intramuscular hemangiosarcoma treated with adjuvant doxorubicin in dogs: 21 cases (2001-2006). J Am Vet Med Assoc 2008;233: 122–8.
132. Shiu KB, Flory AB, Anderson CL, et al. Predictors of outcome in dogs with subcutaneous or intramuscular hemangiosarcoma. J Am Vet Med Assoc 2011;238: 472–9.

133. Hillers KR, Lana SE, Fuller CR, et al. Effects of palliative radiation therapy on nonsplenic hemangiosarcoma in dogs. J Am Anim Hosp Assoc 2007;43(4): 187–92.
134. Nolan MW, Arkans MM, LaVine D, et al. Pilot study to determine the feasibility of radiation therapy for dogs with right atrial masses and hemorrhagic pericardial effusion. J Vet Cardiol 2017;19(2):132–43.
135. Ogilvie GK, Powers BE, Mallinckrodt CH, et al. Surgery and doxorubicin in dogs with hemangiosarcoma. J Vet Intern Med 1996;10(6):379–84.
136. Sorenmo KU, Baez JL, Clifford CA, et al. Efficacy and toxicity of a dose-intensified doxorubicin protocol in canine hemangiosarcoma. J Vet Intern Med 2004;18(2):209–13.
137. Kahn SA, Mullin CM, de Lorimier LP, et al. Doxorubicin and deracoxib adjuvant therapy for canine splenic hemangiosarcoma: a pilot study. Can Vet J 2013; 54(3):237–42.
138. Wiley JL, Rook KA, Clifford CA, et al. Efficacy of doxorubicin-based chemotherapy for non-resectable canine subcutaneous haemangiosarcoma. Vet Comp Oncol 2010;8(3):221–33.
139. Hammer AS, Couto CG, Filppi J, et al. Efficacy and toxicity of VAC chemotherapy (vincristine, doxorubicin, and cyclophosphamide) in dogs with hemangiosarcoma. J Vet Intern Med 1991;5(3):160–6.
140. Dervisis NG, Dominguez PA, Newman RG, et al. Treatment with DAV for advanced-stage hemangiosarcoma in dogs. J Am Anim Hosp Assoc 2011;46: 170–8.
141. Finotello R, Stefanello D, Zini E, et al. Comparison of doxorubicin-cyclophosphamide with doxorubicin-dacarbazine for the adjuvant treatment of canine hemangiosarcoma. Vet Comp Oncol 2017;15(1):25–35.
142. Kim SE, Liptak JM, Gall TT, et al. Epirubicin in the adjuvant treatment of splenic hemangiosarcoma in dogs: 59 cases (1997-2004). J Am Vet Med Assoc 2007; 231(10):1550–7.
143. Payne SE, Rassnick KM, Northrup NC, et al. Treatment of vascular and soft-tissue sarcomas in dogs using an alternating protocol of ifosfamide and doxorubicin. Vet Comp Oncol 2003;1(4):171–9.
144. Lana S, U'Ren L, Plaza S, et al. Continuous low-dose oral chemotherapy for adjuvant therapy of splenic hemangiosarcoma in dogs. J Vet Intern Med 2007;21(4):764–9.
145. Matsuyama A, Poirier VJ, Mantovani F, et al. Adjuvant doxorubicin with or without metronomic cyclophosphamide for canine splenic hemangiosarcoma. J Am Anim Hosp Assoc 2017;53(6):304–12.
146. Finotello R, Henriques J, Sabattini S, et al. A retrospective analysis of chemotherapy switch suggests improved outcome in surgically removed, biologically aggressive canine hemangiosarcoma. Vet Comp Oncol 2017;15(2):493–503.
147. Bray JP, Orbell G, Cave N, et al. Thalidomide prolongs survival in dogs with splenic hemangiosarcoma. J Small Anim Pract 2018;59(2):85–91.
148. Gardner HL, London CA, Portela RA, et al. Maintenance therapy with toceranib following doxorubicin-based chemotherapy for canine splenic hemangiosarcoma. BMC Vet Res 2015;11:131.
149. Borgatti A, Koopmeiners JS, Sarver AL, et al. Safe and effective sarcoma therapy through bispecific targeting of EGFR and uPAR. Mol Cancer Ther 2017; 16(5):956–65.
150. Vail DM, MacEwen EG, Kurzman ID, et al. Liposome-encapsulated muramyl tripeptide phosphatidylethanolamine adjuvant immunotherapy for splenic

hemangiosarcoma in the dog: a randomized multi-institutional clinical trial. Clin Cancer Res 1995;1(10):1165–70.
151. Wirth KA, Kow K, Salute ME, et al. In vitro effects of Yunnan Baiyao on canine hemangiosarcoma cell lines. Vet Comp Oncol 2016;14(3):281–94.
152. Egger C, Gibbs D, Wheeler J, et al. The effect of yunnan baiyao on platelet activation, buccal mucosal bleeding time, prothrombin time, activated partial thromboplastin time, and thromboelastography in healthy dogs: a randomized, controlled, blinded study. Am Jour Trad Chin Vet Med 2016;11(2):27–36.
153. Frederick J, Boysen S, Wagg C, et al. The effects of oral administration of Yunnan Baiyao on blood coagulation in beagle dogs as measured by kaolin-activated thromboelastography and buccal mucosal bleeding times. Can J Vet Res 2017;81(1):41–5.
154. Murphy LA, Panek CM, Bianco D, et al. Use of yunnan baiyao and epsilon aminocaproic acid in dogs with right atrial masses and pericardial effusion. J Vet Emerg Crit Care (San Antonio) 2017;27(1):121–6.
155. Brown DC, Reetz J. Single agent polysaccharopeptide delays metastases and improves survival in naturally occurring hemangiosarcoma. Evid Based Complement Alternat Med 2012;2012:384301.
156. Weisse C, Soares N, Beal MW, et al. Survival times in dogs with right atrial hemangiosarcoma treated by means of surgical resection with or without adjuvant chemotherapy: 23 cases (1986-2000). J Am Vet Med Assoc 2005;226(4):575–9.

Cancer Immunotherapies

Philip J. Bergman, DVM, MS, PhD[a,b,c,*]

KEYWORDS

• Cancer • Immunotherapy • Cancer vaccine • Monoclonal antibody • Canine • Feline

KEY POINTS

- The immune system is generally divided into 2 primary components: the *innate immune response* and the highly specific but more slowly developing *adaptive or acquired immune response.*
- Immune responses can be further separated by whether they are induced by exposure to a foreign antigen (an "active" response) or if they are transferred through serum or lymphocytes from an immunized individual (a "passive" response).
- The ideal cancer immunotherapy agent should be able to discriminate between cancer and normal cells (ie, specificity), be potent enough to kill small or large numbers of tumor cells (ie, sensitivity), and lastly be able to prevent recurrence of the tumor (ie, durability).
- Tumor immunology and immunotherapy is one of the most exciting and rapidly expanding fields, with cancer immunotherapy now recognized as one of the pillars of treatment alongside surgery, radiation, and chemotherapy.

INTRODUCTION

The term "immunity" is derived from the Latin word immunitas, which refers to the legal protection afforded to Roman senators holding office. Although the immune system is normally thought of as providing protection against infectious disease, the immune system's ability to recognize and eliminate cancer is the fundamental rationale for the immunotherapy of cancer. Multiple lines of evidence support a role for the immune system in managing cancer, including (1) spontaneous remissions in patients with cancer without treatment; (2) the presence of tumor-specific cytotoxic T cells within tumor or draining lymph nodes; (3) the presence of monocytic, lymphocytic,

---

Disclosure Statement: Dr P.J. Bergman is a coinventor on patent US7556805B2 and was the veterinary principal investigator for the canine melanoma vaccine Oncept, which received USDA-CVB conditional licensure in 2007 and full licensure in 2009. He also receives a minority royalty stream payment from Merial.

[a] Clinical Studies, VCA; [b] Katonah Bedford Veterinary Center, 546 N Bedford Rd, Bedford Hills, NY 10507, USA; [c] Memorial Sloan-Kettering Cancer Center, New York, NY, USA
* Corresponding author. Katonah Bedford Veterinary Center, 546 N Bedford Rd, Bedford Hills, NY 10507, USA
E-mail address: philip.bergman@vca.com

Vet Clin Small Anim 49 (2019) 881–902
https://doi.org/10.1016/j.cvsm.2019.04.010 vetsmall.theclinics.com
0195-5616/19/

and plasmacytic cellular infiltrates in tumors; (4) the increased incidence of some types of cancer in immunosuppressed patients; and (5) documentation of cancer remissions with the use of immunomodulators.[1,2] With the tools of molecular biology and a greater understanding of mechanisms to harness the immune system, effective tumor immunotherapy is now a reality. This new class of therapeutics offers a more targeted and therefore precise approach to the treatment of cancer. Cancer immunotherapy is now recognized as one of the pillars of treatment alongside surgery, radiation, and chemotherapy.

TUMOR IMMUNOLOGY

Cellular Components

The immune system is generally divided into 2 primary components: the *innate immune response* and, the highly specific but more slowly developing, *adaptive or acquired immune response*. Innate immunity is rapidly acting but typically not very specific and includes physicochemical barriers (eg, skin and mucosa), blood proteins such as complement, phagocytic cells (macrophages, neutrophils, dendritic cells [DCs], and natural killer [NK] cells), and cytokines that coordinate and regulate the cells involved in innate immunity. Adaptive immunity is thought of as the acquired arm of immunity that allows for exquisite specificity, an ability to remember the previous existence of the pathogen (ie, “memory”), differentiate self from nonself, and importantly the ability to respond more vigorously on repeat exposure to the pathogen. Adaptive immunity consists of T and B lymphocytes. The T cells are further divided into CD8 (cluster of differentiation) and major histocompatibility complex (MHC) class I cytotoxic helper T cells (CD4 and MHC class II), NK cells, and regulatory T cells (Tregs). B lymphocytes produce antibodies (humoral system) that may activate complement, enhance phagocytosis of opsonized target cells, and induce antibody-dependent cellular cytotoxicity. B-cell responses to tumors are thought by many investigators to be less important than the development of T-cell–mediated immunity, but there is little evidence to fully support this notion.[3] The innate and adaptive arms of immunity are not mutually exclusive; they are linked by (1) the innate response’s ability to stimulate and influence the nature of the adaptive response and (2) the sharing of effector mechanisms between innate and adaptive immune responses.

Immune responses can be further separated by whether they are induced by exposure to a foreign antigen (an “active” response) or if they are transferred through serum or lymphocytes from an immunized individual (a “passive” response). Although both approaches have the ability to be extremely specific for an antigen of interest, one important difference is the inability of passive approaches to generally confer memory. The principal components of the active/adaptive immune system are lymphocytes, antigen-presenting cells, and effector cells. Furthermore, responses can be subdivided by whether they are specific for a certain antigen or a nonspecific response whereby immunity is attempted to be conferred by upregulating the immune system without a specific target. These definitions are helpful, as they allow methodologies to be more completely characterized, such as active-specific, passive-nonspecific, etc.

Immune Surveillance

The idea that the immune system may actively prevent the development of neoplasia is termed “cancer immunosurveillance.” Sound scientific evidence supports some aspects of this hypothesis[4–7] including the following: (1) interferon gamma (IFNγ) protects mice against the growth of tumors; (2) mice lacking IFNγ receptor were more sensitive to chemically induced sarcomas than normal mice and were more likely to spontaneously develop tumors; (3) mice lacking major components of the adaptive immune response (T and B cells) have a high rate of spontaneous tumors; and (4) mice that lack IFNγ and B/T cells develop tumors, especially at a young age.

Immune Evasion by Tumors

There are significant barriers to the generation of effective antitumor immunity by the host. Many tumors evade surveillance mechanisms and grow in immunocompetent hosts as easily illustrated by the overwhelming numbers of people and animals succumbing to cancer. There are multiple ways in which tumors evade the immune response: (1) immunosuppressive cytokine production (eg, transforming growth factor beta [TGF-β] and interleukin 10 [IL-10])[8,9]; (2) impaired DC function via inactivation ("anergy") and/or poor DC maturation through changes in IL-6/IL-10/vascular endothelial growth factor/granulocyte/macrophage colony-stimulating factor (GM-CSF)[10]; (3) induction of cells called Tregs, which were initially called suppressor T cells (CD4/CD25/cytotoxic T-lymphocyte–associated protein 4 [CTLA-4]/GITR/Foxp3 positive cells that can suppress tumor-specific CD4/CD8+ T cells)[11]; (4) MHC-I loss through structural defects, changes in B2-microglobulin synthesis, defects in transporter-associated antigen processing, or actual MHC-I gene loss (ie, allelic or locus loss); and (5) MHC-I antigen presentation loss through B7-1 attenuation (B7-1 is an important costimulatory molecule for CD28-mediated T-cell receptor and MHC engagement) when the MHC system in #4 remains intact.

Nonspecific Tumor Immunotherapy

Dr William Coley, a New York surgeon in the early 1900s, noted that some patients with cancer developing incidental bacterial infections survived longer than those without infection.[12] Coley developed a bacterial "vaccine" (killed cultures of *Streptococcus marcescens* and *Streptococcus pyogenes* known as "Coley's toxins") to treat people with sarcomas, which provided complete response rates of approximately 15%. Unfortunately, high failure rates and significant side effects lead to discontinuation of this approach. His seminal work laid the foundation for nonspecific modulation of the immune response in the treatment of cancer. There are numerous nonspecific tumor immunotherapy approaches ranging from biological response modifiers (BRMs) to recombinant cytokines as discussed later.

Biological Response Modifiers

BRMs are molecules that can modify the biological response of cells to changes in its external environment, which in the context of cancer immunotherapy could easily span nonspecific and specific immunotherapies. This section discusses nonspecific BRMs (sometimes termed "immunopotentiators"), which are often related to bacteria and/or viruses.

One of the earliest BRM discoveries after Coley's toxin was the use of Bacillus Calmette-Guérin (BCG) (interestingly, Guérin was a veterinarian). BCG is the live attenuated strain of *Mycobacterium bovis*, and intravesical instillation in the urinary bladder causes a significant local inflammatory response that results in antitumor responses.[13] The use of BCG in veterinary patients was first reported by Owen and Bostock in 1974 and has been investigated with numerous types of cancers, including urinary bladder carcinoma, osteosarcoma, lymphoma, prostatic carcinoma, transmissible venereal tumor, mammary tumors, sarcoids, squamous cell carcinoma, and others.[14–18] LDI-100, a product containing BCG and human chorionic gonadotropin, was compared with vinblastine in dogs with measurable grade II or III mast cell tumors.[19] Response rates were 28.6% and 11.7%, respectively, and the LDI-100 group had significantly less neutropenia. It is particularly exciting for veterinary cancer immunotherapy to potentially be able to use a BRM product that has greater efficacy and less toxicity than a chemotherapy standard of care. Unfortunately, LDI-100 is not commercially available at present.

Corynebacterium parvum is another BRM that has been investigated for several tumors in veterinary medicine, including melanoma and mammary carcinoma.[20,21] Other bacterially derived BRMs include attenuated *Salmonella typhimurium* (VNP20009), mycobacterial cell wall DNA complexes (abstracts only at present), and bacterial superantigens.[22,23] Mycobacterial cell walls contain muramyl dipeptide (MDP) that can activate monocytes and tissue macrophages. Muramyl tripeptide phosphatidylethanolamine (MTP-PE) is an analogue of MDP. When encapsulated in multilamellar liposomes (L-MTP-PE), monocytes and macrophages uptake MTP leading to activation and subsequent tumoricidal effects through induction of multiple cytokines, including IL–1a, IL-1b, IL-7, IL-8, IL-12, and tumor necrosis factor.[24] L-MTP-PE has been investigated in numerous tumors in human and veterinary patients, including osteosarcoma, hemangiosarcoma, and mammary carcinoma.[24–28]

Oncolytic viruses have also been used as nonspecific anticancer BRMs in human and veterinary patients.[29] Adenoviruses have been engineered to transcriptionally target canine osteosarcoma cells and have been tested in vitro and in normal dogs with no major signs of virus-associated side effects.[30–32] Similarly, canine distemper virus (CDV), the canine equivalent of human measles virus, has been used in vitro to infect canine lymphocyte cell lines and neoplastic lymphocytes from dogs with B- and T-cell lymphoma,[33] with high infectivity rates, suggesting that CDV may be investigated in the future for treatment of dogs with lymphoma.

Imiquimod (Aldara) is a novel BRM that is a toll-like receptor 7 agonist.[34] Imiquimod has been reported as a successful treatment for Bowen disease (multicentric squamous cell carcinoma in situ) and other skin diseases in humans. Twelve cats with Bowen-like disease were treated topically with imiquimod 5% cream and initial and all subsequent new lesions responded in all cats.[35] An additional cat (with pinnal actinic keratoses and squamous cell carcinoma) and dog with cutaneous melanocytomas has subsequently been reported to have been successfully treated with topical imiquimod 5% cream.[36,37] It therefore seems that Imiquimod 5% cream is well tolerated, and further studies are warranted to further examine its usefulness in cats and dogs with other skin tumors that are not treatable through standardized means.

Recombinant Cytokines, Growth Factors, and Hormones

Several investigations using recombinant cytokines, growth factors, or hormones in various fashions for patients with human and veterinary cancer have been reported to date. Many have investigated the in vitro and/or in vivo effects of the soluble cytokine (eg, IFN, IL-2, IL-12, IL-15, etc. with or without suicide gene therapy)[38–51]; liposome encapsulation of the cytokine (eg, liposomal IL-2)[39,52–55]; or use of a virus, cell, liposome-DNA complex, plasmid, or other mechanism to expresses the cytokine (eg, recombinant poxvirus expressing IL-2).[52,56–63] Important to note, the European Committee for Medicinal Products for Veterinary Use adopted a positive opinion in March, 2013 for the veterinary product Oncept IL-2 (feline pox virus expressing recombinant feline IL-2). This product also received conditional licensure from the USDA Center for Veterinary Biologics (CVB) in 2015. It is labeled for use in addition to surgery and radiation in cats with stage I fibrosarcomas without metastasis or lymph node involvement, to reduce the risk of relapse and increase the time to relapse.

SPECIFIC TUMOR IMMUNOTHERAPY

Overview

The ultimate goal for a tumor immunotherapy with a specific target is elicitation of an antitumor immune response, which results in clinical regression of a tumor and/or its metastases. There are numerous types of specific tumor immunotherapies in phase I–III trials across a wide range of tumor types. Responses to cancer vaccines and other cancer immunotherapies may take several months or more to appear due to the slower speed of induction of the adaptive arm of the immune system as outlined in **Table 1**, and this has necessitated the development of an alternative and more immunotherapeutic-based response system for human studies and this is highly likely necessary in the future for veterinary studies.[64] The ideal cancer immunotherapy agent would be able to discriminate between cancer and normal cells (ie, specificity), be potent enough to kill small or large numbers of tumor cells (ie, sensitivity), and lastly be able to prevent recurrence of the tumor (ie, durability).

The immune system detects tumors through specific tumor-associated antigens (TAAs) and/or abnormal disease-associated antigens (DAAs) that are potentially recognized by both CTLs and antibodies.[65–67] TAAs and/or DAAs may be common to a particular tumor type, be unique to an individual tumor, or may arise from mutated gene products such as ras, p53, p21, and/or others. Although unique TAAs may be more immunogenic than the other aforementioned shared tumor antigens, they are not practical targets because of their narrow specificity. Most shared tumor antigens are normal cellular antigens that are overexpressed in tumors. The first group to be identified was termed "cancer testis antigens" due to expression in normal testes, but they are also found in melanoma and various other solid tumors such as the MAGE/BAGE gene family. This article highlights those approaches that seem to hold particular promise in human clinical trials and many that have been tested to date in veterinary medicine.

A variety of approaches have been taken to date to focus the immune system on the aforementioned targets: (1) whole cell, tumor cell lysate, and/or subunit vaccines (autologous or made from a patient's own tumor tissue; allogeneic or made from individuals within a species bearing the same type of cancer; or whole cell vaccines from γ-irradiated tumor cell lines with or without immunostimulatory cytokines)[58,68–82]; (2) DNA vaccines that immunize with syngeneic and/or xenogeneic (different species than recipient) plasmid DNA designed to elicit antigen-specific

Table 1
Comparison of chemotherapy and various antitumor immunotherapies

Treatment Type	Mechanism of Action	TAA or Target Dependent	Specificity	Sensitivity	Response Time	Durability of Response
Chemotherapy	Cytotoxicity	No	Poor	Variable	Hours–days	Variable
Antitumor vaccine	Immune response	Yes	Good	Good	Weeks–months	Variable–long
Monoclonal antibodies	Immune response	Yes	Good	Good	Weeks	Variable
Checkpoint inhibitors	Immune response	No	Low	Moderate	Weeks–months	Long

humoral and cellular immunity[83–90] (to be discussed in more detail later in this article); (3) viral, viruslike nanoparticle and/or viral vector-based methodologies designed to be oncolytic and/or deliver genes encoding TAAs, telomerase and/or immunostimulatory cytokines[91–101]; and (4) DC or CD40-activated B-cell vaccines (which are commonly loaded or transfected with TAAs, DNA or RNA from TAAs, or tumor lysates)[102–110] and adoptive cell transfer (the "transfer" of specific populations of immune effector cells in order to generate a more powerful and focused antitumor immune response; to be discussed in more detail later in this article with clinically relevant recent advances).[111]

Antibody-Based Therapies

Antibody (Ab) approaches for cancer immunotherapy include monoclonal antibodies (mAbs)[112,113]; antiidiotype Abs (an idiotype is an immunoglobulin sequence unique to each B lymphocyte, and therefore Abs directed against these idiotypes are referred to as antiidiotype)[114]; conjugated Abs (antibody conjugated to a toxin, chemotherapy, radionuclide, etc.)[115]; and engineered Ab "variants"[116,117] such as bispecific mAbs (can bind to 2 different targets at the same time), single-chain variable fragments (often used as artificial T-cell receptors), single-chain Abs, etc.

Rituximab (antihuman CD20 mAb; Rituxan) was the first mAb approved by the Food and Drug Administration (FDA)[118] in 1997, and as of August, 2018 there are more than 75 FDA-approved mAbs for the treatment of various human cancers. In those 20 years a remarkably greater understanding of protein-engineering techniques, reciprocation between the immune system and cancer cells, as well as mechanisms of action and resistance for mAbs have allowed for therapeutic Ab development to explode.[117,119]

Based on the significant improvement in remission and survival length of human patients with B-cell non-Hodgkin lymphoma (NHL) treated with rituximab and standard of care multiagent chemotherapy (and the lack of rituximab binding to canine CD20), numerous groups in veterinary medicine are in pursuit of similar caninized or felinized anti-CD20 mAb approaches.[120–126] Particular initial excitement and promise was noted in early pilot studies with caninized anti-CD20 and CD-52 mAbs for canine B-cell and T-cell NHL, respectively. In 2015 and 2016, each product (Blontress and Tactress, respectively) received USDA-CVB licensure, but subsequent unpublished studies did not show target binding or improvement in clinical outcomes compared with standard of care chemotherapy. Based on rituximab's remarkable track record and continually expanding list of indications (within the previously envisioned area of B-cell neoplasia, but now outside of oncology in the treatment of nononcologic B-cell disorders), this author ardently looks forward to the clinical development of 1E4 (and other anti-CD19/20/21 mAbs) as well as other mAb targets for dogs, cats, and other veterinary species afflicted with cancer and other diseases.[127–132]

Cancer Vaccines

One particularly exciting vaccine approach targets HER-2 with an attenuated listeria therapeutic vaccine or a DNA vaccine approach.[89,133,134] The listeria methodology was used by Mason and colleagues[135] in dogs with appendicular osteosarcoma after being treated with amputation and adjuvant carboplatin chemotherapy. The results from this Phase I study are particularly exciting, as it translated into a median survival time approaching 3 years. It is currently unknown how much of the therapeutic efficacy is from the xenogeneic human HER-2 versus the listeria but may be considered in the future with other HER-2 related histologies. This product from Aratana ("AT-014") received USDA-CVB conditional licensure in early 2018 and is currently undergoing an additional multicenter clinical safety study to potentially move the product to full licensure.

The author has developed a xenogeneic DNA vaccine program for melanoma in collaboration with human investigators from Memorial Sloan-Kettering Cancer Center.[136,137] Preclinical and clinical studies by the author's laboratory and others have shown that xenogeneic DNA vaccination with tyrosinase family members (eg, tyrosinase, GP100, GP75, others) can produce immune responses, resulting in tumor rejection or protection and prolongation of survival, whereas syngeneic vaccination with orthologous DNA does not induce immune responses. Although tyrosinase may not seem to be a preferred target in amelanotic canine melanoma due to poor expression when assessed by immunohistochemistry (IHC),[138] more appropriate/sensitive polymerase chain reaction (PCR)-based studies and other IHC-based studies document significant tyrosinase overexpression in melanotic and amelanotic melanomas across species.[139–144] These studies provided the impetus for development of a xenogeneic tyrosinase (or similar melanosomal glycoproteins) DNA vaccine program in canine malignant melanoma (CMM). Cohorts of dogs received increasing doses of xenogeneic plasmid DNA encoding either human tyrosinase (huTyr), murine GP75 (muGP75), murine tyrosinase (muTyr), muTyr $\pm$ HuGM-CSF (both administered as plasmid DNA), or muTyr "off-study" intramuscularly biweekly for a total of 4 vaccinations. The authors and collaborators have investigated the antibody and T-cell responses in dogs vaccinated with huTyr. Antigen-specific (huTyr) IFNγ T-cells were found along with 2- to 5-fold increases in circulating antibodies to huTyr, which can cross-react to canine tyrosinase, suggesting the breaking of tolerance.[145,146] The clinical results with prolongation in survival have been reported previously.[136,137] The results of these trials demonstrate that xenogeneic DNA vaccination in CMM (1) is safe, (2) leads to the development of antityrosinase antibodies and T cells, (3) is potentially therapeutic, and (4) is an attractive candidate for further evaluation in an adjuvant, minimal residual disease Phase II setting for CMM. Based on these studies a multiinstitutional safety and efficacy trial for USDA licensure in dogs with locally controlled stage II/III oral melanoma was initiated in 2006 with granting of conditional licensure in 2007, which represented the first US governmental regulatory agency approval of a vaccine to treat cancer across species. Results of this licensure trial documented a statistically significant improvement in survival for vaccinates versus controls and a full licensure for the huTyr-based canine melanoma vaccine from USDA-CVB was received in December, 2009 (Oncept, Merial, Inc.).[147] Recently, other investigators have reported safety and feasibility results of a pilot study in dogs with melanoma given huTyr plasmid DNA (ie similar to Oncept), but instead of the typical needle-free transdermal delivery, a novel tattoolike"microseeding" delivery system was used and well tolerated with no toxicity noted in the 6 dogs.[148]

Kaser-Hotz and colleagues[149] reported on concurrent use of Oncept and external beam radiation, as many dogs with oral malignant melanoma may not be able to undergo surgery for local tumor control. This pilot study determined that concurrent use was well tolerated with no unexpected toxicities. Ottnod and colleagues[150] performed a single-site retrospective study on 30 dogs with stage II–III oral malignant melanoma (15 each with and without use of Oncept). They determined that those dogs receiving Oncept did not achieve a greater progression-free survival, disease-free interval, or median survival time than dogs that did not receive the vaccine. Contrary to the aforementioned prospective USDA 5-site licensure trial,[147] this study had less than 35% of cases treated surgically with margins 1 mm or more, suggesting a significant lack of local tumor control. Furthermore, contrary to the aforementioned prospective USDA 5-site licensure trial, the Ottnod and colleagues' study, similar to other noncontrolled retrospective studies, had a wide variety of other treatments used in both the nonvaccinate and vaccinate groups, had small numbers of patients investigated, and/or the cause (in the context of local or distant disease) of death and/or progression of disease was not reported.[151–154] The author reported at the 2016 VCS meeting the outcomes of 320 dogs with malignant melanoma treated with Oncept across VCA oncology centers. The long-term median outcomes noted in that study are extremely similar to those the author reported from the USDA 5-site prospective licensure trial and compare highly favorably with outcomes reported with standardized therapies without Oncept. Not surprisingly, the smaller poorly controlled retrospective studies do not seem to mirror the results seen in larger and more highly controlled studies.

Human clinical trials using various xenogeneic melanosomal antigens as DNA (or peptide with adjuvant) vaccination began in 2005 and the preliminary results look favorable.[155–157] To further highlight xenogeneic DNA vaccination as a platform to target other possible antigens for other histologies, the authors have completed a Phase I trial of murine CD20 for dogs with B-cell lymphoma (USDA-CVB conditionally licensed as Canine Lymphoma Vaccine from Merial Inc. and undergoing currently further efficacy studies in larger numbers of dogs) and have also investigated the efficacy of local tumor control and use of xenogeneic DNA vaccination in dogs with digit malignant melanoma.[158] These investigations led to the development of a canine digit melanoma staging scheme and found an improvement in survival compared with historical outcomes with digit amputation only. The authors also documented a decreased prognosis for dogs with advanced stage disease and/or increased time from digit amputation to the start of vaccination. Phillips and colleagues[139,159] have also reported the overexpression of tyrosinase in equine melanoma, determined the safety and optimal use of the needle-free delivery device into the pectoral region with Oncept, and documented antigen-specific humoral responses after vaccination in all horses. Oncept also seems to be safe for use in cats.[160]

A small subset of dogs with malignant melanoma have exon 11 KIT gene mutations,[161,162] and therefore the more routine use of KIT testing by PCR of CMM and subsequent use of c-kit small molecule inhibitors (particularly in dogs with advanced stage disease and/or lack of response to Oncept), should be considered. Furthermore, with somatic mutations in NRAS and PTEN being found in canine malignant melanoma[163] similar to human melanoma hotspot sites, these may represent logical drugable targets in the future.

The Future of Cancer Immunotherapy

Tumor immunology and immunotherapy is one of the most exciting and rapidly expanding fields at present. Significant resources are focused on mechanisms to simultaneously maximally stimulate an antitumor immune response while minimizing the immunosuppressive aspects of the tumor microenvironment.[8] The recent elucidation and blockade of immunosuppressive cytokines (eg, TGF-β, IL-10 and IL-13) and/or the negative costimulatory molecule CTLA-4[164,165] and PD-1 (Programmed Cell Death 1 or CD279),[166] along with the functional characterization of myeloid derived suppressor cells (MDSC) and Tregs,[167–170] have dramatically improve cell-mediated immunity to tumors by "taking the brake" off the immune system. Immunotherapy is unlikely to become a sole modality in the treatment of cancer, as the traditional modalities of surgery, radiation, and/or chemotherapy are extremely likely to be used in combination with immunotherapy in the future. As any form of anticancer treatment, immunotherapy seems to work best in a minimal residual disease setting, suggesting its most appropriate use will be in an adjuvant setting with local tumor therapies such as surgery and/or radiation.[171] Similarly, the long-held belief that chemotherapy (noncorticosteroid) attenuates immune responses from cancer vaccines is beginning to be disproved through investigations on a variety of levels.[172,173]

The aforementioned greatly expanded molecular understanding of the immune system has recently translated into human cancer immunotherapeutics that confer a survival benefit, such as the use of the checkpoint inhibitor anti-CTLA-4 Ab, ipilimumab (Yervoy), and the selective BRAF inhibitors, vemurafenib (Zelboraf) and dabrafenib (GSK2118436), in patients who are BRAF V600 mutation positive. Currently, FDA-approved Abs directed against another checkpoint inhibitor known as PD-1 receptor or against human PDL-1 (L = ligand) such as nivolumab (Opdivo), pembrolizumab (Keytruda), and others have generated the most excitement due to ~ 20% to 30% of human patients having durable objective tumor responses.[166,174] The highest objective tumor response rates have been seen to date in patients treated with concurrent PD-1 and CTLA-4 checkpoint inhibitors.[166,175,176] Furthermore, pembrolizumab was recently given FDA approval for unresectable or metastatic, microsatellite instability–high (MSI-H), or mismatch repair–deficient (dMMR) solid tumors that have progressed following prior treatment.[177] This is truly revolutionary as it represents the first cancer-agnostic FDA approval and is one of many recent FDA approvals based on single-arm studies. There are currently more than 100 different checkpoint inhibitors in development and the immunooncology (IO) "pendulum" has swung from the previous primarily target-dependent approaches to the current checkpoint inhibitor target-independent approach. The IO pendulum over time is highly likely to come back to the middle with a concurrent target-dependent approach (ie, vaccine or similar) alongside target-independent checkpoint inhibitors.[178,179]

Unfortunately, very few biomarkers of response with these clinically important agents have been found to date except for tumors that generate numerous neoantigens from tumor-specific mutations.[180,181] This further highlights why pembrolizumab was given FDA approval for MSI-H or dMMR solid tumors, as these tumors "throw off" comparatively much higher numbers of neoantigens. A new and highly innovative personalized human cancer vaccine taking advantage of this biomarker-based approach uses the neoantigens specific to that individual's cancer, as they are not present in normal tissues and are highly immunogenic.[182]

Another area of extreme promise in IO is a form of adoptive cell therapy called chimeric antigen receptor T cells (CAR-T). T cells are harvested from a patient and then genetically engineered to express a CAR on their cell surface with expansion in vitro before being reinfused back into the patient.[183] This CAR is specifically designed to recognize a specific TAA with a domain responsible for activating the T cell when the CAR-T binds its TAA. The latest generations of CAR-T are engineered to contain important costimulatory domains that further enhance the immune response against the cancer cell containing the TAA. In 2017, an expert panel of the FDA called Oncologic Drugs Advisory Committee unanimously (10-0) recommended approval of CTL019 (tisagenlecleucel), an investigational CAR-T therapy using CD19 as its CAR of choice for patients with B-cell acute lymphoblastic leukemia. Many CAR-T studies have found greater than 80% to 90% objective tumor responses, but side effects, including death, can occur.[183] Furthermore, CAR-Ts are currently difficult to make and carry a high cost of goods to produce, making for a difficult, but not impossible, commercial development path in veterinary medicine.

Checkpoints, checkpoint inhibitors, and other adoptive cell transfer technologies such as CAR-T and others are also starting to be better understood and pursued in veterinary diseases.[111,184–200] Furthermore, the exciting race to develop commercial veterinary-specific IO therapeutics such as checkpoint inhibitors and CAR-T is currently ongoing with a handful of animal health companies. Because these therapeutics reduce immune tolerance and more easily generate specific antitumor immune responses in patients, pathologic autoimmunity was predicted and is now being seen clinically in human patients as a side effect.[175,201,202]

In summary, the future looks extremely bright for immunotherapy. Similarly, the veterinary oncology profession is uniquely able to greatly contribute to the many advances to come in this field. Unfortunately, what works in a mouse will often not reflect the outcome in patients with human cancer. Therefore, comparative immunotherapy studies using veterinary patients may be able better "bridge" murine and human studies. To this end, a large number of cancers in dogs and cats seem to be remarkably stronger models for counterpart human tumors than presently available murine model systems.[163,203–210] This is likely due to a variety of reasons including, but not limited to, extreme similarities in the biology of the tumors (eg, chemoresistance, radioresistance, sharing metastatic phenotypes and site selectivity, etc.), spontaneous syngeneic cancer (vs typically an induced and/or xenogeneic cancer in murine models), and finally that the dogs and cats that are spontaneously developing these tumors are outbred, immune-competent, and live in the same environment that humans do. The author ardently looks forward to the time when cancer immunotherapy plays the same significant role in the treatment and/or prevention of cancers in veterinary patients as it currently does in human cancers.

REFERENCES

1. Bergman PJ. Biologic response modification. In: Rosenthal RC, editor. Veterinary oncology secrets. 1 edition. Philadelphia: Hanley &Belfus, Inc.; 2001. p. 79–82.
2. Baxevanis CN, Perez SA, Papamichail M. Cancer immunotherapy. Crit Rev Clin Lab Sci 2009;46:167–89.
3. Reilly RT, Emens LA, Jaffee EM. Humoral and cellular immune responses: independent forces or collaborators in the fight against cancer? Curr Opin Investig Drugs 2001;2(1):133–5.
4. Smyth MJ, Godfrey DI, Trapani JA. A fresh look at tumor immunosurveillance and immunotherapy. Nat Immunol 2001;2(4):293–9.
5. Wallace ME, Smyth MJ. The role of natural killer cells in tumor control–effectors and regulators of adaptive immunity. Springer Semin Immunopathol 2005;27(1): 49–64.
6. Itoh H, Horiuchi Y, Nagasaki T, et al. Evaluation of immunological status in tumor-bearing dogs. Vet Immunol Immunopathol 2009;132(2–4):85–90.
7. Schmiedt CW, Grimes JA, Holzman G, et al. Incidence and risk factors for development of malignant neoplasia after feline renal transplantation and cyclosporine-based immunosuppression. Vet Comp Oncol 2009;7:45–53.
8. Catchpole B, Gould SM, Kellett-Gregory LM, et al. Immunosuppressive cytokines in the regional lymph node of a dog suffering from oral malignant melanoma. J Small Anim Pract 2002;43(10):464–7.
9. Zagury D, Gallo RC. Anti-cytokine Ab immune therapy: present status and perspectives. Drug Discov Today 2004;9(2):72–81.
10. Morse MA, Mosca PJ, Clay TM, et al. Dendritic cell maturation in active immunotherapy strategies. Expert Opin Biol Ther 2002;2(1):35–43.
11. Yamaguchi T, Sakaguchi S. Regulatory T cells in immune surveillance and treatment of cancer. Semin Cancer Biol 2006;16(2):115–23.

12. Richardson MA, Ramirez T, Russell NC, et al. Coley toxins immunotherapy: a retrospective review. Altern Ther Health Med 1999;5(3):42–7.
13. Herr HW, Morales A. History of bacillus Calmette-Guerin and bladder cancer: an immunotherapy success story. J Urol 2008;179:53–6.
14. Owen LN, Bostock DE. Proceedings: tumour therapy in dogs using B.C.G. Br J Cancer 1974;29:95.
15. MacEwen EG. An immunologic approach to the treatment of cancer. Vet Clin North Am 1977;7:65–75.
16. Theilen GH, Hills D. Comparative aspects of cancer immunotherapy: immunologic methods used for treatment of spontaneous cancer in animals. J Am Vet Med Assoc 1982;181:1134–41.
17. MacEwen EG. Approaches to cancer therapy using biological response modifiers. Vet Clin North Am Small Anim Pract 1985;15:667–88.
18. Klein WR, Rutten VP, Steerenberg PA, et al. The present status of BCG treatment in the veterinary practice. In Vivo 1991;5:605–8.
19. Henry CJ, Downing S, Rosenthal RC, et al. Evaluation of a novel immunomodulator composed of human chorionic gonadotropin and bacillus Calmette-Guerin for treatment of canine mast cell tumors in clinically affected dogs. Am J Vet Res 2007;68:1246–51.
20. Parodi AL, Misdorp W, Mialot JP, et al. Intratumoral BCG and Corynebacterium parvum therapy of canine mammary tumours before radical mastectomy. Cancer Immunol Immunother 1983;15:172–7.
21. MacEwen EG, Patnaik AK, Harvey HJ, et al. Canine oral melanoma: comparison of surgery versus surgery plus corynebacterium parvum. Cancer Invest 1986; 4(5):397–402.
22. Thamm DH, Kurzman ID, King I, et al. Systemic administration of an attenuated, tumor-targeting Salmonella typhimurium to dogs with spontaneous neoplasia: phase I evaluation. Clin Cancer Res 2005;11:4827–34.
23. Dow SW, Elmslie RE, Willson AP, et al. In vivo tumor transfection with superantigen plus cytokine genes induces tumor regression and prolongs survival in dogs with malignant melanoma. J Clin Invest 1998;101:2406–14.
24. Kleinerman ES, Jia S-F, Griffin J, et al. Phase II study of liposomal muramyl tripeptide in osteosarcoma: the cytokine cascade and monocyte activation following administration. J Clin Oncol 1992;10:1310–6.
25. MacEwen EG, Kurzman ID, Vail DM, et al. Adjuvant therapy for melanoma in dogs: results of randomized clinical trials using surgery, liposome-encapsulated muramyl tripeptide, and granulocyte macrophage colony-stimulating factor. Clin Cancer Res 1999;5:4249–58.
26. Teske E, Rutteman GR, vd Ingh TS, et al. Liposome-encapsulated muramyl tripeptide phosphatidylethanolamine (L-MTP-PE): a randomized clinical trial in dogs with mammary carcinoma. Anticancer Res 1998;18:1015–9.
27. Kurzman ID, MacEwen EG, Rosenthal RC, et al. Adjuvant therapy for osteosarcoma in dogs: results of randomized clinical trials using combined liposome-encapsulated muramyl tripeptide and cisplatin. Clin Cancer Res 1995;1: 1595–601.
28. Vail DM, MacEwen EG, Kurzman ID, et al. Liposome-encapsulated muramyl tripeptide phosphatidylethanolamine adjuvant immunotherapy for splenic hemangiosarcoma in the dog: a randomized multi-institutional clinical trial. Clin Cancer Res 1995;1:1165–70.
29. Arendt M, Nasir L, Morgan IM. Oncolytic gene therapy for canine cancers: teaching old dog viruses new tricks. Vet Comp Oncol 2009;7:153–61.

30. Smith BF, Curiel DT, Ternovoi VV, et al. Administration of a conditionally replicative oncolytic canine adenovirus in normal dogs. Cancer Biother Radiopharm 2006;21:601–6.
31. Le LP, Rivera AA, Glasgow JN, et al. Infectivity enhancement for adenoviral transduction of canine osteosarcoma cells. Gene Ther 2006;13:389–99.
32. Hemminki A, Kanerva A, Kremer EJ, et al. A canine conditionally replicating adenovirus for evaluating oncolytic virotherapy in a syngeneic animal model. Mol Ther 2003;7:163–73.
33. Suter SE, Chein MB, von M, et al. In vitro canine distemper virus infection of canine lymphoid cells: a prelude to oncolytic therapy for lymphoma. Clin Cancer Res 2005;11:1579–87.
34. Meyer T, Stockfleth E. Clinical investigations of Toll-like receptor agonists. Expert Opin Investig Drugs 2008;17:1051–65.
35. Gill VL, Bergman PJ, Baer KE, et al. Use of imiquimod 5% cream (Aldara™) in cats with multicentric squamous cell carcinoma *in situ*: 12 cases (2002-2005). Vet Comp Oncol 2008;6:55–64.
36. Peters-Kennedy J, Scott DW, Miller WH Jr. Apparent clinical resolution of pinnal actinic keratoses and squamous cell carcinoma in a cat using topical imiquimod 5% cream. J Feline Med Surg 2008;10(6):593–9.
37. Coyner K, Loeffler D. Topical imiquimod in the treatment of two cutaneous melanocytomas in a dog. Vet Dermatol 2012;23(2):145–9, e31.
38. Tateyama S, Priosoeryanto BP, Yamaguchi R, et al. In vitro growth inhibition activities of recombinant feline interferon on all lines derived from canine tumors. Res Vet Sci 1995;59:275–7.
39. Kruth SA. Biological response modifiers: interferons, interleukins, recombinant products, liposomal products. Vet Clin North Am Small Anim Pract 1998;28:269–95.
40. Whitley EM, Bird AC, Zucker KE, et al. Modulation by canine interferon-gamma of major histocompatibility complex and tumor-associated antigen expression in canine mammary tumor and melanoma cell lines. Anticancer Res 1995;15:923–9.
41. Hampel V, Schwarz B, Kempf C, et al. Adjuvant immunotherapy of feline fibrosarcoma with recombinant feline interferon-omega. J Vet Intern Med 2007;21:1340–6.
42. Finocchiaro LM, Glikin GC. Cytokine-enhanced vaccine and suicide gene therapy as surgery adjuvant treatments for spontaneous canine melanoma. Gene Ther 2008;15:267–76.
43. Cutrera J, Torrero M, Shiomitsu K, et al. Intratumoral bleomycin and IL-12 electrochemogenetherapy for treating head and neck tumors in dogs. Methods Mol Biol 2008;423:319–25.
44. Finocchiaro LM, Fiszman GL, Karara AL, et al. Suicide gene and cytokines combined nonviral gene therapy for spontaneous canine melanoma. CancerGene Ther 2008;15:165–72.
45. Akhtar N, Padilla ML, Dickerson EB, et al. Interleukin-12 inhibits tumor growth in a novel angiogenesis canine hemangiosarcoma xenograft model. Neoplasia 2004;6:106–16.
46. Dickerson EB, Fosmire S, Padilla ML, et al. Potential to target dysregulated interleukin-2 receptor expression in canine lymphoid and hematopoietic malignancies as a model for human cancer. J Immunother 2002;25:36–45.

47. Okano F, Yamada K. Canine interleukin-18 induces apoptosis and enhances Fas ligand mRNA expression in a canine carcinoma cell line. Anticancer Res 2000; 20:3411–5.
48. Jahnke A, Hirschberger J, Fischer C, et al. Intra-tumoral gene delivery of felL-2, felFN-gamma and feGM-CSF using magnetofection as a neoadjuvant treatment option for feline fibrosarcomas: a phase-I study. J Vet Med A Physiol Pathol Clin Med 2007;54:599–606.
49. Dickerson EB, Akhtar N, Steinberg H, et al. Enhancement of the antiangiogenic activity of interleukin-12 by peptide targeted delivery of the cytokine to alphav-beta3 integrin. Mol Cancer Res 2004;2:663–73.
50. Finocchiaro LM, Fondello C, Gil-Cardeza ML, et al. Cytokine-enhanced vaccine and interferon-beta plus suicide gene therapy as surgery adjuvant treatments for spontaneous canine melanoma. Hum Gene Ther 2015;26:367–76.
51. Finocchiaro LME, Spector AIM, Agnetti L, et al. Combination of suicide and cytokine gene therapies as surgery adjuvant for canine mammary carcinoma. Vet Sci 2018;5 [pii:E70].
52. Dow S, Elmslie R, Kurzman I, et al. Phase I study of liposome-DNA complexes encoding the interleukin-2 gene in dogs with osteosarcoma lung metastases. Hum Gene Ther 2005;16:937–46.
53. Skubitz KM, Anderson PM. Inhalational interleukin-2 liposomes for pulmonary metastases: a phase I clinical trial. Anticancer Drugs 2000;11:555–63.
54. Khanna C, Anderson PM, Hasz DE, et al. Interleukin-2 liposome inhalation therapy is safe and effective for dogs with spontaneous pulmonary metastases. Cancer 1997;79:1409–21.
55. Khanna C, Hasz DE, Klausner JS, et al. Aerosol delivery of interleukin 2 liposomes is nontoxic and biologically effective: canine studies. Clin Cancer Res 1996;2:721–34.
56. Jourdier TM, Moste C, Bonnet MC, et al. Local immunotherapy of spontaneous feline fibrosarcomas using recombinant poxviruses expressing interleukin 2 (IL2). Gene Ther 2003;10(26):2126–32.
57. Siddiqui F, Li CY, Zhang X, et al. Characterization of a recombinant adenovirus vector encoding heat-inducible feline interleukin-12 for use in hyperthermia-induced gene-therapy. Int J Hyperthermia 2006;22:117–34.
58. Quintin-Colonna F, Devauchelle P, Fradelizi D, et al. Gene therapy of spontaneous canine melanoma and feline fibrosarcoma by intratumoral administration of histoincompatible cells expressing human interleukin-2. Gene Ther 1996; 3(12):1104–12.
59. Kamstock D, Guth A, Elmslie R, et al. Liposome-DNA complexes infused intravenously inhibit tumor angiogenesis and elicit antitumor activity in dogs with soft tissue sarcoma. CancerGene Ther 2006;13:306–17.
60. Junco JA, Basalto R, Fuentes F, et al. Gonadotrophin releasing hormone-based vaccine, an effective candidate for prostate cancer and other hormone-sensitive neoplasms. Adv Exp Med Biol 2008;617:581–7.
61. Chou PC, Chuang TF, Jan TR, et al. Effects of immunotherapy of IL-6 and IL-15 plasmids on transmissible venereal tumor in beagles. Vet Immunol Immunopathol 2009;130(1–2):25–34.
62. Chuang TF, Lee SC, Liao KW, et al. Electroporation-mediated IL-12 gene therapy in a transplantable canine cancer model. Int J Cancer 2009;125(3): 698–707.

63. Finocchiaro LM, Glikin GC. Cytokine-enhanced vaccine and suicide gene therapy as surgery adjuvant treatments for spontaneous canine melanoma: 9 years of follow-up. CancerGene Ther 2012;19(12):852–61.
64. Seymour L, Bogaerts J, Perrone A, et al. iRECIST: guidelines for response criteria for use in trials testing immunotherapeutics. Lancet Oncol 2017;18: e143–52.
65. Bergman PJ. Anticancer vaccines. Vet Clin North Am Small Anim Pract 2007;37: 1111–9.
66. Beatty PL, Finn OJ. Preventing cancer by targeting abnormally expressed self-antigens: MUC1 vaccines for prevention of epithelial adenocarcinomas. Ann N Y Acad Sci 2013;1284:52–6.
67. Regan D, Guth A, Coy J, et al. Cancer immunotherapy in veterinary medicine: Current options and new developments. Vet J 2016;207:20–8.
68. Hogge GS, Burkholder JK, Culp J, et al. Preclinical development of human granulocyte-macrophage colony-stimulating factor-transfected melanoma cell vaccine using established canine cell lines and normal dogs. CancerGene Ther 1999;6(1):26–36.
69. Alexander AN, Huelsmeyer MK, Mitzey A, et al. Development of an allogeneic whole-cell tumor vaccine expressing xenogeneic gp100 and its implementation in a phase II clinical trial in canine patients with malignant melanoma. Cancer Immunol Immunother 2006;55(4):433–42.
70. U'Ren LW, Biller BJ, Elmslie RE, et al. Evaluation of a novel tumor vaccine in dogs with hemangiosarcoma. J Vet Intern Med 2007;21:113–20.
71. Bird RC, Deinnocentes P, Lenz S, et al. An allogeneic hybrid-cell fusion vaccine against canine mammary cancer. Vet Immunol Immunopathol 2008;123: 289–304.
72. Turek MM, Thamm DH, Mitzey A, et al. Human granulocyte & macrophage colony-stimulating factor DNA cationic-lipid complexed autologous tumour cell vaccination in the treatment of canine B-cell multicentric lymphoma. Vet Comp Oncol 2007;5:219–31.
73. Kuntsi-Vaattovaara H, Verstraete FJM, Newsome JT, et al. Resolution of persistent oral papillomatosis in a dog after treatment with a recombinant canine oral papillomavirus vaccine. Vet Comp Oncol 2003;1:57–63.
74. Milner RJ, Salute M, Crawford C, et al. The immune response to disialoganglioside GD3 vaccination in normal dogs: a melanoma surface antigen vaccine. Vet Immunol Immunopathol 2006;114:273–84.
75. Marconato L, Frayssinet P, Rouquet N, et al. Randomized, placebo-controlled, double-blinded chemo-immunotherapy clinical trial in a pet dog model of diffuse large B-cell lymphoma. Clin Cancer Res 2013;20(3):668–77.
76. Suckow MA. Cancer vaccines: harnessing the potential of anti-tumor immunity. Vet J 2013;198(1):28–33.
77. Epple LM, Bemis LT, Cavanaugh RP, et al. Prolonged remission of advanced bronchoalveolar adenocarcinoma in a dog treated with autologous, tumour-derived chaperone-rich cell lysate (CRCL) vaccine. Int J Hyperthermia 2013; 29(5):390–8.
78. Andersen BM, Pluhar GE, Seiler CE, et al. Vaccination for invasive canine meningioma induces in situ production of antibodies capable of antibody-dependent cell-mediated cytotoxicity. Cancer Res 2013;73(10):2987–97.
79. Yannelli JR, Wouda R, Masterson TJ, et al. Development of an autologous canine cancer vaccine system for resectable malignant tumors in dogs. Vet Immunol Immunopathol 2016;182:95–100.

80. Marconato L, Stefanello D, Sabattini S, et al. Enhanced therapeutic effect of APAVAC immunotherapy in combination with dose-intense chemotherapy in dogs with advanced indolent B-cell lymphoma. Vaccine 2015;33:5080–6.
81. Weir C, Hudson AL, Moon E, et al. Streptavidin: a novel immunostimulant for the selection and delivery of autologous and syngeneic tumor vaccines. Cancer Immunol Res 2014;2:469–79.
82. Weir C, Oksa A, Millar J, et al. The safety of an adjuvanted autologous cancer vaccine platform in canine cancer patients. Vet Sci 2018;5 [pii:E87].
83. Kamstock D, Elmslie R, Thamm D, et al. Evaluation of a xenogeneic VEGF vaccine in dogs with soft tissue sarcoma. Cancer Immunol Immunother 2007;56:1299–309.
84. Yu WY, Chuang TF, Guichard C, et al. Chicken HSP70 DNA vaccine inhibits tumor growth in a canine cancer model. Vaccine 2011;29(18):3489–500.
85. Impellizeri JA, Ciliberto G, Aurisicchio L. Electro-gene-transfer as a new tool for cancer immunotherapy in animals. Vet Comp Oncol 2012;12(4):310–8.
86. Denies S, Cicchelero L, Polis I, et al. Immunogenicity and safety of xenogeneic vascular endothelial growth factor receptor-2 DNA vaccination in mice and dogs. Oncotarget 2016;7:10905–16.
87. Gabai V, Venanzi FM, Bagashova E, et al. Pilot study of p62 DNA vaccine in dogs with mammary tumors. Oncotarget 2014;5:12803–10.
88. Riccardo F, Iussich S, Maniscalco L, et al. CSPG4-specific immunity and survival prolongation in dogs with oral malignant melanoma immunized with human CSPG4 DNA. Clin Cancer Res 2014;20:3753–62.
89. Gibson HM, Veenstra JJ, Jones R, et al. Induction of HER2 Immunity in Outbred Domestic Cats by DNA Electrovaccination. Cancer Immunol Res 2015;3:777–86.
90. Piras LA, Riccardo F, Iussich S, et al. Prolongation of survival of dogs with oral malignant melanoma treated by en bloc surgical resection and adjuvant CSPG4-antigen electrovaccination. Vet Comp Oncol 2017;15:996–1013.
91. von EH, Sadeghi A, Carlsson B, et al. Efficient adenovector CD40 ligand immunotherapy of canine malignant melanoma. J Immunother 2008;31:377–84.
92. Johnston KB, Monteiro JM, Schultz LD, et al. Protection of beagle dogs from mucosal challenge with canine oral papillomavirus by immunization with recombinant adenoviruses expressing codon-optimized early genes. Virology 2005;336:208–18.
93. Thacker EE, Nakayama M, Smith BF, et al. A genetically engineered adenovirus vector targeted to CD40 mediates transduction of canine dendritic cells and promotes antigen-specific immune responses in vivo. Vaccine 2009;27(50):7116–24.
94. Peruzzi D, Mesiti G, Ciliberto G, et al. Telomerase and HER-2/neu as targets of genetic cancer vaccines in dogs. Vaccine 2010;28(5):1201–8.
95. Gavazza A, Lubas G, Fridman A, et al. Safety and efficacy of a genetic vaccine targeting telomerase plus chemotherapy for the therapy of canine B-cell lymphoma. Hum Gene Ther 2013;24(8):728–38.
96. Autio KP, Ruotsalainen JJ, Anttila MO, et al. Attenuated Semliki Forest virus for cancer treatment in dogs: safety assessment in two laboratory Beagles. BMC Vet Res 2015;11:170.
97. Impellizeri JA, Gavazza A, Greissworth E, et al. Tel-eVax: a genetic vaccine targeting telomerase for treatment of canine lymphoma. J Transl Med 2018;16:349.

98. Hoopes PJ, Wagner RJ, Duval K, et al. Treatment of canine oral melanoma with nanotechnology-based immunotherapy and radiation. Mol Pharm 2018;15: 3717–22.
99. Sanchez D, Cesarman-Maus G, Amador-Molina A, et al. Oncolytic viruses for canine cancer treatment. Cancers (Basel) 2018;10 [pii:E404].
100. Cejalvo T, Perise-Barrios AJ, Del P, et al. Remission of spontaneous canine tumors after systemic cellular viroimmunotherapy. Cancer Res 2018;78:4891–901.
101. Hoopes PJ, Moodie KL, Petryk AA, et al. Hypo-fractionated radiation, magnetic nanoparticle hyperthermia and a viral immunotherapy treatment of spontaneous canine cancer. Proc SPIE Int Soc Opt Eng 2017;10066 [pii:1006605].
102. Gyorffy S, Rodriguez-Lecompte JC, Woods JP, et al. Bone marrow-derived dendritic cell vaccination of dogs with naturally occurring melanoma by using human gp100 antigen. J Vet Intern Med 2005;19(1):56–63.
103. Tamura K, Arai H, Ueno E, et al. Comparison of dendritic cell-mediated immune responses among canine malignant cells. J Vet Med Sci 2007;69:925–30.
104. Tamura K, Yamada M, Isotani M, et al. Induction of dendritic cell-mediated immune responses against canine malignant melanoma cells. Vet J 2008;175: 126–9.
105. Rodriguez-Lecompte JC, Kruth S, Gyorffy S, et al. Cell-based cancer gene therapy: breaking tolerance or inducing autoimmunity? Anim Health Res Rev 2004; 5:227–34.
106. Kyte JA, Mu L, Aamdal S, et al. Phase I/II trial of melanoma therapy with dendritic cells transfected with autologous tumor-mRNA. CancerGene Ther 2006; 13:905–18.
107. Mason NJ, Coughlin CM, Overley B, et al. RNA-loaded CD40-activated B cells stimulate antigen-specific T-cell responses in dogs with spontaneous lymphoma. Gene Ther 2008;15:955–65.
108. Sorenmo KU, Krick E, Coughlin CM, et al. CD40-activated B cell cancer vaccine improves second clinical remission and survival in privately owned dogs with non-Hodgkin's lymphoma. PLoS One 2011;6(8):e24167.
109. Bird RC, Deinnocentes P, Church Bird AE, et al. An autologous dendritic cell canine mammary tumor hybrid-cell fusion vaccine. Cancer Immunol Immunother 2011;60(1):87–97.
110. Hernandez-Granados AJ, Franco-Molina MA, Coronado-Cerda EE, et al. Immunogenic potential of three transmissible venereal tumor cell lysates to prime canine-dendritic cells for cancer immunotherapy. Res Vet Sci 2018;121:23–30.
111. O'Connor CM, Sheppard S, Hartline CA, et al. Adoptive T-cell therapy improves treatment of canine non-Hodgkin lymphoma post chemotherapy. Sci Rep 2012; 2:249.
112. Sharma P, Wagner K, Wolchok JD, et al. Novel cancer immunotherapy agents with survival benefit: recent successes and next steps. Nat Rev Cancer 2011; 11:805–12.
113. Singh S, Kumar N, Dwiwedi P, et al. Monoclonal antibodies: a review. Curr Clin Pharmacol 2018;13(2):85–99.
114. Ladjemi MZ. Anti-idiotypic antibodies as cancer vaccines: achievements and future improvements. Front Oncol 2012;2:158.
115. Thomas A, Teicher BA, Hassan R. Antibody-drug conjugates for cancer therapy. Lancet Oncol 2016;17:e254–62.
116. Ross SL, Sherman M, McElroy PL, et al. Bispecific T cell engager (BiTE(R)) antibody constructs can mediate bystander tumor cell killing. PLoS One 2017;12: e0183390.

117. Strohl WR. Current progress in innovative engineered antibodies. Protein Cell 2018;9(1):86–120.
118. Grillo-Lopez AJ, Hedrick E, Rashford M, et al. Rituximab: ongoing and future clinical development. Semin Oncol 2002;29:105–12.
119. Saxena A, Wu D. Advances in therapeutic Fc engineering - modulation of IgG-associated effector functions and serum half-life. Front Immunol 2016;7:580.
120. Weiskopf K, Anderson KL, Ito D, et al. Eradication of canine diffuse large B-cell lymphoma in a murine xenograft model with CD47 blockade and anti-CD20. Cancer Immunol Res 2016;4:1072–87.
121. Jain S, Aresu L, Comazzi S, et al. The development of a recombinant scFv monoclonal antibody targeting canine CD20 for use in comparative medicine. PLoS One 2016;11:e0148366.
122. Ito D, Brewer S, Modiano JF, et al. Development of a novel anti-canine CD20 monoclonal antibody with diagnostic and therapeutic potential. Leuk Lymphoma 2015;56:219–25.
123. Rue SM, Eckelman BP, Efe JA, et al. Identification of a candidate therapeutic antibody for treatment of canine B-cell lymphoma. Vet Immunol Immunopathol 2015;164:148–59.
124. Kano R, Inoiue C, Okano H, et al. Canine CD20 gene. Vet Immunol Immunopathol 2005;108:265–8.
125. Jubala CM, Wojcieszyn JW, Valli VE, et al. CD20 expression in normal canine B cells and in canine non-Hodgkin lymphoma. Vet Pathol 2005;42:468–76.
126. Impellizeri JA, Howell K, McKeever KP, et al. The role of rituximab in the treatment of canine lymphoma: an ex vivo evaluation. Vet J 2006;171:556–8.
127. London CA, Gardner HL, Rippy S, et al. KTN0158, a humanized anti-KIT monoclonal antibody, demonstrates biologic activity against both normal and malignant canine mast cells. Clin Cancer Res 2017;23:2565–74.
128. Adelfinger M, Bessler S, Frentzen A, et al. Preclinical testing oncolytic vaccinia virus strain GLV-5b451 expressing an anti-VEGF single-chain antibody for canine cancer therapy. Viruses 2015;7:4075–92.
129. Wagner S, Maibaum D, Pich A, et al. Verification of a canine PSMA (FolH1) antibody. Anticancer Res 2015;35:145–8.
130. Singer J, Fazekas J, Wang W, et al. Generation of a canine anti-EGFR (ErbB-1) antibody for passive immunotherapy in dog cancer patients. Mol Cancer Ther 2014;13:1777–90.
131. Michishita M, Uto T, Nakazawa R, et al. Antitumor effect of bevacizumab in a xenograft model of canine hemangiopericytoma. J Pharmacol Sci 2013;121:339–42.
132. Michishita M, Ohtsuka A, Nakahira R, et al. Anti-tumor effect of bevacizumab on a xenograft model of feline mammary carcinoma. J Vet Med Sci 2016;78:685–9.
133. Shahabi V, Seavey MM, Maciag PC, et al. Development of a live and highly attenuated Listeria monocytogenes-based vaccine for the treatment of Her2/neu-overexpressing cancers in human. CancerGene Ther 2011;18:53–62.
134. Fazekas J, Furdos I, Singer J, et al. Why man's best friend, the dog, could also benefit from an anti-HER-2 vaccine. Oncol Lett 2016;12:2271–6.
135. Mason NJ, Gnanandarajah JS, Engiles JB, et al. Immunotherapy with a HER2-targeting listeria induces HER2-specific immunity and demonstrates potential therapeutic effects in a phase I trial in canine osteosarcoma. Clin Cancer Res 2016;22:4380–90.

136. Bergman PJ, Camps-Palau MA, McKnight JA, et al. Development of a xenogeneic DNA vaccine program for canine malignant melanoma at the Animal Medical Center. Vaccine 2006;24(21):4582–5.
137. Bergman PJ, McKnight J, Novosad A, et al. Long-term survival of dogs with advanced malignant melanoma after DNA vaccination with xenogeneic human tyrosinase: a phase I trial. Clin Cancer Res 2003;9(4):1284–90.
138. Smedley RC, Lamoureux J, Sledge DG, et al. Immunohistochemical diagnosis of canine oral amelanotic melanocytic neoplasms. Vet Pathol 2011;48(1):32–40.
139. Phillips JC, Lembcke LM, Noltenius CE, et al. Evaluation of tyrosinase expression in canine and equine melanocytic tumors. Am J Vet Res 2012;73(2):272–8.
140. Cangul IT, van Garderen E, van der Poel HJ, et al. Tyrosinase gene expression in clear cell sarcoma indicates a melanocytic origin: insight from the first reported canine case. APMIS 1999;107(11):982–8.
141. Ramos-Vara JA, Beissenherz ME, Miller MA, et al. Retrospective study of 338 canine oral melanomas with clinical, histologic, and immunohistochemical review of 129 cases. Vet Pathol 2000;37(6):597–608.
142. Ramos-Vara JA, Miller MA. Immunohistochemical identification of canine melanocytic neoplasms with antibodies to melanocytic antigen PNL2 and tyrosinase: comparison with Melan A. Vet Pathol 2011;48(2):443–50.
143. de Vries TJ, Smeets M, de Graaf R, et al. Expression of gp100, MART-1, tyrosinase, and S100 in paraffin-embedded primary melanomas and locoregional, lymph node, and visceral metastases: implications for diagnosis and immunotherapy. A study conducted by the EORTC Melanoma Cooperative Group. J Pathol 2001;193(1):13–20.
144. Gradilone A, Gazzaniga P, Ribuffo D, et al. Prognostic significance of tyrosinase expression in sentinel lymph node biopsy for ultra-thin, thin, and thick melanomas. Eur Rev Med Pharmacol Sci 2012;16(10):1367–76.
145. Liao JC, Gregor P, Wolchok JD, et al. Vaccination with human tyrosinase DNA induces antibody responses in dogs with advanced melanoma. Cancer Immun 2006;6:8.
146. Goubier A, Fuhrmann L, Forest L, et al. Superiority of needle-free transdermal plasmid delivery for the induction of antigen-specific IFNgamma T cell responses in the dog. Vaccine 2008;26:2186–90.
147. Grosenbaugh DA, Leard AT, Bergman PJ, et al. Safety and efficacy of a xenogeneic DNA vaccine encoding for human tyrosinase as adjunctive treatment for oral malignant melanoma in dogs following surgical excision of the primary tumor. Am J Vet Res 2011;72(12):1631–8.
148. Zuleger CL, Kang C, Ranheim EA, et al. Pilot study of safety and feasibility of DNA microseeding for treatment of spontaneous canine melanoma. Vet Med Sci 2017;3:134–45.
149. Herzog A, Buchholz J, Ruess-Melzer K, et al. Concurrent irradiation and DNA tumor vaccination in canine oral malignant melanoma: a pilot study. Schweiz Arch Tierheilkd 2013;155(2):135–42 [in German].
150. Ottnod JM, Smedley RC, Walshaw R, et al. A retrospective analysis of the efficacy of Oncept vaccine for the adjunct treatment of canine oral malignant melanoma. Vet Comp Oncol 2013;11(3):219–29.
151. Verganti S, Berlato D, Blackwood L, et al. Use of Oncept melanoma vaccine in 69 canine oral malignant melanomas in the UK. J Small Anim Pract 2017;58:10–6.

152. Treggiari E, Grant JP, North SM. A retrospective review of outcome and survival following surgery and adjuvant xenogeneic DNA vaccination in 32 dogs with oral malignant melanoma. J Vet Med Sci 2016;78:845–50.
153. McLean JL, Lobetti RG. Use of the melanoma vaccine in 38 dogs: The South African experience. J S Afr Vet Assoc 2015;86:1246.
154. Boston SE, Lu X, Culp WT, et al. Efficacy of systemic adjuvant therapies administered to dogs after excision of oral malignant melanomas: 151 cases (2001-2012). J Am Vet Med Assoc 2014;245:401–7.
155. Wolchok JD, Yuan J, Houghton AN, et al. Safety and immunogenicity of tyrosinase DNA vaccines in patients with melanoma. Mol Ther 2007;15:2044–50.
156. Perales MA, Yuan J, Powel S, et al. Phase I/II study of GM-CSF DNA as an adjuvant for a multipeptide cancer vaccine in patients with advanced melanoma. Mol Ther 2008;16:2022–9.
157. Yuan J, Ku GY, Gallardo HF, et al. Safety and immunogenicity of a human and mouse gp100 DNA vaccine in a phase I trial of patients with melanoma. Cancer Immun 2009;9:5.
158. Manley CA, Leibman NF, Wolchok JD, et al. Xenogeneic murine tyrosinase DNA vaccine for malignant melanoma of the digit of dogs. J Vet Intern Med 2011;25(1):94–9.
159. Phillips JC, Blackford JT, Lembcke LM, et al. Evaluation of needle-free injection devices for intramuscular vaccination in horses. J Equine Vet Sci 2011;31:738–43.
160. Sarbu L, Kitchell BE, Bergman PJ. Safety of administering the canine melanoma DNA vaccine (Oncept) to cats with malignant melanoma - a retrospective study. J Feline Med Surg 2017;19(2):224–30.
161. Chu PY, Pan SL, Liu CH, et al. KIT gene exon 11 mutations in canine malignant melanoma. Vet J 2013;196(2):226–30.
162. Murakami A, Mori T, Sakai H, et al. Analysis of KIT expression and KIT exon 11 mutations in canine oral malignant melanomas. Vet Comp Oncol 2011;9(3):219–24.
163. Gillard M, Cadieu E, De BC, et al. Naturally occurring melanomas in dogs as models for non-UV pathways of human melanomas. Pigment CellMelanoma Res 2014;27(1):90–102.
164. Peggs KS, Quezada SA, Korman AJ, et al. Principles and use of anti-CTLA4 antibody in human cancer immunotherapy. Curr Opin Immunol 2006;18(2):206–13.
165. Graves SS, Stone D, Loretz C, et al. Establishment of long-term tolerance to SRBC in dogs by recombinant canine CTLA4-Ig. Transplantation 2009;88:317–22.
166. Callahan MK, Wolchok JD. At the bedside: CTLA-4- and PD-1-blocking antibodies in cancer immunotherapy. J Leukoc Biol 2013;94:41–53.
167. Biller BJ, Elmslie RE, Burnett RC, et al. Use of FoxP3 expression to identify regulatory T cells in healthy dogs and dogs with cancer. Vet Immunol Immunopathol 2007;116:69–78.
168. Horiuchi Y, Tominaga M, Ichikawa M, et al. Increase of regulatory T cells in the peripheral blood of dogs with metastatic tumors. Microbiol Immunol 2009;53:468–74.
169. O'Neill K, Guth A, Biller B, et al. Changes in regulatory T cells in dogs with cancer and associations with tumor type. J Vet Intern Med 2009;23:875–81.

170. Sherger M, Kisseberth W, London C, et al. Identification of myeloid derived suppressor cells in the peripheral blood of tumor bearing dogs. BMC Vet Res 2012; 8:209.
171. Thamm DH. Interactions between radiation therapy and immunotherapy: the best of two worlds? Vet Comp Oncol 2006;4:189–97.
172. Walter CU, Biller BJ, Lana SE, et al. Effects of chemotherapy on immune responses in dogs with cancer. J Vet Intern Med 2006;20(2):342–7.
173. Emens LA, Jaffee EM. Leveraging the activity of tumor vaccines with cytotoxic chemotherapy. Cancer Res 2005;65(18):8059–64.
174. Wolchok JD, Kluger H, Callahan MK, et al. Nivolumab plus ipilimumab in advanced melanoma. N Engl J Med 2013;369(2):122–33.
175. Ott PA, Hodi FS, Kaufman HL, et al. Combination immunotherapy: a road map. J Immunother Cancer 2017;5:16.
176. Hellmann MD, Friedman CF, Wolchok JD. Combinatorial cancer immunotherapies. Adv Immunol 2016;130:251–77.
177. Le D, Uram J, Wang H, et al. PD-1 blockade in tumors with mismatch-repair deficiency. N Engl J Med 2015;372:2509–20.
178. Karaki S, Anson M, Tran T, et al. Is there still room for cancer vaccines at the era of checkpoint inhibitors. Vaccines (Basel) 2016;4 [pii:E37].
179. Lai X, Friedman A. Combination therapy of cancer with cancer vaccine and immune checkpoint inhibitors: a mathematical model. PLoS One 2017;12: e0178479.
180. Yuasa T, Masuda H, Yamamoto S, et al. Biomarkers to predict prognosis and response to checkpoint inhibitors. Int J Clin Oncol 2017;22:629–34.
181. Khagi Y, Kurzrock R, Patel SP. Next generation predictive biomarkers for immune checkpoint inhibition. CancerMetastasis Rev 2017;36:179–90.
182. Ott PA, Hu Z, Keskin DB, et al. An immunogenic personal neoantigen vaccine for patients with melanoma. Nature 2017;547:217–21.
183. Jackson HJ, Rafiq S, Brentjens RJ. Driving CAR T-cells forward. Nat Rev Clin Oncol 2016;13:370–83.
184. Coy J, Caldwell A, Chow L, et al. PD-1 expression by canine T cells and functional effects of PD-1 blockade. Vet Comp Oncol 2017;15(4):1487–502.
185. Maekawa N, Konnai S, Okagawa T, et al. Immunohistochemical analysis of PD-L1 expression in canine malignant cancers and PD-1 expression on lymphocytes in canine oral melanoma. PLoS One 2016;11:e0157176.
186. Maekawa N, Konnai S, Takagi S, et al. A canine chimeric monoclonal antibody targeting PD-L1 and its clinical efficacy in canine oral malignant melanoma or undifferentiated sarcoma. Sci Rep 2017;7:8951.
187. Shosu K, Sakurai M, Inoue K, et al. Programmed cell death ligand 1 expression in canine cancer. In Vivo 2016;30:195–204.
188. Chiku VM, Silva KL, de Almeida BF, et al. PD-1 function in apoptosis of T lymphocytes in canine visceral leishmaniasis. Immunobiology 2016;221:879–88.
189. Tagawa M, Maekawa N, Konnai S, et al. Evaluation of costimulatory molecules in peripheral blood lymphocytes of canine patients with histiocytic sarcoma. PLoS One 2016;11:e0150030.
190. Esch KJ, Juelsgaard R, Martinez PA, et al. Programmed death 1-mediated T cell exhaustion during visceral leishmaniasis impairs phagocyte function. J Immunol 2013;191:5542–50.
191. Folkl A, Wen X, Kuczynski E, et al. Feline programmed death and its ligand: characterization and changes with feline immunodeficiency virus infection. Vet Immunol Immunopathol 2010;134:107–14.

192. Kumar SR, Kim DY, Henry CJ, et al. Programmed death ligand 1 is expressed in canine B cell lymphoma and downregulated by MEK inhibitors. Vet Comp Oncol 2017;15(4):1527–36.
193. Smith JB, Panjwani MK, Schutsky K, et al. Feasibility and safety of cCD20 RNA CAR-bearing T cell therapy for the treatment of canine B cell malignancies. J Immunother Cancer 2015;3:123.
194. Anderson KL, Modiano JF. Progress in adaptive immunotherapy for cancer in companion animals: success on the path to a cure. Vet Sci 2015;2:363–87.
195. Mata M, Vera J, Gerken C, et al. Towards immunotherapy with redirected T cells in a large animal model: Ex vivo activation, expansion, and genetic modification of canine T cells. J Immunother 2014;37:407–15.
196. Mie K, Shimada T, Akiyoshi H, et al. Change in peripheral blood lymphocyte count in dogs following adoptive immunotherapy using lymphokine-activated T killer cells combined with palliative tumor resection. Vet Immunol Immunopathol 2016;177:58–63.
197. Panjwani MK, Smith JB, Schutsky K, et al. Feasibility and safety of RNA-transfected CD20-specific chimeric antigen receptor T cells in dogs with spontaneous B cell lymphoma. Mol Ther 2016;24:1602–14.
198. Kurupati RK, Zhou X, Xiang Z, et al. Safety and immunogenicity of a potential checkpoint blockade vaccine for canine melanoma. Cancer Immunol Immunother 2018;67:1533–44.
199. Nemoto Y, Shosu K, Okuda M, et al. Development and characterization of monoclonal antibodies against canine PD-1 and PD-L1. Vet Immunol Immunopathol 2018;198:19–25.
200. Canter RJ, Grossenbacher SK, Foltz JA, et al. Radiotherapy enhances natural killer cell cytotoxicity and localization in pre-clinical canine sarcomas and first-in-dog clinical trial. J Immunother Cancer 2017;5:98.
201. Heinzerling L, Goldinger SM. A review of serious adverse effects under treatment with checkpoint inhibitors. Curr Opin Oncol 2017;29:136–44.
202. Kumar V, Chaudhary N, Garg M, et al. Current diagnosis and management of immune related adverse events (irAEs) induced by immune checkpoint inhibitor therapy. Front Pharmacol 2017;8:49.
203. Khanna C, London C, Vail D, et al. Guiding the optimal translation of new cancer treatments from canine to human cancer patients. Clin Cancer Res 2009;15: 5671–7.
204. Paoloni M, Khanna C. Translation of new cancer treatments from pet dogs to humans. Nat Rev Cancer 2008;8:147–56.
205. Ranieri G, Gadaleta CD, Patruno R, et al. A model of study for human cancer: spontaneous occurring tumors in dogs. Biological features and translation for new anticancer therapies. Crit Rev Oncol Hematol 2013;88(1):187–97.
206. Angstadt AY, Thayanithy V, Subramanian S, et al. A genome-wide approach to comparative oncology: high-resolution oligonucleotide aCGH of canine and human osteosarcoma pinpoints shared microaberrations. Cancer Genet 2012; 205(11):572–87.
207. LeBlanc AK, Breen M, Choyke P, et al. Perspectives from man's best friend: National Academy of Medicine's workshop on comparative oncology. Sci Transl Med 2016;8:324ps5.
208. LeBlanc AK, Mazcko C, Brown DE, et al. Creation of an NCI comparative brain tumor consortium: informing the translation of new knowledge from canine to human brain tumor patients. Neuro Oncol 2016;18:1209–18.

209. Seelig DM, Avery AC, Ehrhart EJ, et al. The comparative diagnostic features of canine and human lymphoma. Vet Sci 2016;3 [pii:11].
210. Fulkerson CM, Dhawan D, Ratliff TL, et al. Naturally occurring canine invasive urinary bladder cancer: a complementary animal model to improve the success rate in human clinical trials of new cancer drugs. Int J Genomics 2017;2017: 6589529.

Novel Treatments for Lymphoma

Douglas H. Thamm, VMD

KEYWORDS

• Chemotherapy • Canine • Feline • Cancer

KEY POINTS

- Conventional CHOP-based chemotherapy results in high response rates in dogs, but the vast majority of dogs will eventually relapse.
- Response rates to CHOP-based chemotherapy are lower in cats with intermediate- to high-grade lymphoma than in dogs, but low-grade lymphoma, which has a more favorable outcome with conservative treatment, is more common.
- A variety of alterations in conventional CHOP-based protocols, such as omission of asparaginase or corticosteroids and substituting oral for injectable cyclophosphamide, can be used in dogs with lymphoma without impact on efficacy.
- Several novel immunotherapy approaches, including monoclonal antibodies, vaccines, and cell-based therapies, are in varying stages of clinical development for the treatment of canine lymphoma.
- Three novel small molecules, RV-1001, KPT-335 (verdinexor), and rabacfosadine succinate (Tanovea-CA1), have demonstrated meaningful antitumor activity and reasonable safety in dogs with lymphoma, leading to MUMS (minor use in a major species) designation for the treatment of lymphoma by the US Food and Drug Administration Center for Veterinary Medicine (FDA-CVM). Rabacfosadine succinate has been granted conditional approval by the FDA-CVM for the treatment of canine lymphoma.

INTRODUCTION

Lymphoma is a common disease in companion animals. Although conventional chemotherapy has the potential to induce remission and prolong life, relapse is common and novel treatments are needed to improve outcome. This review will cover the basics of canine and feline lymphoma treatment, then discuss recent advances in standard of care therapy as well as new treatments that are in varying stages of regulatory approval.

Disclosure Statement: Dr D.H. Thamm is a shareholder in and has received research funding from VetDC, Inc, the developer of rabacfosadine, which is discussed in this review.
Flint Animal Cancer Center, College of Veterinary Medicine and Biomedical Sciences, Colorado State University, 300 West Drake Road, Fort Collins, CO 80523-1620, USA
E-mail address: dthamm@colostate.edu

Vet Clin Small Anim 49 (2019) 903–915
https://doi.org/10.1016/j.cvsm.2019.04.004
vetsmall.theclinics.com

REVIEW OF CONVENTIONAL TREATMENTS FOR LYMPHOMA

Canine Lymphoma

Owing to lymphoma's systemic presentation, chemotherapy is the mainstay of treatment. A large number of single-agent and multiagent chemotherapy protocols have been investigated over the last 40 years; however, one optimal chemotherapy protocol has not been identified that integrates positive outcome, toxicity, and cost.

Corticosteroids alone have been shown to induce at least partial remission in many dogs with lymphoma by their direct cytotoxic effect, as well as being associated with symptomatic improvement. Oral corticosteroids (most commonly prednisone/prednisolone at 2 mg/kg/d by mouth initially, then tapered over 1–3 weeks to 0.5–1 mg/kg/d) are a reasonable treatment for some owners if chemotherapy is declined. Although most dogs and cats will experience meaningful short-term improvement, its duration is typically 1 to 2 months, and corticosteroids seem to induce chemotherapy resistance; thus, attempting chemotherapy after prednisone has failed, while not impossible, may be considerably less successful than in a patient that has not been pretreated.

A relatively simple, inexpensive chemotherapy protocol with intermediate efficacy is single-agent doxorubicin (DOX). This has become more affordable because DOX is available in generic form, and requires only one injection every 3 weeks. Furthermore, if a side effect is encountered the drug responsible is easy to identify. Approximately 65% to 85% of dogs will respond to single-agent DOX, with reported median response durations (MRDs) of 100 to 170 days.[1–4] Two unique effects of DOX are its potential for cumulative cardiac toxicity in dogs, and its potential to cause severe skin necrosis if extravasated.

Generally, the most successful chemotherapy protocols are multiagent protocols that include DOX. These protocols, referred to generically as CHOP (cyclophosphamide, doxorubicin, vincristine, and prednisone)-based protocols, are used at most institutions. This treatment uses sequential injections of vincristine, cyclophosphamide (CYC), and DOX, combined with daily prednisone for the first 4 weeks. Published CHOP-based protocols generally range from 15 to 25 weeks in duration (**Table 1**). Complete response (CR) rates are 85% to 95%, median progression-free survival (MPFS) times are 5 to 9 months, and median survival times (MST) are approximately 12 months, with 20% to 25% of dogs living to 2 years.[5–12] Unfortunately, all but approximately 5% of patients will eventually relapse.

Most current CHOP protocols suspend therapy following 4 to 6 months of treatment: monthly rechecks are then pursued to assess remission status, and a recent study confirmed an apparent lack of benefit to "maintenance" therapy following completion of this initial period of intensive treatment.[13]

Factors that have historically carried the most prognostic significance for remission duration and survival include clinical signs at presentation (substage b), hypercalcemia, mediastinal lymphadenopathy, and significant bone marrow infiltration.[14–17] Both hypercalcemia and mediastinal lymphadenopathy are likely surrogate markers for lymphomas with a T-cell immunophenotype, a powerful predictor of outcome. Most veterinary pathology laboratories are capable of immunophenotyping lymphomas through immunohistochemistry. Immunophenotyping alternatively can be performed on fine-needle aspirates using immunocytochemistry, flow cytometry, or PCR for antigen receptor rearrangement.[18–20]

Feline Lymphoma

The basic tenets of treatment for feline intermediate- to high-grade lymphoma are very similar to canine. One important difference, however, is that single-agent DOX seems

Table 1
Select published CHOP-based protocols for canine lymphoma

	Week															
"UW-25" Protocol	**1**	**2**	**3**	**4**	**6**	**7**	**8**	**9**	**11**	**13**	**15**	**17**	**19**	**21**	**23**	**25**
Vincristine 0.7 mg/m^2 IV	X		X		X		X		X		X		X		X	
Cyclophosphamide 250 mg/m^2 PO or IV		X				X				X				X		
Doxorubicin 30 mg/m^2 IV[a]				X				X				X				X
Prednisone (mg/kg/d) PO	2	1.5	1	0.5	Discontinue											

	Week															
"UW-19" Protocol	**1**	**2**	**3**	**4**	**6**	**7**	**8**	**9**	**11**	**12**	**13**	**14**	**16**	**17**	**18**	**19**
Vincristine 0.7 mg/m^2 IV	X		X		X		X		X		X		X		X	
Cyclophosphamide 250 mg/m^2 PO or IV		X				X				X				X		
Doxorubicin 30 mg/m^2 IV[a]				X				X				X				X
Prednisone (mg/kg/d) PO	2	1.5	1	0.5	Discontinue											

	Week											
15-wk CHOP Protocol	**1**	**2**	**3**	**5**	**6**	**7**	**9**	**10**	**11**	**13**	**14**	**15**
Vincristine 0.7 mg/m^2 IV	X			X			X			X		
Cyclophosphamide 250 mg/m^2 PO or IV		X			X			X			X	
Doxorubicin 30 mg/m^2 IV[a]			X			X			X			X
Prednisone (mg/kg/d) PO	2	1.5	1	0.5	Discontinue							

Abbreviations: IV, intravenous; PO, by mouth.
[a] Doxorubicin is often administered at a dose of 1 mg/kg in dogs weighing less than 15 kg.

to have less activity in cats.[21,22] Even with CHOP-based chemotherapy, response and survival rates are lower in cats than in dogs, with approximately 40% to 45% of cats achieving a CR, and approximately 25% experiencing a partial response (PR). Median CR durations are 200 to 400 days and median PR durations are approximately 80 days.[23,24]

Recent reports suggest that most cats with low-grade, small-cell gastrointestinal (GI) lymphoma may respond favorably and enjoy MSTs in the 2 to 3 year range when a protocol using oral chlorambucil and prednisone is used. Three different dosing strategies have been reported: 15 mg/m^2 by mouth daily for 4 days repeated every 3 weeks, 20 mg/m^2 by mouth once every 2 weeks, and 2 mg/cat by mouth every 2 to 3 days continuously.[25–27] Importantly, a designation of low-grade, small-cell lymphoma can only be made histologically.

NEW DATA WITH CONVENTIONAL DRUGS

Asparaginase Versus No Asparaginase

Older publications routinely included a single injection of asparaginase at the beginning of multiagent treatment; however, 2 studies have demonstrated no improvement in any measure of outcome in dogs receiving asparaginase.[10,28] For this reason, the author chooses to omit asparaginase from initial treatment and save it for use as a potential therapy at relapse.

Oral Versus Intravenous Cyclophosphamide

Although most of the statistics generated regarding the efficacy of multiagent lymphoma chemotherapy protocols have used injectable CYC, many clinicians substitute oral CYC at the same dose. Until recently it was not clear whether this was equally efficacious, owing to CYC's unknown oral bioavailability in dogs and cats. Pharmacokinetic analysis comparing oral versus injectable CYC in dogs and cats suggests that, while there is a significant difference in plasma exposure to the parent drug, exposure to the active metabolite of CYC, 4-hydroxycyclophosphamide, is quite similar between the 2 routes of administration. This suggests probable equal efficacy.[29,30] One remaining advantage to injectable CYC is that the appropriate dose can be administered with greater precision that can be attained with tablets, especially in cats and smaller dogs.

Prednisone Versus No Prednisone

There are certain patients in whom corticosteroid therapy may be contraindicated; for example, patients with unregulated hyperadrenocorticism or diabetes mellitus. Until recently, the outcome in canine patients with lymphoma treated with multiagent chemotherapy but without prednisone was unknown. Two recent randomized trials evaluated CYC-vincristine-DOX-based protocols with or without prednisone and found no difference in any measure of outcome.[31,32]

Is There an All-Oral Chemotherapy Protocol that Is Effective for Canine Lymphoma?

Some owners may be uncomfortable with the idea of injectable chemotherapy but may be more comfortable with the concept of oral chemotherapy. Although education regarding the excellent tolerability of most injectable chemotherapy protocols and the potential for side effects and need for careful monitoring, even with oral medications, may help to change some owners' minds, there remain some owners for whom an oral chemotherapy protocol is the only acceptable choice. Oral chemotherapy can be efficacious for 1 very specific form of canine lymphoma: cutaneous T-cell lymphoma (CTCL) in dogs (lomustine ± prednisone); approximately 75% to 85% of dogs with CTCL will have at least a PR to lomustine, although most of the responses are incomplete and the MRD is only approximately 3 months.[33,34] Dogs diagnosed with low-grade or indolent lymphomas may respond well to a conservative oral protocol such as prednisone and chlorambucil[35,36]; however, for most intermediate- or high-grade multicentric lymphoma in dogs, no efficacious oral protocol has been identified. One study evaluated the efficacy of prednisone and lomustine as first-line therapy for canine multicentric lymphoma and found it to be no better than prednisone alone.[37]

Should Dogs with T-Cell Lymphoma Be Treated Differently than Dogs with B-Cell Lymphoma?

With the exception of low-grade/indolent subtypes, dogs with T-cell lymphoma generally have inferior outcomes when treated CHOP-based chemotherapy compared with dogs with B-cell lymphoma. Beaver and colleagues[38] evaluated initial response to a single dose of DOX in dogs with either B-cell or T-cell lymphoma, and found a significantly lower overall response rate (ORR) in dogs with T-cell lymphoma (50% vs 100%). At roughly the same time, a retrospective study was published evaluating a MOPP (mechlorethamine-vincristine-procarbazine-prednisone)-based protocol in dogs with T-cell lymphoma. An ORR of 98% (78% CR), an MPFS of 189 days and an MST of 270 days was reported[39]; however, a contemporary report documented a similarly high ORR (96%) and relatively similar MPFS (146 days) and MST

(235 days) in dogs with T-cell lymphoma treated with a CHOP-based protocol.[40] More recently, 3 additional reports have described outcomes in dogs with T-cell lymphoma treated with so-called "alkylator rich" chemotherapy protocols; either LOPP (lomustine-vincristine-procarbazine-prednisone) or VELCAP-TSC (asparaginase-vincristine-CYC-DOX-actinomycin D-procarbazine-lomustine). In these reports, ORRs ranged from 73% to 97% (64%–90% CR), MPFS was 175 to 431 days and MST was 237 to 507 days.[41–43] Thus, while definitive evidence of a survival advantage is lacking with these alternative protocols, it is possible that they may result in improved outcomes over more conventional CHOP-based chemotherapy for dogs with nonindolent T-cell lymphoma.

Lomustine for Feline Lymphoma

Given that single-agent DOX seems to be a less effective "middle of the road" chemotherapy protocol for cats with intermediate- to high-grade lymphoma, the default for decades has been a COP (cyclophosphamide-vincristine-prednisone) protocol.[44–46] Although efficacy is improved over prednisone alone but inferior to CHOP, there is limited cost savings versus CHOP, and the initial induction period of treatment still requires weekly visits. Furthermore, it is often continued longer-term than CHOP protocols are. Given these considerations, there has been a search for a less-intensive chemotherapy protocol that still retains some efficacy. Recently, results of a retrospective study investigating lomustine and prednisone for the first-line treatment of cats with intermediate to large cell GI lymphoma was reported.[47] The ORR was 50% (22% CR), with an MRD of approximately 300 days. The overall MST was approximately 100 days.

Vincristine Versus Vinblastine for Feline Lymphoma

Contrary to what is typically observed in dogs, some degree of GI disturbance following vincristine administration seems to be more common in cats with lymphoma. A recent prospective study in cats with lymphoma evaluated the use of vincristine or vinblastine within the context of a COP-based protocol.[44] There was no difference in response rate, progression-free interval (PFI) or survival time between the arms, but the incidence of GI toxicity was significantly lower in cats receiving vinblastine than those receiving vincristine (10% vs 44%).

NEW THERAPIES

Radiation Therapy

Since lymphoma is considered a systemic disease in most circumstances, radiation therapy (RT) is not used commonly; however, lymphoma can be very sensitive to RT, and thus is can be useful as a palliative treatment in animals with clinical signs related to lymphoma at a specific site (eg, pleural effusion from mediastinal disease, solitary nasal tumors in cats).[48,49] Several studies have been published recently evaluating the outcomes of dogs treated with chemotherapy followed by half-body RT, and some studies have suggested possible improvement over patients treated with chemotherapy alone.[50,51] Definitive evidence of improvement in outcome is lacking. Two recent studies have evaluated the role of whole-abdomen RT in the treatment of feline GI lymphoma. One used RT as "consolidation" therapy following completion of an abbreviated course of CHOP-based chemotherapy. Although the number of cats treated was too small to draw firm efficacy conclusions, the treatment (10 daily fractions of 1.5 Gy) seemed will tolerated.[52] A second study evaluated whole-abdomen RT (2 daily fractions of 4 Gy) as rescue therapy following chemotherapy relapse. Clinical improvement was noted in 10 of 11 cats treated, and the MST postirradiation was approximately 7 months.[53]

Bone marrow/stem cell transplant

One treatment that is commonly used in some forms of human lymphoma and leukemia is high-dose chemotherapy and/or whole-body RT followed by autologous hematopoietic stem cell (HSC) or bone marrow transplant to "rescue" the patient from fatal myelosuppression. A combination chemotherapy protocol incorporating high-dose CYC and autologous bone marrow rescue has been evaluated in pilot studies in dogs, with encouraging preliminary results.[54] Several specialty groups have HSC or bone marrow transplant programs for dogs with lymphoma. Early data suggest acceptable tolerability,[55–57] but definitive evidence of efficacy remains lacking. Based on human experience, a more profound antitumor effect may be observed following allogeneic, rather than autologous, transplants, owing to the development of a "graft versus tumor" effect. There is a single case report of long-term survival of a dog with an aggressive T-cell lymphoma following allogeneic transplant[58]; however, broad deployment of this approach is hampered by challenges identifying haplocompatible donors.

Immunotherapy

Monoclonal antibodies

Monoclonal antibodies directed against the CD20 antigen expressed on most human B-cell lymphomas (eg, rituximab) have changed the standard of care for the treatment of many forms of B-cell malignancy in humans. Significant single-agent antitumor activity is observed in patients with indolent B-cell lymphoma/leukemia,[59] and when combined with standard of care chemotherapy, improvements in outcome are observed in patients with intermediate- to high-grade disease as well, without an increase in toxicity.[60–62] Surprisingly, after more than 20 years of use, mechanisms responsible for the antitumor effects of anti-CD20 antibody therapy remain incompletely understood. Binding to the lymphoma cell and activation of host immune cells via the Fc component (so-called antibody-dependent cellular cytotoxicity), complement fixation, and crosslinking of CD20 on the cell surface leading to apoptosis are all possible mechanisms.[62] In 2014, a canine-specific anti-CD20 antibody received full licensure through the US Department of Agriculture (USDA) (canine lymphoma monoclonal antibody, B cell; Blontress). Unpublished studies performed following USDA approval failed to demonstrate improvements in outcome over dogs receiving conventional therapy alone, and there were concerns regarding the specificity of the antibody, leading to its withdrawal from the market.

A second anti-canine CD20 monoclonal antibody has been developed. This antibody shows good binding characteristics to canine CD20 and demonstrates evidence of B-cell depletion in vivo in laboratory dogs, as well as evidence of antitumor activity in canine lymphoma mouse xenograft models.[63,64] The current development status of this antibody is unknown.

Lymphoma vaccines

A xenogeneic DNA vaccine targeting CD20 has been granted conditional approval through the USDA for the treatment of canine B-cell lymphoma, and is intended to generate a "rituximab-like" anti-CD20 antibody response. The efficacy of this product is unknown, but is the subject of an ongoing randomized, placebo-controlled trial.

In a nonrandomized, noncontrolled 2-arm study of 42 dogs, Gavazza and colleagues[65] evaluated COP-based chemotherapy $\pm$ a telomerase reverse transcriptase (TERT)-based vaccine. Dogs in remission after an 8-week induction COP protocol went on to maintenance chemotherapy ± vaccination. Interestingly, while there was no difference in first remission duration between the groups, the MST was significantly improved in the vaccinated group (76.1 vs 29.3 weeks). Most of the vaccinated dogs mounted detectable T-cell responses to TERT, and there was a potential correlation between tumor TERT expression and survival in vaccinated patients. Caveats include lack of randomization or an active control arm, nonstandardized rescue therapy, and a lack of comparison of known prognostic factors between groups. Furthermore, it is unclear whether a similar benefit would be realized in dogs treated with a more "optimal" (eg, CHOP based) chemotherapy protocol. The regulatory status of this vaccine is unknown.

A second study evaluated an autologous heat shock protein peptide chaperone (HSPPC)-based vaccine in conjunction with chemotherapy in dogs with B-cell lymphoma through a randomized, placebo-controlled, double-blinded trial.[66] Nineteen dogs were randomized to receive CHOP-based chemotherapy with HSPPC vaccine or placebo. The placebo arm contained more stage V patients and more substage b patients; these differences were not statistically significant, probably owing to the small N. The vaccinated patients had longer median first and second PFIs (304 vs 41 days and 127 vs 32 days, respectively), and there were no differences in adverse effects between the groups. The very small N and unequal distribution of some known powerful prognostic factors in favor of the vaccinated group likely contributed to the unexpectedly poor outcome in the placebo arm. The regulatory status of this vaccine is unknown.

T-cell-based therapies

One of the most recent advances in the treatment of human lymphoid malignancy is the use of chimeric antigen receptor-engineered T cells (CAR-Ts). CAR-Ts are genetically engineered to express a synthetic T-cell receptor that is targeted to a lymphoma-related surface antigen and possesses an inherent activation domain. This allows the recognition of target antigen in an MHC-unrestricted fashion, and does not require a second signal for cell activation. CAR-Ts targeting the B-cell surface antigens CD19, CD22, and CD30 have been described,[67–69] and the significant ORR, even in heavily pretreated patients, has led to the Food and Drug Administration (FDA) approval of a CD19 CAR-T product (tisagenlecleucel, Kymriah) for the treatment of relapsed/refractory large B-cell lymphoma in humans. In the single-arm pivotal trial, the ORR was 50% (32% CR), and the MRD was not reached with a median follow-up time of 9.4 months.[70]

A preliminary study has generated canine CAR-Ts targeting CD20, and demonstrated the specificity and cytotoxic activity of these cells ex vivo. Evidence of clinical antitumor effects has yet to be published, however.[71] Another study has evaluated the safety and efficacy of untransfected but activated and expanded canine autologous T cells for the treatment of a small number of dogs with B-cell lymphoma.[72] These cells persisted in vivo and homed to tumor tissue, and when compared with historical control dogs treated with chemotherapy alone, the addition of these cells to conventional CHOP-based seemed to improve outcome.

Small Molecules

Phosphatidylinositol 3-kinase (PI3K) is an intracellular kinase that is a key signaling node in many forms of cancer, and evidence of PI3K pathway dysregulation is present in canine lymphoma.[73–75] The drug idelalisib (Zydelig) is an orally available inhibitor of the delta isoform of PI3K (PI3Kδ), which was approved for the treatment of human B-cell neoplasia in 2014.[76] RV1001 is an orally available inhibitor of PI3Kδ, which has been evaluated in a phase I/II study in dogs with lymphoma. At the optimal biologic dose, the ORR was 77% (3% CR) with an overall median time to progression of 25.5 days. Activity was observed in both B-cell and T-cell lymphomas. Hepatobiliary and GI adverse events were most frequent.[77] RV1001 has been granted MUMS (minor use in a major species) designation for the treatment of canine lymphoma by the US Food and Drug Administration Center for Veterinary Medicine (FDA-CVM) but is not currently approved.

Verdinexor (KPT-335) is an orally available inhibitor of a protein called exportin-1 (XPO-1), which is responsible for the binding and nuclear export of a large variety of important tumor suppressor genes. In vitro, verdinexor demonstrated particular efficacy against canine lymphoma cells, and in a clinical trial, objective responses were observed in 2 of 17 dogs in the initial dose-finding study, both of which were dogs with lymphoma. In a small expansion cohort in lymphoma, responses were observed in an additional 2 of 6 dogs, which persisted for 35 and 354 days.[78] A recent phase II study reported an ORR of 37% (71% in dogs with T-cell lymphoma), with an MRD of 18 days.[79] GI toxicity, including hyporexia, diarrhea, vomiting, and weight loss, were the most commonly observed adverse effects. Verdinexor has been granted MUMS designation for canine lymphoma treatment by the FDA-CVM but is not currently approved.

In 2017, the FDA-CVM conditionally approved rabacfosadine succinate (Tanovea-CA1), for the treatment of lymphoma in dogs. Rabacfosadine is a double prodrug of the guanine nucleotide analog 9-(2-phosphonylmethoxyethyl) guanine (PMEG). Rabacfosadine is hydrolyzed intracellularly to cPrPMEDAP and subsequently deaminated to PMEG. PMEG is then phosphorylated to PMEG diphosphate (PMEGpp), which is a potent inhibitor of the major DNA polymerases. Rabacfosadine has been demonstrated to inhibit DNA synthesis, resulting in S phase arrest and induction of apoptosis in lymphoid tumor cells.[80] Rabacfosadine is given as a 30-minute intravenous infusion once every 3 weeks. Response rates of 50% to 85% are reported depending on the immunophenotype and degree of pretreatment,[80–82] and a combination of alternating rabacfosadine and DOX resulted in outcomes similar to those obtained with conventional CHOP-based therapy for naïve canine lymphoma: the ORR was 84% (68% CR), and the overall median PFI was 194 days.[83] As with many cytotoxic drugs for lymphoma, improved outcomes are observed in dogs with B-cell disease.[81,82] Activity has also been observed in dogs with CTCL.[84] In addition to GI and hematologic adverse effects similar to those seen with other cytotoxic agents, a cumulative dermatopathy can occur, and rare, presumed idiosyncratic, delayed pulmonary fibrosis can also be observed. Rabacfosadine is not an MDR substrate and does not penetrate the blood-brain barrier (VetDC, Inc, information on file).

SUMMARY

In summary, although companion animal lymphoma is a disease that can rarely be cured, it can be managed effectively in most cases. Therapy is typically very well tolerated, and patients experience an excellent quality of life. Significant improvements have been made in recent years with regard to the treatment of this common disease, and we are hopeful that the coming years will bring equally great improvements.

REFERENCES

1. Lori JC, Stein TJ, Thamm DH. Doxorubicin and cyclophosphamide for the treatment of canine lymphoma: a randomized, placebo-controlled study. Vet Comp Oncol 2010;8:188–95.

2. Mutsaers AJ, Glickman NW, DeNicola DB, et al. Evaluation of treatment with doxorubicin and piroxicam or doxorubicin alone for multicentric lymphoma in dogs. J Am Vet Med Assoc 2002;220:1813–7.
3. Valerius KD, Ogilvie GK, Mallinckrodt CH, et al. Doxorubicin alone or in combination with asparaginase, followed by cyclophosphamide, vincristine, and prednisone for treatment of multicentric lymphoma in dogs: 121 cases (1987-1995). J Am Vet Med Assoc 1997;210:512–6.
4. Postorino NC, Susaneck SJ, Withrow SJ, et al. Single agent therapy with Adriamycin for canine lymphosarcoma. J Am Vet Med Assoc 1989;25:221–5.
5. Burton JH, Garrett-Mayer E, Thamm DH. Evaluation of a 15-week CHOP protocol for the treatment of canine multicentric lymphoma. Vet Comp Oncol 2013;11: 306–15.
6. Curran K, Thamm DH. Retrospective analysis for treatment of naive canine multicentric lymphoma with a 15-week, maintenance-free CHOP protocol. Vet Comp Oncol 2016;14(Suppl 1):147–55.
7. Elliott JW, Cripps P, Marrington AM, et al. Epirubicin as part of a multi-agent chemotherapy protocol for canine lymphoma. Vet Comp Oncol 2013;11:185–98.
8. Greenberg CB, Boria PA, Borgatti-Jeffreys A, et al. Phase II clinical trial of combination chemotherapy with dexamethasone for lymphoma in dogs. J Am Anim Hosp Assoc 2007;43:27–32.
9. Hosoya K, Kisseberth WC, Lord LK, et al. Comparison of COAP and UW-19 protocols for dogs with multicentric lymphoma. J Vet Intern Med 2007;21:1355–63.
10. MacDonald VS, Thamm DH, Kurzman ID, et al. Does L-asparaginase influence efficacy or toxicity when added to a standard CHOP protocol for dogs with lymphoma? J Vet Intern Med 2005;19:732–6.
11. Sorenmo K, Overley B, Krick E, et al. Outcome and toxicity associated with a dose-intensified, maintenance-free CHOP-based chemotherapy protocol in canine lymphoma: 130 cases. Vet Comp Oncol 2010;8:196–208.
12. Garrett LD, Thamm DH, Chun R, et al. Evaluation of a 6-month chemotherapy protocol with no maintenance therapy for dogs with lymphoma. J Vet Intern Med 2002;16:704–9.
13. Lautscham EM, Kessler M, Ernst T, et al. Comparison of a CHOP-LAsp-based protocol with and without maintenance for canine multicentric lymphoma. Vet Rec 2017;180:303.
14. Greenlee PG, Filippa DA, Quimby FW, et al. Lymphomas in dogs. A morphologic, immunologic, and clinical study. Cancer 1990;66:480–90.
15. Marconato L, Stefanello D, Valenti P, et al. Predictors of long-term survival in dogs with high-grade multicentric lymphoma. J Am Vet Med Assoc 2011;238:480–5.
16. Ruslander DA, Gebhard DH, Tompkins MB, et al. Immunophenotypic characterization of canine lymphoproliferative disorders. In Vivo 1997;11:169–72.
17. Teske E. Prognostic factors for malignant lymphoma in the dog: an update. Vet Q 1994;16(Suppl 1):29S–31S.
18. Sapierzynski R. Practical aspects of immunocytochemistry in canine lymphomas. Pol J Vet Sci 2010;13:661–8.
19. Rout ED, Avery PR. Lymphoid neoplasia: correlations between morphology and flow cytometry. Vet Clin North Am Small Anim Pract 2017;47:53–70.
20. Lana SE, Jackson TL, Burnett RC, et al. Utility of polymerase chain reaction for analysis of antigen receptor rearrangement in staging and predicting prognosis in dogs with lymphoma. J Vet Intern Med 2006;20:329–34.

21. Kristal O, Lana SE, Ogilvie GK, et al. Single agent chemotherapy with doxorubicin for feline lymphoma: a retrospective study of 19 cases (1994-1997). J Vet Intern Med 2001;15:125–30.
22. Peaston AE, Maddison JE. Efficacy of doxorubicin as an induction agent for cats with lymphosarcoma. Aust Vet J 1999;77:442–4.
23. Collette SA, Allstadt SD, Chon EM, et al. Treatment of feline intermediate- to high-grade lymphoma with a modified university of Wisconsin-Madison protocol: 119 cases (2004-2012). Vet Comp Oncol 2016;14(Suppl 1):136–46.
24. Limmer S, Eberle N, Nerschbach V, et al. Treatment of feline lymphoma using a 12-week, maintenance-free combination chemotherapy protocol in 26 cats. Vet Comp Oncol 2016;14(Suppl 1):21–31.
25. Kiselow MA, Rassnick KM, McDonough SP, et al. Outcome of cats with low-grade lymphocytic lymphoma: 41 cases (1995-2005). J Am Vet Med Assoc 2008;232:405–10.
26. Pope KV, Tun AE, McNeill CJ, et al. Outcome and toxicity assessment of feline small cell lymphoma: 56 cases (2000-2010). Vet Med Sci 2015;1:51–62.
27. Stein TJ, Pellin M, Steinberg H, et al. Treatment of feline gastrointestinal small-cell lymphoma with chlorambucil and glucocorticoids. J Am Anim Hosp Assoc 2010;46:413–7.
28. Jeffreys AB, Knapp DW, Carlton WW, et al. Influence of asparaginase on a combination chemotherapy protocol for canine multicentric lymphoma. J Am Anim Hosp Assoc 2005;41:221–6.
29. Warry E, Hansen RJ, Gustafson DL, et al. Pharmacokinetics of cyclophosphamide after oral and intravenous administration to dogs with lymphoma. J Vet Intern Med 2011;25:903–8.
30. Stroda KA, Murphy JD, Hansen RJ, et al. Pharmacokinetics of cyclophosphamide and 4-hydroxycyclophosphamide in cats after oral, intravenous, and intraperitoneal administration of cyclophosphamide. Am J Vet Res 2017;78:862–6.
31. Childress MO, Ramos-Vara JA, Ruple A. A randomized controlled trial of the effect of prednisone omission from a multidrug chemotherapy protocol on treatment outcome in dogs with peripheral nodal lymphomas. J Am Vet Med Assoc 2016;249:1067–78.
32. Zandvliet M, Rutteman GR, Teske E. Prednisolone inclusion in a first-line multidrug cytostatic protocol for the treatment of canine lymphoma does not affect therapy results. Vet J 2013;197:656–61.
33. Risbon RE, de Lorimier LP, Skorupski K, et al. Response of canine cutaneous epitheliotropic lymphoma to lomustine (CCNU): a retrospective study of 46 cases (1999-2004). J Vet Intern Med 2006;20:1389–97.
34. Williams LE, Rassnick KM, Power HT, et al. CCNU in the treatment of canine epitheliotropic lymphoma. J Vet Intern Med 2006;20:136–43.
35. Flood-Knapik KE, Durham AC, Gregor TP, et al. Clinical, histopathological and immunohistochemical characterization of canine indolent lymphoma. Vet Comp Oncol 2013;11:272–86.
36. Lane J, Price J, Moore A, et al. Low-grade gastrointestinal lymphoma in dogs: 20 cases (2010 to 2016). J Small Anim Pract 2018;59:147–53.
37. Sauerbrey ML, Mullins MN, Bannink EO, et al. Lomustine and prednisone as a first-line treatment for dogs with multicentric lymphoma: 17 cases (2004-2005). J Am Vet Med Assoc 2007;230:1866–9.
38. Beaver LM, Strottner G, Klein MK. Response rate after administration of a single dose of doxorubicin in dogs with B-cell or T-cell lymphoma: 41 cases (2006-2008). J Am Vet Med Assoc 2010;237:1052–5.

39. Brodsky EM, Maudlin GN, Lachowicz JL, et al. Asparaginase and MOPP treatment of dogs with lymphoma. J Vet Intern Med 2009;23:578–84.
40. Rebhun RB, Kent MS, Borrofka SA, et al. CHOP chemotherapy for the treatment of canine multicentric T-cell lymphoma. Vet Comp Oncol 2011;9:38–44.
41. Brown PM, Tzannes S, Nguyen S, et al. LOPP chemotherapy as a first-line treatment for dogs with T-cell lymphoma. Vet Comp Oncol 2018;16:108–13.
42. Goodman IH, Moore AS, Frimberger AE. Treatment of canine non-indolent T cell lymphoma using the VELCAP-TSC protocol: a retrospective evaluation of 70 dogs (2003-2013). Vet J 2016;211:39–44.
43. Morgan E, O'Connell K, Thomson M, et al. Canine T cell lymphoma treated with lomustine, vincristine, procarbazine, and prednisolone chemotherapy in 35 dogs. Vet Comp Oncol 2018;16(4):622–9.
44. Krick EL, Cohen RB, Gregor TP, et al. Prospective clinical trial to compare vincristine and vinblastine in a COP-based protocol for lymphoma in cats. J Vet Intern Med 2013;27:134–40.
45. Mahony OM, Moore AS, Cotter SM, et al. Alimentary lymphoma in cats: 28 cases (1988-1993). J Am Vet Med Assoc 1995;207:1593–8.
46. Waite AH, Jackson K, Gregor TP, et al. Lymphoma in cats treated with a weekly cyclophosphamide-, vincristine-, and prednisone-based protocol: 114 cases (1998-2008). J Am Vet Med Assoc 2013;242:1104–9.
47. Rau SE, Burgess KE. A retrospective evaluation of lomustine (CeeNU) in 32 treatment naive cats with intermediate to large cell gastrointestinal lymphoma (2006-2013). Vet Comp Oncol 2017;15:1019–28.
48. Fujiwara-Igarashi A, Fujimori T, Oka M, et al. Evaluation of outcomes and radiation complications in 65 cats with nasal tumours treated with palliative hypofractionated radiotherapy. Vet J 2014;202:455–61.
49. Haney SM, Beaver L, Turrel J, et al. Survival analysis of 97 cats with nasal lymphoma: a multi-institutional retrospective study (1986-2006). J Vet Intern Med 2009;23:287–94.
50. Lurie DM, Gordon IK, Theon AP, et al. Sequential low-dose rate half-body irradiation and chemotherapy for the treatment of canine multicentric lymphoma. J Vet Intern Med 2009;23:1064–70.
51. Williams LE, Johnson JL, Hauck ML, et al. Chemotherapy followed by half-body radiation therapy for canine lymphoma. J Vet Intern Med 2004;18:703–9.
52. Williams LE, Pruitt AF, Thrall DE. Chemotherapy followed by abdominal cavity irradiation for feline lymphoblastic lymphoma. Vet Radiol Ultrasound 2010;51:681–7.
53. Parshley DL, Larue SM, Kitchell B, et al. Abdominal irradiation as a rescue therapy for feline gastrointestinal lymphoma: a retrospective study of 11 cats (2001-2008). J Feline Med Surg 2011;13:63–8.
54. Frimberger AE, Moore AS, Rassnick KM, et al. A combination chemotherapy protocol with dose intensification and autologous bone marrow transplant (VELCAP-HDC) for canine lymphoma. J Vet Intern Med 2006;20:355–64.
55. Warry EE, Willcox JL, Suter SE. Autologous peripheral blood hematopoietic cell transplantation in dogs with T-cell lymphoma. J Vet Intern Med 2014;28:529–37.
56. Willcox JL, Pruitt A, Suter SE. Autologous peripheral blood hematopoietic cell transplantation in dogs with B-cell lymphoma. J Vet Intern Med 2012;26:1155–63.
57. Escobar C, Grindem C, Neel JA, et al. Hematologic changes after total body irradiation and autologous transplantation of hematopoietic peripheral blood progenitor cells in dogs with lymphoma. Vet Pathol 2012;49:341–3.

58. Lupu M, Sullivan EW, Westfall TE, et al. Use of multigeneration-family molecular dog leukocyte antigen typing to select a hematopoietic cell transplant donor for a dog with T-cell lymphoma. J Am Vet Med Assoc 2006;228:728–32.
59. McLaughlin P, Grillo-Lopez AJ, Link BK, et al. Rituximab chimeric anti-CD20 monoclonal antibody therapy for relapsed indolent lymphoma: half of patients respond to a four-dose treatment program. J Clin Oncol 1998;16:2825–33.
60. Coiffier B, Lepage E, Briere J, et al. CHOP chemotherapy plus rituximab compared with CHOP alone in elderly patients with diffuse large-B-cell lymphoma. N Engl J Med 2002;346:235–42.
61. Pfreundschuh M, Trumper L, Osterborg A, et al. CHOP-like chemotherapy plus rituximab versus CHOP-like chemotherapy alone in young patients with good-prognosis diffuse large-B-cell lymphoma: a randomised controlled trial by the MabThera International Trial (MInT) Group. Lancet Oncol 2006;7:379–91.
62. Lim SH, Levy R. Translational medicine in action: anti-CD20 therapy in lymphoma. J Immunol 2014;193:1519–24.
63. Rue SM, Eckelman BP, Efe JA, et al. Identification of a candidate therapeutic antibody for treatment of canine B-cell lymphoma. Vet Immunol Immunopathol 2015; 164:148–59.
64. Weiskopf K, Anderson KL, Ito D, et al. Eradication of canine diffuse large B-cell lymphoma in a murine xenograft model with CD47 blockade and anti-CD20. Cancer Immunol Res 2016;4:1072–87.
65. Gavazza A, Lubas G, Fridman A, et al. Safety and efficacy of a genetic vaccine targeting telomerase plus chemotherapy for the therapy of canine B-cell lymphoma. Hum Gene Ther 2013;24:728–38.
66. Marconato L, Frayssinet P, Rouquet N, et al. Randomized, placebo-controlled, double-blinded chemoimmunotherapy clinical trial in a pet dog model of diffuse large B-cell lymphoma. Clin Cancer Res 2014;20:668–77.
67. Fry TJ, Shah NN, Orentas RJ, et al. CD22-targeted CAR T cells induce remission in B-ALL that is naive or resistant to CD19-targeted CAR immunotherapy. Nat Med 2018;24:20–8.
68. Maude SL, Frey N, Shaw PA, et al. Chimeric antigen receptor T cells for sustained remissions in leukemia. N Engl J Med 2014;371:1507–17.
69. Ramos CA, Ballard B, Zhang H, et al. Clinical and immunological responses after CD30-specific chimeric antigen receptor-redirected lymphocytes. J Clin Invest 2017;127:3462–71.
70. Schuster SJ, Bishop MR, Tam CS, et al. Primary analysis of Juliet: a global, pivotal, phase 2 trial of CTL019 in adult patients with relapsed or refractory diffuse large B-cell lymphoma. Blood 2017;130:577.
71. Panjwani MK, Smith JB, Schutsky K, et al. Feasibility and safety of RNA-transfected CD20-specific chimeric antigen receptor T cells in dogs with spontaneous B cell lymphoma. Mol Ther 2016;24:1602–14.
72. O'Connor CM, Sheppard S, Hartline CA, et al. Adoptive T-cell therapy improves treatment of canine non-Hodgkin lymphoma post chemotherapy. Sci Rep 2012; 2:249.
73. Elvers I, Turner-Maier J, Swofford R, et al. Exome sequencing of lymphomas from three dog breeds reveals somatic mutation patterns reflecting genetic background. Genome Res 2015;25:1634–45.
74. Zamani-Ahmadmahmudi M, Najafi A, Nassiri SM. Reconstruction of canine diffuse large B-cell lymphoma gene regulatory network: detection of functional modules and hub genes. J Comp Pathol 2015;152:119–30.

75. Mooney M, Bond J, Monks N, et al. Comparative RNA-Seq and microarray analysis of gene expression changes in B-cell lymphomas of *Canis familiaris*. PLoS One 2013;8:e61088.
76. Furman RR, Sharman JP, Coutre SE, et al. Idelalisib and rituximab in relapsed chronic lymphocytic leukemia. N Engl J Med 2014;370:997–1007.
77. Gardner HL, Rippy SB, Bear MD, et al. Phase I/II evaluation of RV1001, a novel PI3Kdelta inhibitor, in spontaneous canine lymphoma. PLoS One 2018;13:e0195357.
78. London CA, Bernabe LF, Barnard S, et al. Preclinical evaluation of the novel, orally bioavailable selective inhibitor of nuclear export (SINE) KPT-335 in spontaneous canine cancer: results of a phase I study. PLoS One 2014;9:e87585.
79. Sadowski AR, Gardner HL, Borgatti A, et al. Phase II study of the oral selective inhibitor of nuclear export (SINE) KPT-335 (verdinexor) in dogs with lymphoma. BMC Vet Res 2018;14:250.
80. Reiser H, Wang J, Chong L, et al. GS-9219–a novel acyclic nucleotide analogue with potent antineoplastic activity in dogs with spontaneous non-Hodgkin's lymphoma. Clin Cancer Res 2008;14:2824–32.
81. Saba CF, Vickery KR, Clifford CA, et al. Rabacfosadine for relapsed canine B-cell lymphoma: efficacy and adverse event profiles of 2 different doses. Vet Comp Oncol 2018;16:E76–82.
82. Vail DM, Thamm DH, Reiser H, et al. Assessment of GS-9219 in a pet dog model of non-Hodgkin's lymphoma. Clin Cancer Res 2009;15:3503–10.
83. Thamm DH, Vail DM, Post GS, et al. Alternating rabacfosadine/doxorubicin: efficacy and tolerability in naive canine multicentric lymphoma. J Vet Intern Med 2017;31:872–8.
84. Morges MA, Burton JH, Saba CF, et al. Phase II evaluation of VDC-1101 in canine cutaneous T-cell lymphoma. J Vet Intern Med 2014;28:1569–74.

Targeted Therapies in Veterinary Oncology

Priya Londhe, PhD[a], Megan Gutwillig[b], Cheryl London, DVM, PhD[c,*]

KEYWORDS

- Inhibitor • Small molecule • Cancer • Targeted therapy

KEY POINTS

- Recent advances in molecular biology have permitted the identification and characterization of specific abnormalities regarding cell signaling and function in cancer cells.
- Proteins that are found to be dysregulated in cancer cells can serve as relevant targets for therapeutic intervention.
- Although there are several approaches to block proteins that contribute to cellular dysfunction, the one most commonly used involves a class of therapeutics called small molecule inhibitors.
- Such inhibitors work by disrupting critical pathways/processes in cancer cells, thereby disrupting their ability to grow and survive.
- Although only a few small molecule inhibitors are currently approved for use in veterinary medicine, it is likely their use will increase substantially over the next decade given the marked incorporation of such agents into human cancer treatment.

INTRODUCTION

Advances in genetic and molecular techniques have permitted the identification and characterization of key proteins that contribute to dysregulation of cancer through their roles in regulating cell survival, growth, differentiation, and migration, among other critical processes. Although many of these are kinases that phosphorylate other proteins in the cell and are integral components of signaling, others include transcription factors, antiapoptotic proteins, heat shock proteins, and regulators of nuclear export. Given their known role in driving the malignant phenotype, substantial effort has been directed at blocking the function of these proteins. Several approaches

Disclosure Statement: Dr C. London has received honoraria from Rhizen Pharmaceuticals, Zoeits, Karyopharm Therapeutics, and Anivive. The other 2 authors have nothing to disclose.
[a] Tufts University School of Medicine, Boston, MA 02111, USA; [b] Sackler School of Graduate Biomedical Sciences, Tufts University, Boston, MA 02111, USA; [c] Cummings School of Veterinary Medicine and School of Medicine, Tufts University, Jaharis Building, Room 814, 150 Harrison Avenue, Boston, MA 0211, USA
* Corresponding author.
E-mail address: cheryl.london@tufts.edu

Vet Clin Small Anim 49 (2019) 917–931
https://doi.org/10.1016/j.cvsm.2019.04.005
vetsmall.theclinics.com

have been used, including monoclonal antibodies and small molecule inhibitors. Although antibodies are primarily directed at cell surface proteins, small molecule inhibitors are capable of targeting protein on the cell surface, in the cytoplasm, and in the nucleus. Over the past 2 decades, a variety of small molecule inhibitors and antibodies have been approved to treat human cancers, and many of these have markedly impacted patient outcomes. In veterinary medicine the use of small molecule inhibitors and antibodies to treat cancer is relatively recent, with only one, toceranib (Palladia; Zoetis, Madison, NJ, USA), currently approved by the Food and Drug Administration (FDA) for use in dogs.[1,2] Several other inhibitors are under development, and the use of human-approved targeted therapeutics has also expanded. This article provides an overview of protein dysfunction in cancer, describes the impact small molecule inhibitors have had on human oncology, and summarizes data with respect to use of small molecule inhibitors in veterinary oncology.

DYSREGULATION OF CELL SIGNALING IN CANCER

Cells receive a multitude of signals from their environment from growth factors (GFs), cytokines, adjacent cells, and extracellular matrix, among others, that are continuously processed over time to determine cell fate. These signals influence cell function by promoting the induction or repression of gene expression, changing the status of proteins critical to regulation of cell cycling, and modulating the genome itself via epigenetic changes with the ultimate goal of maintaining cellular homeostasis.

One of the best characterized components of signaling involves protein kinases that use ATP to phosphorylate themselves and other proteins.[3] They are termed tyrosine kinases (TKs) if they phosphorylate proteins on the amino acid tyrosine or serine/threonine kinases if they phosphorylate proteins on the amino acids serine and threonine. Receptor tyrosine kinases (RTKs) are those TKs expressed on the cell surface that are stimulated by binding of GFs. Signaling generated by kinases is a major driver of normal cell differentiation, survival, and growth. RTKs, including vascular endothelial growth factor receptor (VEGFR), platelet-derived growth factor receptor (PDGFR), fibroblast growth factor receptor (FGFR), and Tie-1 and Tie-2 (receptors for angiopoietin) are also important in the process of angiogenesis, which is critical for tumors to grow beyond a few millimeters in size.[4–7]

The 2 cytoplasmic pathways known to be key players in normal cell signaling are the RAF/MAPK (RAS-RAF-MEK-ERK/p38/JNK family members),[8,9] and the phosphatidyl inositol-3 kinase pathway (PI3K, AKT, NFκB, and mTOR, among others).[10,11] These pathways have previously been reviewed in detail (**Fig. 1**). Specific members of the RAS/MAPK pathway known to be mutated in human tumors include RAS (lung cancer, colon cancer, and several hematologic malignancies) and BRAF (melanomas and thyroid carcinomas, colon cancer).[8,12,13] Abnormalities of PI3K, including mutations and gene amplification, are found in many human cancers, including breast, colorectal, lung, and ovarian carcinomas.[14] Another manner in which this pathway can become activated is through loss of activity of PTEN, a phosphatase that normally acts to regulate AKT and terminate signaling.[11,15,16] PTEN mutations and/or decreased PTEN expression occur in many human cancers (eg, glioblastoma and prostate cancer)[14,15] and have been documented in canine cancers (osteosarcoma, melanoma).[17–19]

Dysfunction of proteins occurs frequently in cancers, typically through mutation, overexpression, the generation of fusion proteins, and/or the presence of autocrine loops of activation. Mutations often alter the structure of a protein, inducing activation in the absence of an appropriate stimulus. In many cases, the protein dysregulated is a kinase, resulting in constitutive intracellular signaling. Other classes of proteins that

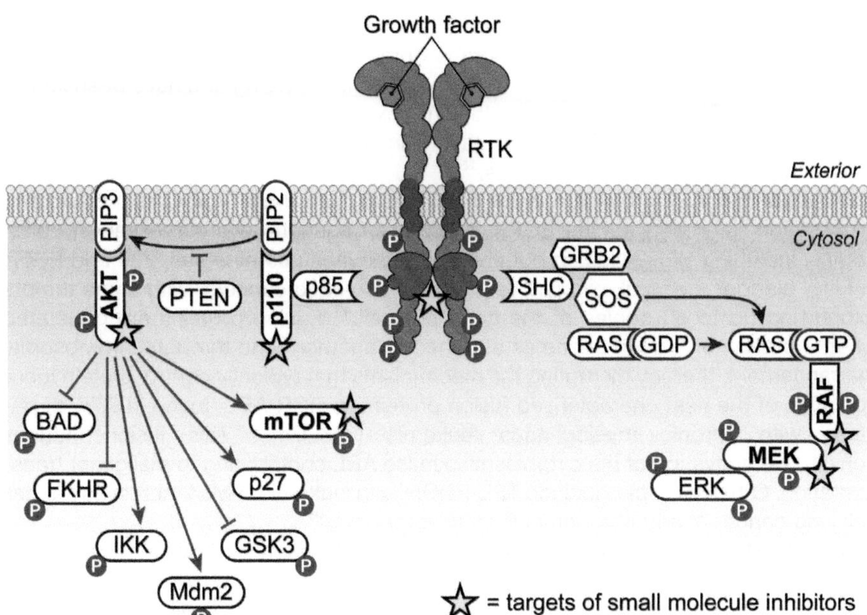

Fig. 1. Cytoplasmic signal transduction. Ras pathway: Activated receptor TKs recruit SOS to the plasma membrane through binding of SHC and GRB2. SOS replaces bound GDP with GTP, thereby activating RAS. The downstream target RAF is then phosphorylated by RAS, leading to subsequent activation of MEK and then ERK. ERK has several substrates both in the nucleus and in the cytoplasm that regulate cell-cycle progression. Current targets of therapeutic intervention are indicated. PI3K pathways: Following RTK activation, PI3 kinase is recruited to the phosphorylated receptor through binding of the p85 adaptor subunit leading to activation of the catalytic subunit (p110). This activation results in the generation of the second messenger phosphatidylinositol-3,4,5-triphosphate (PIP3). PIP3 recruits AKT to the membrane and, following its phosphorylation, several downstream targets are subsequently phosphorylated leading to either their activation or their inhibition. The cumulative effect results in cell survival, growth, and proliferation. Current targets of therapeutic intervention are indicated. (*From* C. London. Small molecule inhibitors in veterinary oncology practice. Advances in Veterinary Oncology 2014;44:895; with permission.)

are frequently altered in tumor cells include transcription factors, regulators of chromatin structure, and inhibitors of apoptosis. Examples of proteins known to be altered in human and canine cancers are discussed later.

Nearly 60% of human cutaneous melanomas possess a point mutation in the BRAF gene[20,21] that induces a conformational change in the protein, resulting in constitutive activation, downstream signaling, and promotion of cell growth and survival.[22,23] Interestingly, orthologous BRAF mutations are found in canine transitional cell carcinomas, with more than 80% of tumors testing positive.[24] RAS is another kinase that is dysregulated through point mutation in several hematopoietic neoplasms, lung cancer, colon cancer, and many others.[8,21,25] KIT, an RTK normally expressed on hematopoietic stem cells, melanocytes, interstitial cells of Cajal, in the central nervous system, and on mast cells, is altered in several cancers.[26] Approximately 30% of high-grade canine mast cell tumors (MCTs) possess internal tandem duplications (ITDs) and point mutations in the juxtamembrane domain of KIT or extracellular ligand binding domain (encoded by exons 11 and 8, respectively), resulting in ligand-independent activation.

These mutations are associated with a higher risk of local recurrence and metastasis.[27–29] Deletions in the juxtamembrane domain of KIT are found in 50% to 80% of human patients with gastrointestinal stromal tumors (GISTs) and have been identified in canine GISTs as well.[30–32] Additional examples include FLT3 ITDs in acute myeloid leukemia,[33–36] EGFR point mutations in lung carcinomas,[37,38] and PI3Kα mutations in several types of carcinomas.[15]

Overexpression of proteins, particularly kinases, can drive tumor cell survival and proliferation. Members of the EGFR family are frequently overexpressed in carcinomas, including HER2/Neu, in both breast and ovarian carcinomas,[39–41] and EGFR in lung, bladder, cervical, ovarian, renal, and pancreatic cancers, with some tumors expressing up to 60 copies of the gene per cell.[42] Fusion proteins are generated when a portion of 1 gene becomes attached to another gene through chromosomal rearrangement, thereby disrupting the mechanisms that typically control protein function. One of the best characterized fusion proteins is BCR-ABL, found in 90% of patients with chronic myelogenous leukemia (CML).[43,44] This fusion induces constitutive activation of the cytoplasmic kinase ABL contributing to malignant transformation. Other examples include TEL-PDGFRα in leukemia, EML4-ALK in non–small cell lung cancer,[45] and Myc-Igh in Burkitt lymphoma.[46]

Autocrine loops of activation occur when tumor cells express both the receptor and the GF, resulting in constitutive signaling. Examples include coexpression of TGF-β and EGFR in glioblastoma and squamous cell carcinoma, insulin-like growth factor (IGF), and its ligand, IGF-1R, in breast and colorectal cancer, and VEGF and VEGFR in melanoma and glioblastoma.[47–50] In canine cancers, possible autocrine loops have been documented in osteosarcoma (OSA, MET, and hepatocyte growth factor) and hemangiosarcoma (HSA, KIT, and stem cell factor).[45,51–53]

Small Molecule Inhibitors

The first small molecule inhibitor to be approved for human use was imatinib, an orally administered drug that binds the ATP pocket of ABL as well as the RTKs KIT and PDGFRα.[54] Imatinib was developed to block the BCR-ABL fusion protein found in humans with CML, with remission rates close to 95%.[55–59] Imatinib also has substantial single-agent activity against human GIST with activating mutations in KIT or PDGFRαa.[60–62]

There are several small molecule inhibitors approved for use in the treatment of human cancers, and many more are undergoing active clinical investigation. Non–small cell lung cancers that possess activating mutations in EGFR typically respond to erlotinib or gefitinib, both small molecule inhibitors of EGFR with response rates reaching 80%.[63–66] A small number of patients with non–small cell lung cancer exhibit ALK activation through its fusion to EML4,[67,68] and there are now 4 small molecule inhibitors (crizotinib, ceritinib, alectinib, and brigatinib) approved to target ALK + lung cancer. BRAF inhibitors alone (vemurafenib, dabrafenib, encorafenib) or in combination with MEK inhibitors (trametinib, binimetinib) have substantial activity in BRAF mutant melanoma with response rates often exceeding 50%.[69] Rapamycin, a drug used for many years as an immunosuppressive agent, is the prototypic mTOR, the downstream target of PI3K signaling.[14,70] More specific rapamycin analogues temsirolimus and everolimus are approved for use in patients with metastatic renal carcinoma, and additional mTOR inhibitors are under investigation for their potential activity in soft tissue sarcomas and bone sarcomas.[14,70]

Although many small molecule inhibitors target a restricted set of proteins, others exhibit far broader activity. These include sunitinib, sorafenib, lenvatinib, axitinib, cabozantinib, pazopanib, regorafenib, and vandetanib that target VEGFR family members with variable activity against additional kinases, including PDGFR, RET, FGFR, and RET, among others.[71–74] The multitargeted nature of these therapeutics may be responsible for observed activity in several types of cancer including GIST, renal cell carcinoma, thyroid carcinoma, and insulinoma, among others.[72–74] Although such agents often have significant clinical activity, they are usually associated with a more substantial range of toxicities that can limit their chronic use.

KINASE INHIBITORS IN VETERINARY MEDICINE

Toceranib (Palladia)

Toceranib phosphate is an orally bioavailable small molecule inhibitor that blocks a variety of RTKs expressed on the cell surface by acting as a reversible competitive inhibitor of ATP binding, thereby preventing receptor phosphorylation and subsequent downstream signaling. Toceranib's published inhibitory profile includes the RTKs, VEGFR2, PDGFRα, and KIT.[2,75–77] However, it is very closely related to another sunitinib that blocks the activity, VEGFR2, 3, PDGFRα/β, KIT, CSF1R, FLT-3, and RET.[74] The combination of antiangiogenic and antitumor activity likely provides more extensive clinical response than that observed with narrowly targeted small molecule inhibitors. Biologic activity of toceranib was first demonstrated in a phase 1 study in dogs with a variety of spontaneous tumors, with 28% of dogs experiencing an objective response and 54% of dogs showing clinical benefit.[75] In a subsequent phase 2 clinical trial in canine MCT, approximately 30% possess activating mutations in KIT targeted by this drug.[2] The objective response rate (ORR; PR and CRs) for dogs receiving toceranib was 42.8%, and MCT bearing activating KIT mutations were more likely to have a CR compared with KIT-mutation negative tumors.[2] A third study demonstrated that toceranib actively inhibits phosphorylation of KIT in canine MCTs, providing direct evidence of a pharmacokinetic/pharmacodynamic relationship.[78]

Following its approval, toceranib has been used off-label to treat several types of canine cancers, often after failure of primary or standard-of-care treatments. Evidence for biologic activity has been found in several solid tumors, including anal sac anal gland adenocarcinoma, thyroid carcinoma, head and neck carcinoma, and nasal carcinoma, among others.[79–81] There has also been substantial effort to combine toceranib with other anticancer therapies, including chemotherapy, radiation therapy, and as part of a metronomic treatment regimen. In a study evaluating toceranib in combination with piroxicam, several antitumor responses were observed.[82] Toceranib was evaluated in combination with vinblastine to treat MCTs, and although substantial clinical activity was observed, significant reductions in vinblastine were required to mitigate enhanced myelosuppression.[83] Toceranib has also been combined with other chemotherapeutics, and in most cases, modifications of chemotherapy dose given have been required.

A few studies have evaluated the activity of toceranib in combination with radiation therapy. In 1 trial, dogs with nonresectable MCTs received prednisone, omeprazole, diphenhydramine, toceranib, and coarse fractionated radiation.[84] The ORR of this combination therapy was 76.4%, and the overall median survival time was not reached with a median follow-up of 374 days. The combination of radiation and toceranib also appears to benefit dogs with nasal carcinoma. Dogs receiving 10 fractions of radiation (total dose 42 Gy) with toceranib had a median survival time of 615 days compared with 371 days for a similarly treated historical control that did not get toceranib.[85]

Toceranib has been demonstrated to have immunomodulatory properties through its modulation of regulatory T cells (Tregs),[86] significantly reducing the number and percentage of Tregs in the peripheral blood of treated dogs, with a concomitant increase in interferon-γ serum concentrations. Despite this activity, there was no added benefit when toceranib was combined with piroxicam and cyclophosphamide following carboplatin in dogs with microscopic metastatic osteosarcoma or in dogs with microscopic hemangiosarcoma following splenectomy and doxorubicin treatment.[87,88]

Although there have been a few studies of toceranib in cats, there have been no large trials that have explored effectiveness in a specific disease entity. It is generally well tolerated when given to cats at doses similar to those used in dogs, and a few reports have demonstrated activity in MCTs.[89–91] However, there does not appear to be substantial efficacy in the setting of other cancers, such as squamous cell carcinoma or injection site sarcoma.[92–94]

Masitinib and Imatinib

Masitinib mesylate (Kinavet), conditionally approved by the FDA in 2010, blocks the activity of KIT, PDGFR, and the cytoplasmic kinase, Lyn. A large placebo controlled clinical trial was performed in more than 200 dogs with MCTs in which masitinib significantly improved time to progression compared with placebo, and outcome was improved in dogs with MCTs possessing KIT mutations.[1] Subsequent follow-up of patients treated with masitinib for 2 years identified an increased number of patients with long-term disease control compared with those treated with placebo.[95] A retrospective analysis of dogs with MCT treated with masitinib showed a response rate of approximately 50%.[96] Masitinib has also been reported to have activity against T-cell lymphoma in dogs, although no formal clinical trials have been undertaken in this disease setting. There have been no specific studies of imatinib mesylate (Gleevec) in veterinary medicine, although a few reports have been published regarding its use in both dogs and cats. In these, imatinib was well tolerated, and objective antitumor responses were observed in dogs with MCTs carrying both mutant and wild-type KIT.[97–99] Responses have also been observed in cats with MCT that have KIT mutations.[100,101]

PI3K Inhibitor

RV1001 is an orally bioavailable inhibitor of the PI3Kδ isoform, the expression of which is typically restricted to hematopoietic cells. Phase 1 and 2 clinical trials of RV1001 in dogs' lymphoma validated target inhibition and established pharmacokinetic/pharmacodynamic relationships, tolerability, and activity of the drug.[102] The ORR was 62% (complete response [CR], n = 3; partial response [PR], n = 10) in the initial phase 1 study, and responses were observed in both naive and chemotherapy-resistant B- and T-cell lymphoma.[102] The ORR in the phase 2 study was 77% (n = 1 CR; n = 26 PR); responses were noted in both naive and relapsed patients, with 86.7% of naive B-cell, 57.1% of relapsed B-cell, 100% of naive T-cell, and 62.5% of relapsed T-cell lymphoma obtaining an objective response to RV1001 administration. Clinical toxicities were primarily hepatobiliary and gastrointestinal and were responsive to dose modifications and/or temporary drug discontinuation. Hepatotoxicity was the primary dose-limiting toxicity.

Bruton Tyrosine Kinase Inhibitors

Ibrutinib and acalabrutinib are Bruton tyrosine kinase (BTK) inhibitors, approved for use to treat B-cell malignancies. BTK is a kinase downstream of the B-cell receptor, associated with proliferation and survival. Ibrutinib was initially evaluated in dogs with B-cell lymphoma whereby objective responses and safety were demonstrated, in addition to high levels of target inhibition.[103] Dogs with spontaneous B-cell lymphoma were subsequently used to evaluate a second-generation BTK inhibitor, acalabrutinib, before clinical studies in people. In this phase 1 clinical trial, acalabrutinib was shown to be both safe and efficacious, with an ORR of 25%.[104] Importantly, twice daily dosing was associated with improved clinical responses and BTK occupancy, a finding not predicted by prior preclinical modeling, helping to guide dosing in the subsequent human trials.

Other Kinase Inhibitors

Several additional small molecule inhibitors are currently being explored for potential clinical utility in veterinary patients with cancer. These include dasatinib (an inhibitor of Src family members, PDGFR, KIT, and BCR-ABL), trametinib (MEK inhibitor), vemurafenib (BRAF inhibitor), and lapatinib (EGFR inhibitor). Although there are limited clinical data regarding efficacy, it is likely the use of these compounds will increase over time as the genetics of veterinary cancers become more clearly defined, and as the drugs transition to generics that may be more affordable.

NONKINASE TARGETS OF SMALL MOLECULE INHIBITORS

Although kinases have represented the major target for therapeutic intervention with small molecule inhibitors, there are several other proteins known to be critical players in cancer cell growth and survival. There are now several small molecule inhibitors of these proteins, including those that target the proteasome, histone deacetylases (HDAC), and heat shock proteins, among others. Some of these have been evaluated in veterinary oncology patients with encouraging results.

Exportin 1 Inhibitors

Exportin 1 (XPO1) is a member of the karyopherin family of transport receptors that binds approximately 220 target proteins through a nuclear export signal (NES) present in the cargo, resulting in nuclear export.[105] XPO1 is the sole nuclear exporter of several major tumor suppressor and growth regulatory proteins,[106,107] and its expression is upregulated in both hematologic malignancies and solid tumors, often correlating with a poor prognosis.[108–110] Verdinexor (KPT-335) and selinexor (KPT-330) are orally bioavailable small molecule inhibitors of XPO1 that induce apoptosis and block proliferation in several cancer cell lines[106,111–113] while sparing normal cells.[114] Verdinexor was evaluated in dogs with spontaneous cancers before the evaluation of selinexor in people, to validate target inhibition, tolerability, and biologic activity. The phase 1 clinical trial of verdinexor demonstrated clinical benefit in 65% of dogs, with most of those in the setting of lymphoma.[115] A subsequent phase 2 clinical trial of verdinexor in dogs with naive or relapsed B- or T-cell lymphoma demonstrated an ORR of 37%, of which dogs with T-cell lymphoma had an ORR of 71%.[116] In both studies, verdinexor was well tolerated with dose-limiting clinical toxicities primarily observed in the gastrointestinal tract (anorexia, weight loss). Clinical development of verdinexor is ongoing.

Heat Shock Protein 90 Inhibitors

STA-1474 is a highly soluble prodrug of ganetespib (formerly STA-9090), a novel small molecule that binds in the ATP-binding domain at the N-terminus of heat shock protein 90 (HSP90) and acts as a potent HSP90 inhibitor.[117] This prevents the stabilization of several client proteins (including KIT, MET, BRAF, and AKT, among others), ultimately resulting in their degradation. A phase 1 clinical trial of STA-1474 was performed in dogs with cancer, resulting in an ORR of 24%; most of these were seen in dogs that received the drug over 8 hours.[118] Toxicities were largely low grade and gastrointestinal in nature. A subsequent regimen-finding clinical trial was conducted in mouse models of cancer and dogs with MCTs, demonstrating that a 2-day-in-a-row dosing regimen was most effective at downregulating HSP90 function and inducing tumor regression.[119] These studies validated HSP90 as a relevant target for therapeutic intervention in canine cancers.

Histone Deacetylase Inhibitors

HDAC enzymes are responsible for the removal of acetyl groups from the NH_2-terminal tails of histone proteins and play a crucial role in the control of gene expression.[120] There has been significant interest in the use of HDAC inhibitors (HDACi) to treat cancer given that this therapy can alter the expression of epigenetically silenced genes in tumor cells and thereby inhibit tumor progression.[121,122] To date, 4 HDACi, vorinostat, romidepsin, panobinostat, and belinostat, have been approved for the treatment of human cancers. There has been limited use of these drugs to date in dogs, with only vorinostat and valproic acid (a drug with off-target effects as an HDACi) tested in canine cancers.[123,124]

RESISTANCE TO SMALL MOLECULE INHIBITORS

In people, small molecule inhibitors are typically associated with ORRs that exceed 50% when the drug targets a known tumor driver. Unfortunately, in most instances, the responses are not durable, lasting on average from 6 to 18 months. The mechanisms responsible for this resistance have been well characterized for many of these therapeutics and include such things as mutations in the ATP binding pocket of the kinase (typically called gatekeeper mutations), overexpression of the target, and mutations in other proteins that circumvent the target, among others. Other mechanisms of resistance to kinase inhibitors that are not as well characterized include epigenetic changes secondary to alterations in histone acetylation/deacetylation and chromatin and histone methylation.[125] Taken together, these observations reinforce the notion that drug-resistant cell populations may be selected via multiple mechanisms, making prevention and treatment of this resistance challenging.

SUMMARY

Progress in molecular biology has permitted a greater understanding of how protein dysregulation in tumor cells drives uncontrolled growth and survival. The development of small molecule inhibitors that target these key proteins has transformed human cancer therapy. The use of such agents is just beginning to be explored in veterinary oncology, and this process has been accelerated through the approval of both toceranib and masitinib and the ongoing development of verdinexor and RV1001. Nevertheless, significant challenges remain, including determining how these therapies can be effectively combined with chemotherapy and radiation therapy to provide optimal anticancer efficacy without enhancing toxicity and identifying strategies that are less likely to result in drug resistance.

REFERENCES

1. Hahn KA, Ogilvie G, Rusk T, et al. Masitinib is safe and effective for the treatment of canine mast cell tumors. J Vet Intern Med 2008;22(6):1301–9.
2. London CA, Malpas PB, Wood-Follis SL, et al. Multi-center, placebo-controlled, double-blind, randomized study of oral toceranib phosphate (SU11654), a

receptor tyrosine kinase inhibitor, for the treatment of dogs with recurrent (either local or distant) mast cell tumor following surgical excision. Clin Cancer Res 2009;15(11):3856–65.

3. Lemmon MA, Schlessinger J. Cell signaling by receptor tyrosine kinases. Cell 2010;141(7):1117–34.
4. Cherrington JM, Strawn LM, Shawver LK. New paradigms for the treatment of cancer: the role of anti- angiogenesis agents. Adv Cancer Res 2000;79:1–38.
5. Eskens FA. Angiogenesis inhibitors in clinical development; where are we now and where are we going? Br J Cancer 2004;90(1):1–7.
6. McCarty MF, Liu W, Fan F, et al. Promises and pitfalls of anti-angiogenic therapy in clinical trials. Trends Mol Med 2003;9(2):53–8.
7. Thurston G. Role of Angiopoietins and Tie receptor tyrosine kinases in angiogenesis and lymphangiogenesis. Cell Tissue Res 2003;314(1):61–8.
8. Downward J. Targeting RAS signalling pathways in cancer therapy. Nat Rev Cancer 2003;3(1):11–22.
9. Johnson GL, Lapadat R. Mitogen-activated protein kinase pathways mediated by ERK, JNK, and p38 protein kinases. Science 2002;298(5600):1911–2.
10. Franke TF, Hornik CP, Segev L, et al. PI3K/Akt and apoptosis: size matters. Oncogene 2003;22(56):8983–98.
11. Fresno Vara JA, Casado E, de Castro J, et al. PI3K/Akt signalling pathway and cancer. Cancer Treat Rev 2004;30(2):193–204.
12. Davies H, Bignell GR, Cox C, et al. Mutations of the BRAF gene in human cancer. Nature 2002;417(6892):949–54.
13. Mercer KE, Pritchard CA. Raf proteins and cancer: B-Raf is identified as a mutational target. Biochim Biophys Acta 2003;1653(1):25–40.
14. Markman B, Atzori F, Perez-Garcia J, et al. Status of PI3K inhibition and biomarker development in cancer therapeutics. Ann Oncol 2010;21(4):683–91.
15. Simpson L, Parsons R. PTEN: life as a tumor suppressor. Exp Cell Res 2001; 264(1):29–41.
16. Weng LP, Smith WM, Dahia PL, et al. PTEN suppresses breast cancer cell growth by phosphatase activity-dependent G1 arrest followed by cell death. Cancer Res 1999;59(22):5808–14.
17. Kanae Y, Endoh D, Yokota H, et al. Expression of the PTEN tumor suppressor gene in malignant mammary gland tumors of dogs. Am J Vet Res 2006;67(1): 127–33.
18. Koenig A, Bianco SR, Fosmire S, et al. Expression and significance of p53, rb, p21/waf-1, p16/ink-4a, and PTEN tumor suppressors in canine melanoma. Vet Pathol 2002;39(4):458–72.
19. Levine RA, Forest T, Smith C. Tumor suppressor PTEN is mutated in canine osteosarcoma cell lines and tumors. Vet Pathol 2002;39(3):372–8.
20. Ma J, Waxman DJ. Collaboration between hepatic and intratumoral prodrug activation in a P450 prodrug-activation gene therapy model for cancer treatment. Mol Cancer Ther 2007;6(11):2879–90.
21. Malumbres M, Barbacid M. RAS oncogenes: the first 30 years. Nat Rev Cancer 2003;3(6):459–65.
22. Dhillon AS, Kolch W. Oncogenic B-Raf mutations: crystal clear at last. Cancer Cell 2004;5(4):303–4.
23. Wan PT, Garnett MJ, Roe SM, et al. Mechanism of activation of the RAF-ERK signaling pathway by oncogenic mutations of B-RAF. Cell 2004;116(6):855–67.
24. Decker B, Parker HG, Dhawan D, et al. Homologous mutation to human BRAF V600E is common in naturally occurring canine bladder cancer–evidence for

a relevant model system and urine-based diagnostic test. Mol Cancer Res 2015;13(6):993–1002.
25. Brose MS, Volpe P, Feldman M, et al. BRAF and RAS mutations in human lung cancer and melanoma. Cancer Res 2002;62(23):6997–7000.
26. Galli SJ, Zsebo KM, Geissler EN. The kit ligand, stem cell factor. Adv Immunol 1994;55:1–95.
27. Downing S, Chien MB, Kass PH, et al. Prevalence and importance of internal tandem duplications in exons 11 and 12 of c-kit in mast cell tumors of dogs. Am J Vet Res 2002;63(12):1718–23.
28. London CA, Galli SJ, Yuuki T, et al. Spontaneous canine mast cell tumors express tandem duplications in the proto-oncogene c-kit. Exp Hematol 1999;27(4):689–97.
29. Zemke D, Yamini B, Yuzbasiyan-Gurkan V. Mutations in the juxtamembrane domain of c-KIT are associated with higher grade mast cell tumors in dogs. Vet Pathol 2002;39(5):529–35.
30. Demetri GD. Targeting the molecular pathophysiology of gastrointestinal stromal tumors with imatinib. Mechanisms, successes, and challenges to rational drug development. Hematol Oncol Clin North Am 2002;16(5):1115–24.
31. Demetri GD. Differential properties of current tyrosine kinase inhibitors in gastrointestinal stromal tumors. Semin Oncol 2011;38(Suppl 1):S10–9.
32. Frost D, Lasota J, Miettinen M. Gastrointestinal stromal tumors and leiomyomas in the dog: a histopathologic, immunohistochemical, and molecular genetic study of 50 cases. Vet Pathol 2003;40(1):42–54.
33. Iwai T, Yokota S, Nakao M, et al. Internal tandem duplication of the FLT3 gene and clinical evaluation in childhood acute myeloid leukemia. The Children's Cancer and Leukemia Study Group, Japan. Leukemia 1999;13(1):38–43.
34. Kondo M, Horibe K, Takahashi Y, et al. Prognostic value of internal tandem duplication of the FLT3 gene in childhood acute myelogenous leukemia. Med Pediatr Oncol 1999;33(6):525–9.
35. Nakao M, Yokota S, Iwai T, et al. Internal tandem duplication of the flt3 gene found in acute myeloid leukemia. Leukemia 1996;10(12):1911–8.
36. Yokota S, Kiyoi H, Nakao M, et al. Internal tandem duplication of the FLT3 gene is preferentially seen in acute myeloid leukemia and myelodysplastic syndrome among various hematological malignancies. A study on a large series of patients and cell lines. Leukemia 1997;11(10):1605–9.
37. Pao W, Chmielecki J. Rational, biologically based treatment of EGFR-mutant non-small-cell lung cancer. Nat Rev Cancer 2010;10(11):760–74.
38. Wen J, Fu J, Zhang W, et al. Genetic and epigenetic changes in lung carcinoma and their clinical implications. Mod Pathol 2011;24(7):932–43.
39. Pacey S, Banerji U, Judson I, et al. Hsp90 inhibitors in the clinic. Handb Exp Pharmacol 2006;(172):331–58.
40. Paik S, Hazan R, Fisher ER, et al. Pathologic findings from the National Surgical Adjuvant Breast and Bowel Project: prognostic significance of erbB-2 protein overexpression in primary breast cancer. J Clin Oncol 1990;8(1):103–12.
41. Slamon DJ, Clark GM, Wong SG, et al. Human breast cancer: correlation of relapse and survival with amplification of the HER-2/neu oncogene. Science 1987;235(4785):177–82.
42. Laskin JJ, Sandler AB. Epidermal growth factor receptor: a promising target in solid tumours. Cancer Treat Rev 2004;30(1):1–17.
43. Melo JV, Hughes TP, Apperley JF. Chronic myeloid leukemia. Hematology Am Soc Hematol Educ Program 2003;132–52.

44. Van Etten RA. Mechanisms of transformation by the BCR-ABL oncogene: new perspectives in the post-imatinib era. Leuk Res 2004;28(Suppl 1):S21–8.
45. Fosmire SP, Dickerson EB, Scott AM, et al. Canine malignant hemangiosarcoma as a model of primitive angiogenic endothelium. Lab Invest 2004;84(5):562–72.
46. Janz S. Myc translocations in B cell and plasma cell neoplasms. DNA Repair (Amst) 2006;5(9–10):1213–24.
47. Ekstrand AJ, James CD, Cavenee WK, et al. Genes for epidermal growth factor receptor, transforming growth factor alpha, and epidermal growth factor and their expression in human gliomas in vivo. Cancer Res 1991;51(8):2164–72.
48. Graeven U, Fiedler W, Karpinski S, et al. Melanoma-associated expression of vascular endothelial growth factor and its receptors FLT-1 and KDR. J Cancer Res Clin Oncol 1999;125(11):621–9.
49. Sciacca L, Costantino A, Pandini G, et al. Insulin receptor activation by IGF-II in breast cancers: evidence for a new autocrine/paracrine mechanism. Oncogene 1999;18(15):2471–9.
50. Zwick E, Bange J, Ullrich A. Receptor tyrosine kinases as targets for anticancer drugs. Trends Mol Med 2002;8(1):17–23.
51. Ferracini R, Angelini P, Cagliero E, et al. MET oncogene aberrant expression in canine osteosarcoma. J Orthop Res 2000;18(2):253–6.
52. Ferracini R, Di Renzo MF, Scotlandi K, et al. The Met/HGF receptor is over-expressed in human osteosarcomas and is activated by either a paracrine or an autocrine circuit. Oncogene 1995;10(4):739–49.
53. MacEwen EG, Kutzke J, Carew J, et al. c-Met tyrosine kinase receptor expression and function in human and canine osteosarcoma cells. Clin Exp Metastasis 2003;20(5):421–30.
54. Hernandez-Boluda JC, Cervantes F. Imatinib mesylate (Gleevec, Glivec): a new therapy for chronic myeloid leukemia and other malignancies. Drugs Today (Barc) 2002;38(9):601–13.
55. Druker BJ, Sawyers CL, Kantarjian H, et al. Activity of a specific inhibitor of the BCR-ABL tyrosine kinase in the blast crisis of chronic myeloid leukemia and acute lymphoblastic leukemia with the Philadelphia chromosome. N Engl J Med 2001;344(14):1038–42.
56. Druker BJ, Talpaz M, Resta DJ, et al. Efficacy and safety of a specific inhibitor of the BCR-ABL tyrosine kinase in chronic myeloid leukemia. N Engl J Med 2001; 344(14):1031–7.
57. Kantarjian HM, Talpaz M. Imatinib mesylate: clinical results in Philadelphia chromosome-positive leukemias. Semin Oncol 2001;28(5 Suppl 17):9–18.
58. Mauro MJ, Druker BJ. STI571: targeting BCR-ABL as therapy for CML. Oncologist 2001;6(3):233–8.
59. Sawyers CL. Rational therapeutic intervention in cancer: kinases as drug targets. Curr Opin Genet Dev 2002;12(1):111–5.
60. Duffaud F, Blay JY. Gastrointestinal stromal tumors: biology and treatment. Oncology 2003;65(3):187–97.
61. Heinrich MC, Corless CL, Duensing A, et al. PDGFRA activating mutations in gastrointestinal stromal tumors. Science 2003;299(5607):708–10.
62. Heinrich MC, Rubin BP, Longley BJ, et al. Biology and genetic aspects of gastrointestinal stromal tumors: KIT activation and cytogenetic alterations. Hum Pathol 2002;33(5):484–95.
63. Bunn PA Jr, Franklin W. Epidermal growth factor receptor expression, signal pathway, and inhibitors in non-small cell lung cancer. Semin Oncol 2002;29(5 Suppl 14):38–44.

64. Chmielecki J, Foo J, Oxnard GR, et al. Optimization of dosing for EGFR-mutant non-small cell lung cancer with evolutionary cancer modeling. Sci Transl Med 2011;3(90):90ra59.
65. Oxnard GR, Arcila ME, Chmielecki J, et al. New strategies in overcoming acquired resistance to epidermal growth factor receptor tyrosine kinase inhibitors in lung cancer. Clin Cancer Res 2011;17(17):5530–7.
66. Paez JG, Janne PA, Lee JC, et al. EGFR mutations in lung cancer: correlation with clinical response to gefitinib therapy. Science 2004;304(5676):1497–500.
67. Bang YJ. The potential for crizotinib in non-small cell lung cancer: a perspective review. Ther Adv Med Oncol 2011;3(6):279–91.
68. Shaw AT, Yeap BY, Solomon BJ, et al. Effect of crizotinib on overall survival in patients with advanced non-small-cell lung cancer harbouring ALK gene rearrangement: a retrospective analysis. Lancet Oncol 2011;12(11):1004–12.
69. Roskoski R Jr. Targeting oncogenic Raf protein-serine/threonine kinases in human cancers. Pharmacol Res 2018;135:239–58.
70. Vilar E, Perez-Garcia J, Tabernero J. Pushing the envelope in the mTOR pathway: the second generation of inhibitors. Mol Cancer Ther 2011;10(3): 395–403.
71. Gentile C, Martorana A, Lauria A, et al. Kinase inhibitors in multitargeted cancer therapy. Curr Med Chem 2017;24(16):1671–86.
72. Chow LQ, Eckhardt SG. Sunitinib: from rational design to clinical efficacy. J Clin Oncol 2007;25(7):884–96.
73. Mena AC, Pulido EG, Guillen-Ponce C. Understanding the molecular-based mechanism of action of the tyrosine kinase inhibitor: sunitinib. Anticancer Drugs 2010;21(Suppl 1):S3–11.
74. Papaetis GS, Syrigos KN. Sunitinib: a multitargeted receptor tyrosine kinase inhibitor in the era of molecular cancer therapies. BioDrugs 2009;23(6):377–89.
75. London CA, Hannah AL, Zadovoskaya R, et al. Phase I dose-escalating study of SU11654, a small molecule receptor tyrosine kinase inhibitor, in dogs with spontaneous malignancies. Clin Cancer Res 2003;9(7):2755–68.
76. Yancey MF, Merritt DA, Lesman SP, et al. Pharmacokinetic properties of toceranib phosphate (Palladia, SU11654), a novel tyrosine kinase inhibitor, in laboratory dogs and dogs with mast cell tumors. J Vet Pharmacol Ther 2010;33(2): 162–71.
77. Yancey MF, Merritt DA, White JA, et al. Distribution, metabolism, and excretion of toceranib phosphate (Palladia, SU11654), a novel tyrosine kinase inhibitor, in dogs. J Vet Pharmacol Ther 2010;33(2):154–61.
78. Pryer NK, Lee LB, Zadovaskaya R, et al. Proof of target for SU11654: inhibition of KIT phosphorylation in canine mast cell tumors. Clin Cancer Res 2003;9(15): 5729–34.
79. London C, Mathie T, Stingle N, et al. Preliminary evidence for biologic activity of toceranib phosphate (Palladia®) in solid tumours. Vet Comp Oncol 2012;10(3): 194–205.
80. Marcinowska A, Warland J, Brearley M, et al. A novel approach to treatment of lymphangiosarcoma in a boxer dog. J Small Anim Pract 2013;54(6):334–7.
81. Perez ML, Culver S, Owen JL, et al. Partial cytogenetic response with toceranib and prednisone treatment in a young dog with chronic monocytic leukemia. Anticancer Drugs 2013;24(10):1098–103.
82. Chon E, McCartan L, Kubicek LN, et al. Safety evaluation of combination toceranib phosphate (Palladia®) and piroxicam in tumour-bearing dogs (excluding

mast cell tumours): a phase I dose-finding study. Vet Comp Oncol 2012;10(3): 184–93.

83. Robat C, London C, Bunting L, et al. Safety evaluation of combination vinblastine and toceranib phosphate (Palladia) in dogs: a phase I dose-finding study. Vet Comp Oncol 2012;10(3):174–83.
84. Carlsten KS, London CA, Haney S, et al. Multicenter prospective trial of hypofractionated radiation treatment, toceranib, and prednisone for measurable canine mast cell tumors. J Vet Intern Med 2012;26(1):135–41.
85. Ehling TJ, Smith L, Farrelly J, et al. A multi-center VRTOG study examining the efficacy of toceranib phosphate (Palladia) as a primary and/or adjuvant agent for the treatment of canine nasal carcinoma. Proceedings from the Annual Conference of the Veterinary Cancer Society, Tysons Corner, Virginia, USA. October 15–17, 2015.
86. Mitchell L, Thamm DH, Biller BJ. Clinical and immunomodulatory effects of toceranib combined with low-dose cyclophosphamide in dogs with cancer. J Vet Intern Med 2012;26(2):355–62.
87. London CA, Gardner HL, Mathie T, et al. Impact of toceranib/piroxicam/cyclophosphamide maintenance therapy on outcome of dogs with appendicular osteosarcoma following amputation and carboplatin chemotherapy: a multi-institutional study. PLoS One 2015;10(4):e0124889.
88. Gardner HL, London CA, Portela RA, et al. Maintenance therapy with toceranib following doxorubicin-based chemotherapy for canine splenic hemangiosarcoma. BMC Vet Res 2015;11:131.
89. Berger EP, Johannes CM, Post GS, et al. Retrospective evaluation of toceranib phosphate (Palladia) use in cats with mast cell neoplasia. J Feline Med Surg 2018;20(2):95–102.
90. Harper A, Blackwood L. Toxicity and response in cats with neoplasia treated with toceranib phosphate. J Feline Med Surg 2017;19(6):619–23.
91. Merrick CH, Pierro J, Schleis SE, et al. Retrospective evaluation of toceranib phosphate (Palladia(R)) toxicity in cats. Vet Comp Oncol 2017;15(3):710–7.
92. Olmsted GA, Farrelly J, Post GS, et al. Tolerability of toceranib phosphate (Palladia) when used in conjunction with other therapies in 35 cats with feline oral squamous cell carcinoma: 2009-2013. J Feline Med Surg 2017;19(6): 568–75.
93. Wiles V, Hohenhaus A, Lamb K, et al. Retrospective evaluation of toceranib phosphate (Palladia) in cats with oral squamous cell carcinoma. J Feline Med Surg 2017;19(2):185–93.
94. Holtermann N, Kiupel M, Hirschberger J. The tyrosine kinase inhibitor toceranib in feline injection site sarcoma: efficacy and side effects. Vet Comp Oncol 2017; 15(2):632–40.
95. Hahn KA, Legendre AM, Shaw NG, et al. Evaluation of 12- and 24-month survival rates after treatment with masitinib in dogs with nonresectable mast cell tumors. Am J Vet Res 2010;71(11):1354–61.
96. Smrkovski OA, Essick L, Rohrbach BW, et al. Masitinib mesylate for metastatic and non-resectable canine cutaneous mast cell tumours. Vet Comp Oncol 2015; 13(3):314–21.
97. Isotani M, Ishida N, Tominaga M, et al. Effect of tyrosine kinase inhibition by imatinib mesylate on mast cell tumors in dogs. J Vet Intern Med 2008;22(4):985–8.
98. Marconato L, Bettini G, Giacoboni C, et al. Clinicopathological features and outcome for dogs with mast cell tumors and bone marrow involvement. J Vet Intern Med 2008;22(4):1001–7.

99. Yamada O, Kobayashi M, Sugisaki O, et al. Imatinib elicited a favorable response in a dog with a mast cell tumor carrying a c-kit c.1523A>T mutation via suppression of constitutive KIT activation. Vet Immunol Immunopathol 2011;142(1–2):101–6.
100. Isotani M, Tamura K, Yagihara H, et al. Identification of a c-kit exon 8 internal tandem duplication in a feline mast cell tumor case and its favorable response to the tyrosine kinase inhibitor imatinib mesylate. Vet Immunol Immunopathol 2006;114(1–2):168–72.
101. Isotani M, Yamada O, Lachowicz JL, et al. Mutations in the fifth immunoglobulin-like domain of kit are common and potentially sensitive to imatinib mesylate in feline mast cell tumours. Br J Haematol 2010;148(1):144–53.
102. Gardner HL, Rippy SB, Bear MD, et al. Phase I/II evaluation of RV1001, a novel PI3Kdelta inhibitor, in spontaneous canine lymphoma. PLoS One 2018;13(4): e0195357.
103. Honigberg LA, Smith AM, Sirisawad M, et al. The Bruton tyrosine kinase inhibitor PCI-32765 blocks B-cell activation and is efficacious in models of autoimmune disease and B-cell malignancy. Proc Natl Acad Sci U S A 2010;107(29): 13075–80.
104. Harrington BK, Gardner HL, Izumi R, et al. Preclinical evaluation of the novel BTK inhibitor acalabrutinib in canine models of B-cell non-Hodgkin lymphoma. PLoS One 2016;11(7):e0159607.
105. Xu D, Grishin NV, Chook YM. NESdb: a database of NES-containing CRM1 cargoes. Mol Biol Cell 2012;23(18):3673–6.
106. Daelemans D, Costes SV, Lockett S, et al. Kinetic and molecular analysis of nuclear export factor CRM1 association with its cargo in vivo. Mol Cell Biol 2005; 25(2):728–39.
107. Fornerod M, Ohno M, Yoshida M, et al. CRM1 is an export receptor for leucine-rich nuclear export signals. Cell 1997;90(6):1051–60.
108. Nguyen KT, Holloway MP, Altura RA. The CRM1 nuclear export protein in normal development and disease. Int J Biochem Mol Biol 2012;3(2):137–51.
109. Turner JG, Dawson J, Sullivan DM. Nuclear export of proteins and drug resistance in cancer. Biochem Pharmacol 2012;83(8):1021–32.
110. Turner JG, Sullivan DM. CRM1-mediated nuclear export of proteins and drug resistance in cancer. Curr Med Chem 2008;15(26):2648–55.
111. Azmi AS, Aboukameel A, Bao B, et al. Selective inhibitors of nuclear export block pancreatic cancer cell proliferation and reduce tumor growth in mice. Gastroenterology 2013;144(2):447–56.
112. McCauley D, Landesman Y, Senapedis W, et al. Preclinical evaluation of selective inhibitors of nuclear export (SINE) in basal-like breast cancer (BLBC). J Clin Oncol 2012;30(Suppl) [abstract: 1055].
113. Lapalombella R, Sun Q, Williams K, et al. Selective inhibitors of nuclear export show that CRM1/XPO1 is a target in chronic lymphocytic leukemia. Blood 2012;120(23):4621–34.
114. Etchin J, Sun Q, Kentsis A, et al. Antileukemic activity of nuclear export inhibitors that spare normal hematopoietic cells. Leukemia 2013;27(1):66–74.
115. London CA, Bernabe LF, Barnard S, et al. Preclinical evaluation of the novel, orally bioavailable Selective Inhibitor of Nuclear Export (SINE) KPT-335 in spontaneous canine cancer: results of a phase I study. PLoS One 2014;9(2):e87585.
116. Sadowski AR, Gardner HL, Borgatti A, et al. Phase II study of the oral selective inhibitor of nuclear export (SINE) KPT-335 (verdinexor) in dogs with lymphoma. BMC Vet Res 2018;14(1):250.

117. Choi HK, Lee K. Recent updates on the development of ganetespib as a Hsp90 inhibitor. Arch Pharm Res 2012;35(11):1855–9.
118. London CA, Bear MD, McCleese J, et al. Phase I evaluation of STA-1474, a prodrug of the novel HSP90 inhibitor ganetespib, in dogs with spontaneous cancer. PLoS One 2011;6(11):e27018.
119. London CA, Acquaviva J, Smith DL, et al. Consecutive day HSP90 inhibitor administration improves efficacy in murine models of KIT-driven malignancies and canine mast cell tumors. Clin Cancer Res 2018;24(24):6396–407.
120. Ropero S, Esteller M. The role of histone deacetylases (HDACs) in human cancer. Mol Oncol 2007;1(1):19–25.
121. Feinberg AP, Tycko B. The history of cancer epigenetics. Nat Rev Cancer 2004; 4(2):143–53.
122. Zhu P, Martin E, Mengwasser J, et al. Induction of HDAC2 expression upon loss of APC in colorectal tumorigenesis. Cancer Cell 2004;5(5):455–63.
123. Cohen LA, Powers B, Amin S, et al. Treatment of canine haemangiosarcoma with suberoylanilide hydroxamic acid, a histone deacetylase inhibitor. Vet Comp Oncol 2004;2(4):243–8.
124. Wittenburg LA, Gustafson DL, Thamm DH. Phase I pharmacokinetic and pharmacodynamic evaluation of combined valproic acid/doxorubicin treatment in dogs with spontaneous cancer. Clin Cancer Res 2010;16(19):4832–42.
125. Rosenzweig SA. Acquired resistance to drugs targeting receptor tyrosine kinases. Biochem Pharmacol 2012;83(8):1041–8.

Update in Veterinary Radiation Oncology

Focus on Stereotactic Radiation Therapy

Michael W. Nolan, DVM, PhD*, Tracy L. Gieger, DVM

KEYWORDS

- Radiotherapy • Radiosurgery • Brain tumors • Nasal tumors • Osteosarcoma
- Radiobiology

KEY POINTS

- Stereotactic radiation therapy (SRT) requires accurate and precise delivery of large radiation doses to a well-defined target in few treatment sessions.
- Common aliases include stereotactic radiosurgery, stereotactic body radiotherapy, stereotactic ablative radiotherapy, radiosurgery, CyberKnife, and Gamma Knife.
- SRT is increasingly accessible and can be delivered with palliative or definitive intent.
- Common indications include nasal, brain, and appendicular tumors. Emerging uses include oral, lung, prostate, and adrenal tumors.
- Even when technically feasible, SRT is not always the optimal radiation treatment modality.

INTRODUCTION

Few dogs and cats with cancer are treated with radiotherapy (RT), despite increasing availability.[1] Pet owners cite finances, distance required to travel to veterinary RT centers, protracted treatment schedules, and the potential for displeasing side effects as deterrents. Stereotactic radiotherapy (SRT) overcomes several of these barriers. With SRT, large doses of radiation are carefully sculpted to match the shape of the target (tumor) and then delivered with exacting precision. This allows intensive courses of cancer treatment to be compressed into 5 or fewer treatment sessions, often with minimal acute toxicity. The purpose of this article is to review key features of SRT's unique radiobiology, describe the evidence base for common and emerging applications of SRT applications, and discuss controversies in the use of SRT.

Disclosure Statement: Neither Dr M.W. Nolan nor Dr T.L.Gieger have relevant commercial or financial conflicts of interest or funding sources that are relevant to this article.
Department of Clinical Sciences, College of Veterinary Medicine, North Carolina State University, 1060 William Moore Drive, Raleigh, NC 27607, USA
* Corresponding author.
E-mail address: mwnolan@ncsu.edu

Vet Clin Small Anim 49 (2019) 933–947
https://doi.org/10.1016/j.cvsm.2019.05.001
vetsmall.theclinics.com

PHYSICS AND BIOLOGY OF STEREOTACTIC RADIOTHERAPY

SRT involves delivery of large fractional doses of radiation to a well-defined target with extreme accuracy (stereotaxis) and with a steep radiation dose gradient that escalates dose in the target, while minimizing dose in adjacent healthy tissues.

A variety of technologies have been developed for SRT planning and delivery. Beginning in 1951, Lars Leksell developed the Gamma Knife system, which combines a stereotactic head frame with 179 sealed cobalt-60 sources that can be collimated to produce favorable radiation dose distributions.[2,3] The Gamma Knife remains in use today. CyberKnife represents another approach, wherein a 6-MV linear accelerator (linac) is mounted on a robotic arm that can literally dance around the patient. Hundreds of small radiation beamlets are delivered from multiple angles and converge on the tumor, whose location is verified with submillimeter accuracy by matching bony landmarks and/or intratumoral gold fiducial markers using orthogonal radiography. Conventional C-arm linacs can also be modified to allow SRT. The best-accepted methodology involves use of either intensity-modulated radiotherapy (IMRT) or volumetric modulated arc therapy (VMAT) plans to achieve adequate conformity and dose gradients, and cone beam computed tomography (CBCT)-based image guidance to achieve stereotaxis. Regardless of the mechanisms used for treatment planning and delivery, equipment that is designed for SRT will generally produce similar dosimetric and clinical outcomes.

In addition to the various mechanical SRT systems, several acronyms are also used to describe this therapeutic modality:

- Stereotactic radiosurgery (SRS) refers to a single fraction protocol, often limited to a central nervous system (CNS) target.
- Stereotactic body radiotherapy (SBRT) refers to treatment of a non-CNS target.[2]
- The term "stereotactic ablative body radiotherapy" reflects the notion that targeted, high-dose radiation can be used to "ablate" a tissue (ie, render it nonfunctional). This concept is founded in the radiobiologic basis of SRT and how it is thought to differ from conventional, finely fractionated radiotherapy (FRT).[3]

In classic radiobiology, DNA is considered the target of ionizing radiation. Unrepaired DNA double-strand breaks halt tumor growth by preventing cell cycle progression and/or inducing cell death. In clinical practice, a margin of normal tissue has conventionally been included in the treatment field to account for microscopic tumor extension, and an additional margin is used to account for inter- and intrafraction motion, comprising the planning target volume (PTV). A homogeneous dose of radiation is then prescribed to the PTV. Even with highly conformal treatment plans, that approach results in delivery of equal doses of radiation to both tumor and normal tissues that lie within the PTV. In FRT, repair of sublethal DNA damage and repopulation of cells between radiation fractions protect normal tissues. Between doses of FRT, reoxygenation of previously hypoxic tumor and redistribution of surviving tumor cells to more sensitive phases of the cell cycle enhance tumor control. The impact of these 4 Rs (repair, repopulation, reoxygenation, and redistribution) can be seen in experiments performed to determine radiation dose-response relationships in vitro. Resultant cell survival curves can be mathematically modeled. The linear-quadratic (LQ) model predicts that for any given dose of radiation, delivery via large fractional doses will be associated with a higher risk of severe late radiation toxicity than if the dose had been given in multiple smaller dose fractions. That is particularly true in certain so-called late-responding normal tissues, such as the spinal cord, heart, bones, and peripheral nerves, which are all characterized by a low alpha-to-beta ratio. Rather than biological sparing, SRT excludes as much normal tissue from the PTV as possible and physically shields tissues that are immediately adjacent. This approach enables delivery of large dose fractions (>6 Gy vs 2.5–3 Gy fractions that are typically used in FRT). Interestingly, clinical and experimental outcomes of SRT often exceed that which would be predicted by LQ modeling. Regardless of whether one trusts the LQ model in the setting of severely hypofractionated RT (>6–8 Gy fractions), it is increasingly clear that ionizing radiation has differential effects at high versus low fractional doses.

SRT biology is perhaps most unique in the tumor microenvironment. Kolesnick and Fuks demonstrated that high-dose irradiation induces translocation of endothelial cell acid sphingomyelinase, which hydrolyzes sphingomyelin to generate ceramide, thus initiating apoptosis and microvascularcollapse.[4] Their results have not been replicated, and conflicting data call into question the importance of this endothelial response.[5] Regardless of mechanism, there are numerous other reports describing severe vascular destruction and dysfunction at doses of greater than or equal to 10 Gy in experimental rodent tumors.[6,7] This vascular dysfunction causes tumor hypoxia that can impair homologous recombination repair of radiation-induced DNA double-strand breaks and produce secondary cell killing.[8] In addition to vascular effects, it is also well established that radiation induces immunogenic cell death and primes T cells to tumor antigens.[9,10] The magnitude and character of these effects are influenced by radiation dose, and interestingly, the "optimal" immunogenic dose of radiation is not necessarily the highest radiation dose.[11] Recent preclinical data indicate that systemic effects of localized radiation are mediated by CD8+ T cells and interferon receptors, but that 1 or 3 daily doses of 8 Gy improve outcomes as compared with single doses of 20 to 30 Gy or less than 8 Gy.[12]

Independent of tumor microenvironment effects, high radiation dose intensity is another key difference between SRT and FRT. Large (6–9 Gy) dose fractions have long been used in palliative care for veterinary patients, but those fractions have most often been delivered at 7-day intervals. Even though the size of SRT dose fractions is similar, SRT uses much shorter (24–48 hour) intrafraction intervals. This difference is impactful because tumors are continually growing. Hence, reduction in total treatment time reduces the number of tumor cells that are "seen" by a given dose of radiation, thus improving the expected efficacy of treatment on a per-Gray basis.

CLINICAL APPROACH TO STEREOTACTIC RADIOTHERAPY

The key components of SRT include (1) clinical evaluation to ensure suitability, (2) optimizing patient immobilization and respiratory motion to enable reproducible positioning, (3) delineating tumor vs nontumor compartments via imaging, (4) treatment planning that generates steep dose gradients between organs at risk (OAR) and target tissues, and (5) verification of precise patient position via on-board imaging, before (6) accurate dose delivery.[4] In veterinary medicine, use of SRT is largely anecdotal, with recent publications focusing on a few specific tumor types.

CLINICAL DATA: BRAIN TUMORS

Canine and feline brain tumors are frequently treated with SRT; recent publications have documented outcomes for individual tumor types (**Table 1**). Survival times are generally similar when comparing SRT and FRT, but it remains unclear whether or not SRT causes more toxicity. Two publications report that approximately one-third of dogs receiving SRT for intracranial meningioma experience neurologic decline in the first 6 months after treatment.[13,14] Although most dogs in those studies improved (typically with steroid administration), these events were sometimes fatal. In most

Table 1
Summary of recent publications regarding stereotactic radiotherapy for intracranial tumors in dogs

Reference	Tumor Type	# Dogs	Radiation Prescription	Overall Survival Time	Toxicity	Comments
Swift et al,[41] 2017	Trigeminal nerve sheath tumor	27 dogs (15 treated with SRT)	8 Gy × 3 = 24 Gy 10 Gy × 3 = 30 Gy	Median 441 d (95% CI 260–518) for dogs treated with SRT	Some dogs developed facial pain after treatment	Because of overlap in the 95% CI between treated and untreated dogs, unknown benefit of SRT as compared with no treatment; clinical signs such as facial pain and ocular deficits did not resolve after treatment in most dogs
Dolera et al,[42] 2018	Trigeminal nerve sheath tumor	7	7.4 Gy × 5 = 37 Gy	Median 952 d (95% CI, 543–1361d)	None reported	MRI after irradiation in all dogs; 1 CR, 4 PR, 2 SD; 4/7 dogs had extracranial extension of the tumor; clinical signs did not resolve in most dogs
Hansen et al,[43] 2016	Trigeminal nerve sheath tumor	8	8 Gy × 3 = 24 Gy	Median 324 d (95% CI: 99–975)	None reported. 6/8 dogs were euthanized due to seizures and progressive neurologic signs, and the remaining 2 dogs experienced accident-related death	Median disease-specific survival time: 745 d

Dolera et al,[44] 2018	Glioma	42	4.2 Gy × 10 = 42 Gy 5.3 Gy × 7 = 37 Gy 6.6 Gy× 5 = 33 Gy 7 Gy× 5 = 35 Gy	RT alone: 50% alive at 1 y, 41% at 2 y RT + temozolomide (TMZ): 65% alive at 1 y, 40% at 2 y	Minimal	Radiation dose was scaled based on tumor grade and volume 22 dogs RT alone; 20 RT + TMZ; no difference in outcomes; RT dose based on size of tumor relative to normal brain
Griffin et al,[14] 2016	Meningioma	30	8 Gy× 3 = 24 Gy	Median 561 d (95% CI 423–875d), 60.8% A1 year survival, 33.2% 2 y	37% worsened neurologically 3–16 wk after SRT; 13% died of neurologic progression within 6 mo	Volume of normal brain treated predicted death
Kelsey et al,[13] 2018	Meningioma	32	16 Gy× 1 = 16 Gy	Median 519 d (95% CI 330–708d), 64% 1 y survival, 24% 2 y	31% worsened neurologically within 6 mo after SRT; 10% died of neuroprogression	Infratentorial tumors and higher-gradient index predicted shorter survival time
Dolera et al,[45] 2018	Meningioma	39 (33 with encephalic meningioma, 6 spinal meningioma)	6.6 Gy × 5 = 33 Gy	2-y overall survival: 74.3%	One dog had mild neurotoxicity	2-y disease-specific survival: 97.4%. 49% of dogs had a partial or complete response at 2 y, when considering both objective follow-up imaging data and clinical status in response evaluation.

Abbreviations: CI, confidence interval; CR, complete response; PR, partial response; RT, radiation therapy; SD, stable disease.

cases, early delayed radiation toxicity was suspected, as opposed to tumor progression, but this could not be confirmed due to lack of reimaging and/or necropsy (**Fig. 1**). It is critical that practitioners treating brain tumors with SRT continue working to identify predictors of toxicity and oncologic response. Future studies should ideally include regularly scheduled and prospectively collected neurologic outcomes assessments/surveys and follow-up imaging and increased use of necropsy such that clinical findings can be correlated with imaging and histopathology data.

Nonresectable intracranial tumors and recurrent feline meningioma can be treated with SRT. Pituitary tumors also commonly affect cats. They typically cause acromegaly with insulin-resistant diabetes mellitus (DM). In a study of 53 cats with insulin-dependent DM and pituitary adenomas, SRT was prescribed at 6 to 17 Gy per fraction for a total dose of 17 to 28 Gy.[15] Adverse effects after SRT occurred in 18% and were typically mild. Hypothyroidism developed in 14% of the cats, typically 4 to 6 months after SRT. Impressively, 95% of cats had decreased insulin requirements (median time to lowest insulin dose was 9.5 months), with 32% achieving diabetic remission. The overall median survival time was 1072 days. Tumor volume did not correlate with survival time.

CLINICAL DATA: NASAL TUMORS

External beam megavoltage RT is the cornerstone of management for canine nonlymphomatous sinonasal tumors. A recent systematic review found that conventional palliative-intent RT protocols were associated with median overall survival times

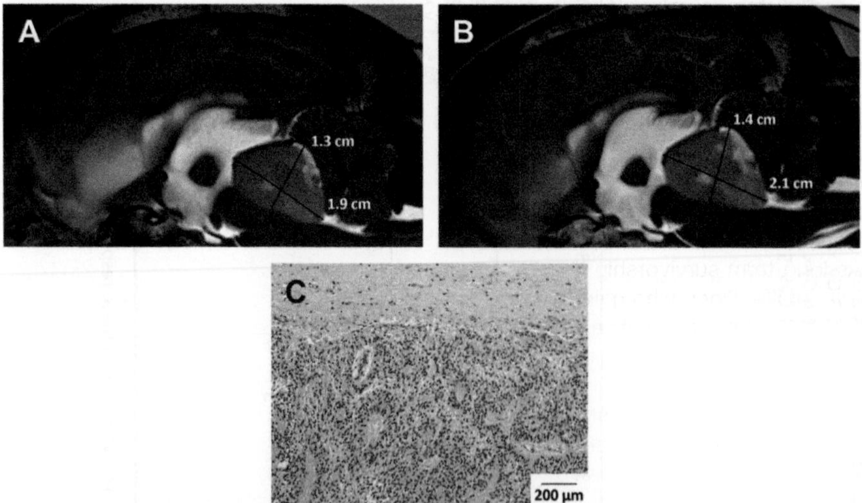

Fig. 1. In the absence of cross-sectional imaging to prove tumor progression, neurologic decline within the first few months after SRT/SRS is typically attributed to early delayed neuro-radiotoxicity in retrospective studies. Objective data are needed to better characterize outcomes. (*A*) A midbrain tumor that was treated with SRS. The dog's neurologic signs worsened a month after SRS and failed to improve with symptomatic treatment for early delayed neurotoxicity. (*B*) Recheck MRI 2 months after SRS revealed tumor enlargement. Progression and pseudoprogression were differential diagnoses. (*C*). Necropsy revealed ependymoma without intratumoral edema, inflammation or degeneration, and without radiation-induced changes in adjacent neuroparenchyma. (*Courtesy of* M. Kent, DVM, Athens, GA.)

ranging from 4.8 to 16.8 months (median 8.5 months), whereas survival ranged from 10.4 to 19.1 months (median 14.0 months) after treatment with definitive-intent FRT.[16]

Stereotactic RT is increasingly used (**Table 2**). Treatment causes few/mild acute side effects. But comparing the oncologic outcomes achieved with SRT versus conventional techniques is confusing. To date, 3 papers have been published.[17–19] Although the median prescribed doses (27–30 Gy) were similar, the reported median overall survival times are strikingly different. This may be related to differences in both irradiation protocols and case characteristics. Both Glasser (2014) and Gieger (2018) used modest fractionation (3-fraction SRT), which should allow improved oxygenation of previously hypoxic tumor cells, redistribution of surviving tumor cells to more sensitive phases of the cell cycle, and generation of a more favorable immune landscape within the irradiated tumor, as compared with the single fraction protocols used by Kubicek and colleagues. There are also differences in how radiation was prescribed. For example, Glasser and colleagues normalized their radiation plans such that the prescribed dose was delivered to at least 95% of the gross tumor volume (GTV), whereas Gieger and Nolan prescribed dose to 99% of the GTV. There were also qualitative differences in how the GTVs were identified, as was recently highlighted by Christensen and colleagues (2016).[20] Case selection may have also influenced these differences in survival. For example, some investigators have associated nasal chondrosarcoma with longer survival times after irradiation versus other tumor types. This could have contributed to longer survival in the cohort treated by Gieger and Nolan; 28% of those dogs had chondrosarcoma, versus 7% to 10% in the other 2 studies. To the contrary, Kubicek's paper included far fewer dogs with stage IV tumors as compared with either Glasser or Gieger (18% vs 42%–45%). If the current nasal tumor staging system is valuable in prognostication of dogs treated with SRT, one would expect Kubicek to have had superior results as compared with Glasser and Gieger. This paradox underscores the need to critically reevaluate the prognostic significance of various patient and tumor characteristics in the context of SRT, as it may be inappropriate to extrapolate knowledge from FRT to SRT. Ultimately, there is not yet enough high-level evidence to consider any one SRT protocol as the new "gold standard" in the care of dogs with nasal cancer. However, it does seem that there is enough evidence to support continued use of certain SRT protocols as a reasonable alternative to FRT.

As long-term survivorship improves, careful attention must be paid to maximizing quality of life. Dogs who gain excellent tumor control from SRT are at risk for developing one or more significant complications of either the disease or its treatment. For example, many dogs will experience chronic rhinosinusitis that develops secondary to tumor and/or radiation-induced damage to the mucociliary apparatus (**Fig. 2**). Other dogs may develop osteoradionecrosis and/or dermal atrophy with subsequent formation of either oronasal or nasocutaneous fistulae. Careful documentation will help determine the actual risk of such complications, and formal scientific investigation is needed to develop strategies that effectively prevent or treat these conditions.

CLINICAL DATA: THORACIC AND ABDOMINAL CAVITY MALIGNANCIES

Intrathoracic tumors present a unique challenge for RT planning and delivery due to constant cardiac and thoracic cavity movement and intimate association of tumors with the great vessels, trachea, esophagus, and heart (which are generally very tolerant of FRT but become dose-limiting in SRT). The process of RT planning begins with a CT scan, for which considerations to delineate organs at risk (such as the esophagus, which may be delineated with assistance of a radiopaque esophageal

Table 2
Overview of the published literature describing stereotactic radiotherapy for canine sinonasal tumors

		Treatment Techniques					
Author	**# Dogs**	**Radiation Dose**	**Position Verification**	**Delivery**	**Response Rate**	**Severe (Late) Adverse Events**	**Median Overall Survival Time**
Glasser et al,[18] 2014	19	24–36 Gy (3 fractions)	Implanted gold fiducials and orthogonal planar radiography	CyberKnife	95% (Subjective)	N = 7 dogs • Oronasal fistula (1) • Seizures (6)	13.1 mo
Kubicek et al,[17] 2016	57	12.5–28 Gy (1 fraction)	Bite plate with array of infrared light-emitting diodes	Cone-based SRT	Not reported	N = 7 dogs • Osteonecrosis (6) • Seizures (2)	8.5 mo
Gieger et al,[19] 2018	29	30 Gy (3 fractions)	CBCT	Intensity-modulated SRT	100% (Subjective); 95% (Objective)	N = 7 dogs • Fistulas (3) • CNS signs (2) • Fungal rhinitis (2)	19.3 mo

Adapted from Ref.[46]

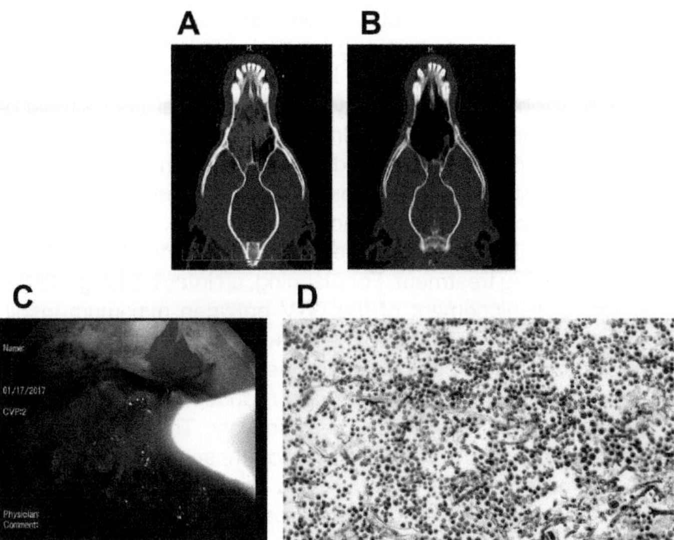

Fig. 2. Chronic rhinitis and sinusitis are relatively common in dogs with nasal tumors that have excellent tumor control after SRT. Sterile inflammation is possible, but secondary infection (with or without osteomyelitis) must also be considered. (*A*) A nasal carcinoma that was treated with SRT. Clinical signs improved, but nasal discharge recurred 22 months later. (*B*) Recheck CT revealed complete resolution of the tumor with progressive osteolysis and complete loss of the nasal septum. (*C*) Rhinoscopy revealed plaques. (*D*) Histopathology revealed pigmented fungal spores and hyphae. Infection resolved with clotrimazole infusions.

feeding tube) as well as management of respiratory motion (using techniques such as high-frequency jet ventilation or respiratory neuroparalytics and breath holding) should be made in advance of the scan.[21]

There is a paucity of literature documenting outcomes with irradiation of intrathoracic tumors in veterinary patients, and a gold standard for treatment of nonsurgically resectable tumors does not exist. In a recent publication, 6 dogs with presumed (N = 5) or confirmed (N = 1) chemodectomas were treated with SBRT (30 Gy in 3 fractions delivered in 3–5 days).[22] Treatments were planned with IMRT, and CBCT was used to verify patient positioning before irradiation. Respiratory motion was managed with neuroparalytics (N = 3) or jet ventilation (N = 3; 180 breaths/minute). The tumor volume decreased by 30% to 70% in all 4 dogs that were reimaged after treatment. Possible treatment-associated toxicities included periprocedural esophageal reflux, cough, tachyarrhythmias, and congestive heart failure. Two dogs died suddenly at 150 and 294 days after SBRT, and the other 4 lived greater than 408 days after treatment. Arrhythmias, heart failure, and sudden death may be attributable to the tumor or radiation injury to the heart. Thus, until more is known about potential treatment-related morbidity and mortality, a conservative approach to case selection is considered prudent. Delaying treatment may be a consideration for tumors that are slow-growing (as assessed by periodic volumetric imaging) and for dogs that are asymptomatic. Also, assessing for arrhythmias via Holter monitor before and after SBRT should be part of the treatment plan. In addition to chemodectomas, primary lung tumors, intrathoracic sarcomas, thymomas and cardiac hemangiosarcomas, and oligometastatic lung tumors have also been treated with SBRT at the authors' institution. Of note, patients with pleural or pericardial effusion may not be candidates for SBRT, because dynamic changes in fluid volumes over the course of treatment can affect dosimetry of radiation treatment plans and respiratory motion management.

Abdomino-pelvic malignancies are also increasingly managed with SBRT. As with the thorax, respiratory motion and proximity to critical normal tissues must be carefully considered for cranial abdominal tumors. In a recent publication describing SBRT for canine adrenocortical tumors, 3/9 dogs had cortisol-secreting tumors, and 6/9 tumors were discovered incidentally.[23] Radiation prescriptions ranged from 30 to 45 Gy in 3 to 5 daily fractions; dose escalations were made based on proximity of the target to OAR. To limit thoracic excursions, the dogs were positioned in lateral recumbency and the abdomen was taped during treatment. For planning, an internal margin (IM) was calculated by determining displacement of the GTV between maximum inspiration and expiration. A setup margin was added to the IM + GTV to create a PTV. No significant side effects were noted. Whole body CT scans were performed 2, 4, and 6 months after SBRT. All dogs had progressive tumor size reduction, with a mean decrease in diameter and volume of 32% and 30%, respectively. The overall median survival time following treatment was 1030 days. Based on these results, treatment of nonresectable adrenal tumors with SBRT could be a consideration. Anecdotally, clinical benefit has been achieved by treatment of retroperitoneal sarcomas, solitary hepatocellular carcinoma, renal cell carcinoma, and prostate-confined neoplasms with SBRT.

Duration of the interfraction interval is an important consideration for abdominopelvic irradiation. Men with prostate cancer are frequently treated with 5 fraction SBRT protocols, to a total of 35 to 36.25 Gy. Their risk of late colorectal complication is decreased by separation of radiation dose fractions by at least 36 hours, and[24] this is done without any apparent impact on tumor control. Similar risk reduction has been reported for dogs and is achieved by decreasing the likelihood of a consequential late effect (ie, the unusual situation wherein a late effect arises secondary to a severe acute effect).[25,26] Recall, however, that total treatment time is not a recognized risk factor for classic late toxicities. Thus, although prolongation of the interfraction interval may prove beneficial for patients when the tumor abuts acutely responding tissue, and when the requisite dose for tumor control exceeds the tolerance of that normal tissue, this strategy is unlikely to provide benefit for patients undergoing SRT at sites such as the brain.

CLINICAL DATA: BONE TUMORS

Although the "gold standard" for treatment of osteosarcoma (OSA) remains complete surgical excision followed by chemotherapy, RT can be an appealing alternative in certain cases. The use of high fractional doses in SBRT may theoretically provide improved tumor control versus FRT, because OSA is thought to be a tumor with a low alpha-to-beta ratio. SBRT may in fact provide a locally curative limb-salvage option.[27,28] Most suitable for SBRT are those dogs who are poor candidates for limb amputation or whose owners decline amputation. It is also a reasonable option for nonresectable axial bone tumors.

Stereotactic RT anecdotally provides potent and lasting analgesia in most dogs with appendicular OSA. Aside from distant metastasis, the biggest concern after SBRT is early treatment failure due to pathologic limb fracture, which generally necessitates amputation, repair, or euthanasia.[29] In a study by Kubicek and colleagues,[30] 46 dogs were treated with SBRT (37.5–52.5 Gy in a single fraction), and 29 dogs (63%) developed fractures, at a median of 5.9 months after irradiation, which is higher than expected for dogs managed without RT.[31] This may be a result of tumor progression after SRT or may reflect increased strain on the limb as activity levels improve with RT-induced analgesia. Boston and colleagues[32] described surgical attempts to prophylactically stabilize limbs and thus reduce fracture risk, but due to their high rate of complications, this is not recommended. Other strategies for improving bone integrity are desperately needed. Until then, careful case selection is paramount. The paper by Kubicek and colleagues[30] identified subchondral bone involvement as a predictor of early fracture (at a median of 4.2 months vs 16.3 months for dogs without). In that study, the overall median survival time of all treated dogs was 9.7 months, which is similar to outcomes achieved with amputation plus carboplatin (10–12 months). Of the dogs that developed fractures, 38% were euthanized and others were treated with amputation or were lost to follow-up. The median survival time of dogs treated with amputation was 13 months following fracture.

A recent case series describes 9 dogs with primary or metastatic vertebral OSA that were treated with SBRT (13.5–36 Gy in 1–5 fractions).[33] Five of six dogs with spinal pain experienced analgesia, with a median clinical response duration of 77 days. The overall survival time for these 9 dogs was 139 days. The investigators acknowledged the difficulty of trying to dosimetrically spare the spinal cord adjacent to the tumor (to reduce risk of radiation-induced myelopathy as a potential late effect) while simultaneously delivering a dose of RT that would be sufficient to afford durable tumor control. Although standard dose tolerance recommendations are often used in SBRT prescriptions, recent animal model data suggest those recommendations may be too conservative and that cautious dose escalation for spinal tumors should be tolerable.[34,35]

CONTROVERSIES IN STEREOTACTIC RADIOTHERAPY

There are significant differences of opinion with regard to optimal application of SRT. Here, some of the most interesting controversies have been summarized.

What Is the Minimum Requirement for Safe and Effective Stereotactic Radiotherapy Delivery?

A growing number of veterinary RT centers have acquired equipment that is designed for SRT planning and delivery. Other centers are meeting the demand by adapting and upgrading older technologies.[36] It is important for clinicians to be aware that it is not simply a matter of combining IMRT with image guidance that enables SRT. SRT treatments require different quality assurance tests and linac tolerances; for example, per the American Association of Physicists in Medicine Task Group report 142, stricter tolerance limits exist for imaging (eg, CBCT), couch position indicators and lasers, and coincidence of the mechanical and radiation isocenters for SRS/SBRT versus non-SRS/SBRT.[37] In addition, target dose conformity and steepness of dose gradients that are acceptable for full-course IMRT may be insufficient for SRT. There is also new anatomy that needs to be learned. For example, the optic chiasm is not commonly contoured for full-course RT but is routinely drawn for SRT of certain calvarial targets. Guidelines for normal tissue contouring are increasingly available to aid practitioners as they learn SRTplanning.[38] Finally, although planar imaging may be sufficient for localization of certain osseous targets, the limitations of such imaging must be carefully considered. For example, the prostate translates in the cranial-to-caudal direction depending on bladder filling. Thus, use of the pelvic bones as a surrogate for prostate location would be insufficient, unless a large expansion of the target volume is used to account for substantial potential setup error. This could be overcome by using intratumorally implanted fiducial markers.

Can Stereotactic Radiotherapy Be Used to Effectively Manage Residual Microscopic Disease Burdens After Surgery?

Conventional FRT is often used after surgery for treatment of brain tumors, cutaneous mast cell tumors and soft tissue sarcomas, and oral tumors. Depending on tumor and patient characteristics, RT fields are usually drawn to encompass the surgical bed plus 1 to 4 cm of surrounding normal tissue. FRT dosing is based on normal tissue tolerance. Some veterinary radiation oncologists now offer SRT in such cases, using ablative doses for large fields that contain mostly normal tissue, and just a few residual tumor cells.[1] Planning and delivering such treatment is straightforward. But a major concern with this approach is that uncomplicated tumor control will be compromised by either excessive toxicity or excessive tumor recurrence that results from application of total radiation doses that are too low or radiation fields that are too small. It is also important to ask, if SRT works via unique radiobiological effects in the tumor microenvironment, is it possible to capitalize on those effects in the absence of a bulky tumor?

Are There Bulky Tumors that Make Poor Candidates with Stereotactic Radiotherapy?

The highly infiltrative and large nature of most canine nasal tumors suggests that they would not be ideal SRT candidates; however, published data regarding linac-based SRT are encouraging.[19] Conversely, pituitary macroadenomas are often thought of as an ideal target for SRT. And indeed, use of SRT for management of feline acromegaly has been rewarding.[15] However, initial experiences regarding SRT for management of canine pituitary macroadenomas are more worrisome. Gieger and Nolan recently presented data regarding use of SRS (16 Gy in a single fraction) for canine pituitary macroadenomas.[39] In their series of 13 dogs, median survival time was 357 days, which does not compare favorably with previously published estimates of survival in nonirradiated dogs (median overall survival time 359 days in a group of 27 dogs),[40] which is interesting because (1) these tumors are extra-axial and usually well demarcated on cross-sectional imaging, thus there is no real concern for invasion into surrounding neuroparenchyma; (2) they are encased within a bony target and thus simple to localize for treatment; and (3) they are usually round/spherical, which simplifies the process of generating a treatment plan that is highly conformal and has steep dose gradients. Nevertheless, based on currently available data, caution is recommended when considering SRT for canine pituitary tumors. Additional data are required to determine whether modest fractionation (eg, 3–5 fraction SRT) may improve outcomes and approximate survival times that are achieved with conventional FRT. This exemplifies just how important it is to develop and share robust clinical outcomes data to guide therapeutic decision-making.

FUTURE DIRECTIONS

Veterinary radiation oncology has undergone incredible growth with regard to adoption of new SRT technologies and protocols. That has been mirrored by increases in the amount of published data describing initial clinical experiences with SRT for various diseases. Yet questions regarding appropriate application of this unique treatment modality still abound. Future studies would ideally focus on further defining recommended OAR dose constraints as well as long-term outcomes for treated patients. And as long-term survivorship improves, we will need significant effort devoted to timely identification of strategies that maximize quality of life in patients who are already enjoying extended quantity of life.

REFERENCES

1. Dunfield EM, Turek MM, Buhr KA, et al. A survey of stereotactic radiation therapy in veterinary medicine. Vet Radiol Ultrasound 2018;59(6):786–95.
2. Yang M, Timmerman R. Stereotactic ablative radiotherapy uncertainties: delineation, setup and motion. SeminRadiatOncol 2018;28(3):207–17.
3. Brown JM, Carlson DJ, Brenner DJ. Dose escalation, not "new biology," can account for the efficacy of stereotactic body radiation therapy with non-small cell lung cancer reply. Int J RadiatOncolBiol Phys 2014;89(3):693–4.
4. Fuks Z, Kolesnick R. Engaging the vascular component of the tumor response. Cancer Cell 2005;8(2):89–91.
5. Moding EJ, Castle KD, Perez BA, et al. Tumor cells, but not endothelial cells, mediate eradication of primary sarcomas by stereotactic body radiation therapy. SciTransl Med 2015;7(278):278ra34.
6. Wong HH, Song CW, Levitt SH. Early changes in functional vasculature of Walker carcinoma 256 following irradiation. Radiology 1973;108(2):429–34.
7. Song CW, Lee YJ, Griffin RJ, et al. Indirect tumor cell death after high-dose hypofractionated irradiation: implications for stereotactic body radiation therapy and stereotactic radiation surgery. Int J RadiatOncolBiol Phys 2015;93(1):166–72.
8. Kumareswaran R, Ludkovski O, Meng A, et al. Chronic hypoxia compromises repair of DNA double-strand breaks to drive genetic instability. J Cell Sci 2012; 125(1):189–99.
9. Stone HB, Peters LJ, Milas L. Effect of host immune capability on radiocurability and subsequent transplantability of a murine fibrosarcoma. J NatlCancer Inst 1979;63(5):1229–35.
10. Lugade AA, Moran JP, Gerber SA, et al. Local radiation therapy of B16 melanoma tumors increases the generation of tumor antigen-specific effector cells that traffic to the tumor. J Immunol 2005;174(12):7516–23.
11. Dewan MZ, Galloway AE, Kawashima N, et al. Fractionated but not single-dose radiotherapy induces an immune-mediated abscopal effect when combined with anti-CTLA-4 antibody. Clin Cancer Res 2009;15(17):5379–88.
12. Vanpouille-Box C, Alard A, Aryankalayil MJ, et al. DNA exonucleaseTrex1 regulates radiotherapy-induced tumour immunogenicity. Nat Commun 2017;8:15618.
13. Kelsey KL, Gieger TL, Nolan MW. Single fraction stereotactic radiation therapy (stereotactic radiosurgery) is a feasible method for treating intracranial meningiomas in dogs. Vet RadiolUltrasound 2018;59(5):632–8.
14. Griffin LR, Nolan MW, Selmic LE, et al. Stereotactic radiation therapy for treatment of canine intracranial meningiomas. Vet Comp Oncol 2016;14(4):E158–70.
15. Wormhoudt TL, Boss MK, Lunn K, et al. Stereotactic radiation therapy for the treatment of functional pituitary adenomas associated with feline acromegaly. J Vet Intern Med 2018;32(4):1383–91.
16. Nolan MW, Dobson JM. The future of radiotherapy in small animals - should the fractions be coarse or fine? J Small AnimPract 2018;59(9):521–30.
17. Kubicek L, Milner R, An Q, et al. Outcomes and prognostic factors associated with canine sinonasal tumors treated with curative intent cone-based stereotactic radiosurgery (1999-2013). Vet RadiolUltrasound 2016;57(3):331–40.
18. Glasser SA, Charney S, Dervisis NG, et al. Use of an image-guided robotic radiosurgery system for the treatment of canine nonlymphomatous nasal tumors. J Am AnimHosp Assoc 2014;50(2):96–104.

19. Gieger TL, Nolan MW. Linac-based stereotactic radiation therapy for canine non-lymphomatous nasal tumours: 29 cases (2013-2016). Vet Comp Oncol 2018; 16(1):E68–75.
20. Christensen NI, Forrest LJ, White PJ, et al. Single institution variability in intensity modulated radiation target delineation for canine nasal neoplasia. Vet Radiol Ultrasound 2016;57(6):639–45.
21. Kelsey KL, Kubicek LN, Bacon NJ, et al. Neuromuscular blockade and inspiratory breath hold during stereotactic body radiation therapy for treatment of heart base tumors in four dogs. J Am Vet Med Assoc 2017;250(2):199–204.
22. Magestro LM, Gieger TL, Nolan MW. Stereotactic body radiation therapy for heart-base tumors in six dogs. J Vet Cardiol 2018;20(3):186–97.
23. Dolera M, Malfassi L, Pavesi S, et al. Volumetric-modulated arc stereotactic radiotherapy for canine adrenocortical tumours with vascular invasion. J small Anim Pract 2016;57(12):710–7.
24. King CR, Brooks JD, Gill H, et al. Long-term outcomes from a prospective trial of stereotactic body radiotherapy for low-risk prostate cancer. Int J RadiatOncolBiol Phys 2012;82(2):877–82.
25. Nolan MW, Marolf AJ, Ehrhart EJ, et al. Pudendalnerve and internal pudendal artery damage may contribute to radiation-induced erectile dysfunction. Int J RadiatOncolBiol Phys 2015;91(4):796–806.
26. Langberg CW, Waldron JA, Baker ML, et al. Significance of overall treatment time for the development of radiation-induced intestinal complications. An experimental study in the rat. Cancer 1994;73(10):2663–8.
27. Fitzpatrick CL, Farese JP, Milner RJ, et al. Intrinsic radiosensitivity and repair of sublethal radiation-induced damage in canine osteosarcoma cell lines. Am J Vet Res 2008;69(9):1197–202.
28. Farese JP, Milner R, Thompson MS, et al. Stereotactic radiosurgery for treatment of osteosarcomas involving the distal portions of the limbs in dogs. J Am Vet Med Assoc 2004;225(10):1567–72, 1548.
29. Covey JL, Farese JP, Bacon NJ, et al. Stereotactic radiosurgery and fracture fixation in 6 dogs with appendicular osteosarcoma. Vet Surg 2014;43(2):174–81.
30. Kubicek L, Vanderhart D, Wirth K, et al. Association between computed tomographic characteristics and fractures following stereotactic radiosurgery in dogs with appendicular osteosarcoma. Vet RadiolUltrasound 2016;57(3):321–30.
31. Rubin JA, Suran JN, Brown DC, et al. Factors associated with pathological fractures in dogs with appendicular primary bone neoplasia: 84 cases (2007-2013). J Am Vet Med Assoc 2015;247(8):917–23.
32. Boston SE, Vinayak A, Lu X, et al. Outcome and complications in dogs with appendicular primary bone tumors treated with stereotactic radiotherapy and concurrent surgical stabilization. Vet Surg 2017;46(6):829–37.
33. Swift KE, LaRue SM. Outcome of 9 dogs treated with stereotactic radiation therapy for primary or metastatic vertebral osteosarcoma. Vet Comp Oncol 2018; 16(1):E152–8.
34. Medin PM, Foster RD, van der Kogel AJ, et al. Spinal cord tolerance to single-session uniform irradiation in pigs: implications for a dose-volume effect. RadiotherOncol 2013;106(1):101–5.
35. Benedict SH, Yenice KM, Followill D, et al. Stereotactic body radiation therapy: the report of AAPM Task Group 101. Med Phys 2010;37(8):4078–101.
36. Rancilio NJ, Bentley RT, Plantenga JP, et al. Safety and feasibility of stereotactic radiotherapy using computed portal radiography for canine intracranial tumors. Vet RadiolUltrasound 2018;59(2):212–20.

37. Klein EE, Hanley J, Bayouth J, et al. Task Group 142 report: quality assurance of medical accelerators. Med Phys 2009;36(9):4197–212.
38. Nolan MW, Randall EK, LaRue SM, et al. Accuracy of CT and MRI for contouring the feline optic apparatus for radiation therapy planning. Vet RadiolUltrasound 2013;54(5):560–6.
39. Gieger TL, Nolan MW. Stereotactic radiation therapy for the treatment of canine pituitary tumors: 13 cases (2014-2018). Paper presented at: ACVR/IVRA Joint Scientific Conference; Fort Worth, Texas, October 14-19, 2018.
40. Kent MS, Bommarito D, Feldman E, et al. Survival, neurologic response, and prognostic factors in dogs with pituitary masses treated with radiation therapy and untreated dogs. J Vet Intern Med 2007;21(5):1027–33.
41. Swift KE, McGrath S, Nolan MW, et al. Clinical and imaging findings, treatments, and outcomes in 27 dogs with imaging diagnosed trigeminal nerve sheath tumors: A multi-center study. Vet RadiolUltrasound 2017;58(6):679–89.
42. Dolera M, Malfassi L, Marcarini S, et al. High dose hypofractionated frameless volumetric modulated arc radiotherapy is a feasible method for treating canine trigeminal nerve sheath tumors. Vet RadiolUltrasound 2018;59(5):624–31.
43. Hansen KS, Zwingenberger AL, Theon AP, et al. Treatment of MRI-diagnosed trigeminal peripheral nerve sheath tumors by stereotactic radiotherapy in dogs. J Vet Intern Med 2016;30(4):1112–20.
44. Dolera M, Malfassi L, Bianchi C, et al. Frameless stereotactic radiotherapy alone and combined with temozolomide for presumed canine gliomas. Vet Comp Oncol 2018;16(1):90–101.
45. Dolera M, Malfassi L, Pavesi S, et al. Stereotactic volume modulated arc radiotherapy in canine meningiomas: imaging-based and clinical neurological post-treatment evaluation. J Am AnimHosp Assoc 2018;54(2):77–84.
46. Nolan MW. Canine Nasal Tumors: An Assessment of the Evidence Base for Stereotactic Radiotherapy. Paper presented at: ACVIM Forum2018; Seattle, Washington, June 13-16, 2018.

Veterinary Clinics

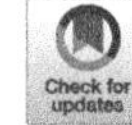

Tumor Ablation

William T.N. Culp, VMD[a,*], Maureen A. Griffin, DVM[b]

KEYWORDS

• Locoregional therapy • Interventional oncology • Image-guidance

KEY POINTS

- With any form of ablation, the use of image guidance is deemed mandatory to optimize tumor localization and placement of instrumentation.
- When considering which ablation technique (if any) may be best for a particular patient, many factors need to be considered, including (but not limited to) target organ, location of tumor within the organ, and tumor size.
- Although ablation may be considered for many tumors in companion animals, reported outcomes are rare and significant assessment is still required.

BACKGROUND

Image-guided tumor ablation has become an established treatment modality for the control of neoplastic disease in human medicine. Tumor ablation is a highly evolving field of interventional oncology with a growing breadth of ablation techniques and equipment. As such, consensus statements regarding standardization of terminology and reporting recently have been proposed.[1,2] Tumor ablation is defined as the direct application of chemical (nonenergy) or energy-based (including both thermal and nonthermal) therapies to a focal tumor (or tumors) in an attempt to eradicate or substantially destroy the tumor(s).[1–5] These therapies importantly are direct in nature, which distinguishes them from other interventional oncology techniques that are performed intravascularly or endoscopically.[1] In order to provide effective and safe tumor ablation therapy, image-based planning and guidance (via ultrasound, computed tomography [CT], magnetic resonance [MR], positron emission tomography-computed tomography, and/or fluoroscopy) throughout the procedure are critical.[1,4,5] Tumor ablation techniques have the potential of being performed minimally invasively or as an adjuvant to open surgery.[1,6–12]

[a] Department of Surgical and Radiological Sciences, University of California, Davis, 1 Shields Avenue, Davis, CA 95616, USA; [b] 1 Shields Avenue, Davis, CA 95616, USA
* Corresponding author.
E-mail address: wculp@ucdavis.edu

Vet Clin Small Anim 49 (2019) 949–966
https://doi.org/10.1016/j.cvsm.2019.04.007
0195-5616/19/
vetsmall.theclinics.com

Historically, the main tumor ablation categories (based on mechanism of action) consisted of chemical and thermal ablation.[1,2] Recently, however, tumor ablation techniques have expanded to include therapeutic strategies that do not fit into either category, such as irreversible electroporation (IRE), an energy-based ablative technique that is nonthermal and also nonchemical.[1] Therefore, a newer classification scheme for tumor ablation incorporates all current ablative modalities into the subgroups of chemical (nonenergy) ablation and energy-based (both thermal and nonthermal) ablation.[1] Chemical ablation involves instillation of a chemical compound into a lesion, thereby inducing necrosis due to direct toxicity of the agent.[1,13] Energy-based thermal ablation includes both hyperthermic-based strategies, such as radiofrequency (RF) ablation, microwave ablation, ultrasound ablation, and laser ablation, and hypothermic-based strategies (i.e. cryoablation) that cause tumor cell death.[13] Energy-based, nonthermal tumor destruction modalities, such as IRE, involve energy application without significant thermal contribution to cause tumor destruction.[1] It is possible that some tumor ablation modalities may have aspects of both ablation categories based on mechanism of tissue damage.[1,14,15] Ultimately, the consensus guidelines recommend assignment of a tumor ablation classification in association with the predominant mechanism of action.[1,15]

Common indications for tumor ablation in human medicine include hepatic, renal, skeletal, and pulmonary tumors.[12] Tumor ablation is an important local disease treatment modality option for people who have failed chemotherapy or radiation therapy and/or are not appropriate surgical candidates (due to tumor characteristics or patient comorbidities).[12] Tumor ablation is used as a first-line treatment in human patients with small tumors that can be easily targeted.[12,16] In general, the primary goal of tumor ablation is to eradicate all neoplastic cells within a specified target volume while concurrently sparing normal surrounding tissues as much as possible.[3] In most cases, recommended ablation treatment margins of grossly normal tissue beyond the apparent tumor boundaries are 0.5 cm to 1.0 cm.[3,4,17] Due to the ability for treatment precision with maximal sparing of normal surrounding tissues, tumor ablation has emerged as an important neoplastic treatment option in many patients.[3,18–21] Tumor ablation also has become an important therapeutic method in palliation for patients with skeletal metastasis and hormonally active neuroendocrine tumors.[3,22,23] Factors that are important in decision making regarding tumor ablation modality include organ involvement, tumor type, size, and pattern of distribution, tumor proximity to vulnerable structures, patient factors, system availability, and operator experience.[3,12,24]

The use of ablation techniques in companion animals is still rare and available literature on these treatments is scarce. Many of the earliest reports of ablation in companion animals evaluated techniques used to treat benign disease (eg, parathyroid nodules) or experimentally induced lesions. Although the focus of this article is on ablation of neoplastic disease, descriptions and outcomes associated with the use of ablation for benign disease are included. New information is emerging regarding the use of ablation techniques for the treatment of spontaneously occurring tumors in dogs and cats, and this database will continue to grow as these modalities become used more regularly.

CHEMICAL ABLATION

Chemical ablation was one of the earliest tumor ablation modalities described, and, although thermal ablation techniques recently have become more widespread, chemical ablation remains an effective treatment option for small tumors and clinical cases in which thermal ablation techniques are contraindicated. Moreover, the simplicity and reduced costs associated with chemical ablation make this an attractive alternative in developing regions.[3] The most commonly used chemical ablation substance is ethanol, with acetic acid being a less frequently used alternative.[13] Chemical ablation causes tumor necrosis via both direct and indirect mechanisms.[13] Direct tumor cellular necrosis occurs due to cytoplasmic dehydration and protein denaturation secondary to chemical instillation into the tumor bed; indirect tumor necrosis occurs due to uptake into the local circulation and subsequent vascular endothelium necrosis and platelet aggregation, resulting in vascular thrombosis and ischemic necrosis of the tumor.[3,13,25,26]

Equipment required to perform chemical ablation includes imaging guidance (typically via ultrasound or CT), a 20-gauge to 22-gauge single end-hole or multi–side-hole needle of appropriate length to reach the distal tumor aspect, and the chemical agent.[13] The volume of chemical agent to be instilled is calculated on the basis of a spherical volume; 0.5 cm typically is added to the tumor radius used in this equation to attain adequate margins of tumor treatment.[13] The needle can be repositioned as the chemical is instilled, or several needles can be placed for multiple locations of chemical instillation.[13] If CT is used, the chemical ablative compound typically is combined with a small volume of iodinated contrast material to enhance visualization of treatment.[13] Chemical ablation can be performed via a single treatment or as a staged procedure over multiple treatment sessions.[13]

Chemical ablation is considered more effective for the treatment of primary hepatocellular carcinoma than for hepatic metastatic disease due to differences in tumor characteristics (softer tissue composition for primary hepatic tumors compared with the typically dense fibrous structure of metastatic disease) and a common tumor capsule or pseudocapsule surrounding primary hepatocellular tumors (and not metastatic lesions) that can limit diffusion and increase concentration of the chemical compound within the desired tumor target.[3,27] Due to limited diffusion capabilities and a limited extent of small vessel thrombosis, tumors greater than 3 cm in diameter represent a contraindication for use of chemical ablation in humans.[13] Ultimately, due to poor efficacy rates of ethanol instillation for treatment of hepatic metastatic disease, ethanol ablation is not recommended.[3] Another disadvantage of ethanol ablation entails its poor and uneven distribution and limited efficacy in a wide range of tumor types.[3]

The main indication for ethanol ablation in companion animals has been in the treatment of thyroid and parathyroid tissue.[28–31] The earliest study evaluated the response of parathyroid nodules to ethanol ablation in eight dogs.[28] In that study, a needle was inserted into the mass, and 96% ethanol was injected. Adverse effects were rare in this cohort.[28] In a larger, more recent study, 27 dogs that were presumed to have functional parathyroid nodules were treated with percutaneous ethanol ablation.[31] In these dogs, 95% ethanol was injected percutaneously into the parathyroid nodules.[31] A second treatment was necessary in three dogs due to failure of the initial treatment or development of an additional nodule.[31] In total, 23 of 27 procedures resulted in resolution of hypercalcemia.[31] There were no periprocedural or immediate postprocedural adverse effects; complications included transient dysphagia and hypersalivation that resolved two days after the procedure in one dog and a cyst in a dog's neck that did not recur after lancing and drainage.[31] In a separate study, 15 dogs underwent ethanol ablation as treatment of hyperparathyroidism.[30] Of those dogs, 87% were considered to have been treated successfully; however, this percentage was less than that for dogs that underwent surgical parathyroidectomy or RF ablation.[30]

In a study on seven cats that underwent ethanol ablation of thyroid nodules as treatment of hyperthyroidism, outcomes were considered poor.[29] One cat that underwent bilateral thyroid ethanol injection died.[29] In the other six cats, hyperthyroidism was only transiently controlled and many adverse effects, including dysphonia and laryngeal paralysis, were encountered.[29]

Other masses and/or cystic lesions have been percutaneously treated with ethanol ablation in dogs.[32,33] In one dog with a renal cyst that was treated with 95% ethanol, the procedure was performed successfully and no adverse effects were encountered.[32] Hypotensive shock and death occurred, however, after ethanol infusion into a pancreatic pseudocyst in another dog.[33] Further investigation is needed to determine if ethanol ablation can be considered as a safe and effective adjunctive treatment modality for tumors that are highly cystic or cyst lesions in other locations.

ENERGY-BASED ABLATION—THERMAL

Thermal ablation modalities aim to cause tumor cell death by increasing or decreasing local temperature sufficiently to cause irreversible cellular injury.[3] Hyperthermic ablation modalities result in heat generation via electromagnetic (eg, RF, microwave, or laser) energy or ultrasonic energy.[3] Cryoablation techniques result in subfreezing local temperatures that cause tumor cell death. Several general factors are important in the ability to heat or cool large tissue volumes in different environments to result in coagulative necrosis of tumor cells, including magnitude of energy deposited, local tissue interactions, and extent of heat loss prior to inducing thermal damage.[3,5] Ultimately, the complex relationship between cellular temperature and cellular death is multifactorial and is affected by temperature, exposure time, perfusion, vascular coagulation, adjunctive treatments, and cellular fragility.[24,34]

In general, for hyperthermic ablation, the typical goal temperature in the target tissue to cause coagulative necrosis is greater than 50°C to 55°C, with rapid reduction of temperature outside the target volume to spare normal tissues.[3,24] At temperatures greater than 45°C, cellular protein denaturation and dysfunction of the cellular membrane occur, resulting in irreversible coagulative necrosis.[13,35] Studies have demonstrated an exponential relationship between temperature rise beyond 45°C and rate of coagulative necrosis; necrosis occurs within 20 minutes to 30 minutes at 45°C, within 5 minutes at 50°C to 55°C, and immediately at 60°C to 110°C; at temperatures greater than 100°C to 110°C, tissue vaporization and carbonization occur.[13,35–38] A hyperthermic ablation zone within tissues results from both active and passive heating.[13] Active heating occurs when heat is created by the thermal ablation source directly at the location, where it results in cell death; passive heating occurs when conduction from the thermal ablation source through tissues results in cell death.[13] Factors that reduce heat production within a tissue target volume include tissue charring, significant local blood flow, and greater distance from the heat source.[13,35,38]

Radiofrequency Ablation

RF ablation uses a generator to create alternating electrical current (generally between 200 Hz and 1200 Hz) between interstitial electrodes; if monopolar RF ablation is used, the current is transmitted through an insterstitial electrode and returns through grounding pads on the skin, whereas if bipolar RF ablation is used, the current oscillates between two interstitial electrodes without the use of a grounding pad.[3,13,24,39–41] Due to electrical impedance associated with tissues, the electric current flow causes rapid oscillation of ions within adjacent tissue, thereby resulting in frictional heating in regions of high current density near the electrode(s); this is known as the Joule effect.[3,24,39] Thermal diffusion via conduction enables additional growth of the ablation zone.[13,24,42,43] Thus, RF ablation functions as a closed electrical circuit in which the current loop is composed of a generator, cabling, electrode(s), tissue that acts as a resistive element, and grounding pads (in the case of the most commonly used monopolar RF ablation).[3,13] Sufficient heat via this technique results in coagulative necrosis of tumor cells with the goal of incorporating a 0.5 cm to 1 cm tumor-free margin.[13] Because rapid and excessive heating can result in desiccation and charring of tissues, thereby limiting the number of ions capable of generating heat, the generator needs to undergo multiple cycles of controlled increases in power, current, and temperature to control and limit excessive heating.[13]

Equipment required to perform RF ablation includes imaging guidance (generally ultrasound and/or CT), electrodes within needles that are placed into the tumor tissue, generator, and grounding pad.[13] Multiple commercial RF ablation devices are available.[13] Generators provide the important functions of power generation, control, and user interface.[3] Electrode designs are varied and include both straight insulated needles with an exposed metallic tip component and multitined electrodes; multiple tines may enable larger ablation zones as well as more rapid heating.[3,44] Ground pads used in monopolar RF ablation are designed to provide a large dissipative surface for flow of electrical current through skin; if uneven placement or insufficient numbers of pads are used, dermal burn wounds can result.[3,45–47]

Two main disadvantages of RF ablation have been described and have reduced the applicability of RF ablation to effectively treat several tumors. First, the nature of RF ablation involves a self-limiting process. RF ablation creates water vapor, desiccation, and charring, which gradually cause an increased tissue impedance, thereby reducing the ability to apply additional electrical current and limiting temperatures that can be reached in the ablation zone.[24] Second, heat transfer via conduction is a slow process in most tissues that has a limited ability to overcome even minor countering processes (such as local tissue perfusion and ventilation); subsequently, RF ablation zones can vary significantly based on the local tissue environment.[24,48,49] For instance, aerated lung has a high impedance to flow of electrical current and poor transfer of heat relative to solid tissues, thereby reducing power delivery and growth of the RF ablation zone.[24,50,51] Increases in power and ablation time can help to counter these limitations, but ultimately RF ablation is generally not recommended for ablation of pulmonary tumors.[24,52] Multiple alterations have been pursued in an effort to overcome these physical deficiencies of RF ablation, including methods to enhance the ablation zone size (via internal electrode cooling; expandable, multitined, or clustered electrodes; and rapidly altering multielectrode approaches) and also have incorporated use of saline infusion and high-power generators.[24,53–58] Although these methods have resulted in an improvement in the overall performance of RF ablation, they also can be associated with an increased risk for complications, such as skin burns and collateral damage.[24]

As with ethanol ablation, evaluation of the efficacy of RF ablation has been performed predominantly in canine and feline patients as treatment of parathyroid and thyroid disease.[30,59–63] Currently, five studies describing the use of percutaneous RF ablation of parathyroid nodules are available in the veterinary literature.[30,59,61–63] Overall, the results for control of hypercalcemia are promising, but proper case selection is needed because larger mass size and hypothyroidism may be contraindications for this treatment.[61]

The use of RF ablation in the treatment of pulmonary and prostatic neoplasia also has been described in the veterinary literature.[64,65] In a study on experimentally induced pulmonary tumors in dogs, RF ablation was performed percutaneously to treat five solitary pulmonary nodules and three clusters of three pulmonary nodules each (14 total tumors).[64] Percutaneous RF ablation was technically successful in all cases; however, pneumothorax was encountered postablation and became life-threatening in one dog. On histopathologic evaluation of resected lung lobes, no viable tumor was noted after RF ablation.[64] In one dog that was diagnosed with prostatic carcinoma (with a mass measuring 1 cm × 1 cm × 1.1 cm), the dog underwent celiotomy for lymph node extirpation (metastatic from a previously diagnosed anal sac adenocarcinoma), and RF ablation was performed via direct visualization of the prostate tumor.[65] The RF ablation electrode was placed intraoperatively, and ablation was successfully performed; no complications were encountered perioperatively in this dog.[65]

Microwave Ablation

Microwave ablation entails transmission of microwave electromagnetic energy (300 MHz to 300 GHz but most often 915 MHz or 2.45 GHz) through an antenna into a tumor.[3] Formation of an electromagnetic field results in water molecule orientation within the field (due to the weak unequal dipole nature of water molecules).[13] When an oscillating microwave field is applied, polar molecules (predominantly water) continuously realign with the oscillating field, thereby increasing kinetic energy and temperature and causing coagulative necrosis of the tumor.[13,24] Thus, microwave heating is produced via dielectric hysteresis (rotating dipoles), rather than the Joule heating mechanism with RF ablation.[3] Heat is further generated with microwave ablation as polarized ions gain kinetic energy within the magnetic field and collide with other ions.[13]

Equipment required to perform microwave ablation includes imaging guidance (generally ultrasound and/or CT), a microwave generator, flexible coaxial cable, and microwave antenna; no grounding pads are required.[13] Multiple commercially available microwave ablation devices are present, and three types of microwave systems exist: first-generation systems that lack active antenna cooling, second-generation systems that incorporate active antenna cooling but have limited generator power, and third-generation systems that have both active antenna cooling and high-power generators.[13,24] Microwave antenna design has an important effect on size and shape of the ablation zone, and multiple antenna forms have been created to control energy delivery in various ways.[24,66,67]

In contrast to electrical currents, microwave energy radiates through all biological tissues regardless of impedance to electrical current (such as skeletal, pulmonary, and charred or desiccated tissues).[3,24,68] Thus, microwave ablation may be a more ideal ablative modality than RF ablation for tumors in tissues with high impedance, such as lung and bone, and for tissues with high water content, such as solid organs and tumors.[69,70] Microwaves can continuously generate heat in a larger tissue volume surrounding an applicator relative to RF current, and microwave energy is capable of producing faster, higher temperature, and larger ablation zones in multiple tissue types compared with RF current.[3,24,71,72] With microwave ablation, tissues are heated more efficiently than with RF ablation, grounding pads are not required, and multiple antennas can be used simultaneously to amplify the ablative effect in a synergistic fashion.[3,69,73,74] The thermal profile achieved with microwave ablation can also more readily overcome the heat-sink effect from large vessels near tumors.[13] These findings represent significant clinical advantages of microwave ablation compared with RF ablation. In general, microwave ablation is faster, achieves higher temperatures, attains more consistent results regardless of tissue type, is relatively insensitive to heat-sinks, and has the ability to create larger ablation zones compared with RF ablation.[24,67–70,75,76] Challenges associated with microwave ablation include fewer clinical data and experience with this ablation technique due to its more recent introduction in the field of tumor ablation (although this is rapidly changing with the institution of many clinical studies), potentially larger ablation zones achievable resulting in a learning curve with the safe use of microwave ablation, and significant differences in clinical microwave ablation systems with resulting differences in performance characteristics.[24] Furthermore, microwave systems use larger cables than RF systems, and the microwave antennas are prone to overheating such that cooling mechanisms to protect the superficial structures along the antenna are recommended.[69,70]

Much of the recent veterinary ablation literature has focused on the use of microwave ablation. Relative to RF ablation, microwave ablation may offer advantages in companion animals, such as the ability to generate higher intratumoral temperatures, larger tumor ablation volumes, and faster ablation times. Additionally, with microwave ablation, multiple applicators can be placed simultaneously into larger tumors, and no grounding pads are necessary, which is particularly beneficial in smaller patients.

Microwave ablation has been described in conjunction with surgical techniques in two recent studies.[77,78] A metastatic pulmonary lesion secondary to appendicular osteosarcoma in a dog was successfully treated with microwave ablation using thoracoscopic assistance, and no procedural complications occurred.[78] In this dog, hypertrophic osteopathy was present prior to treatment, and this resolved within 40 days post-treatment.[78] In five dogs with liver tumors, microwave ablation antennas were placed in the tumors after ventral midline laparotomy; no complications associated with microwave ablation were encountered in these dogs.[77] Further investigation of the use of microwave ablation for the treatment of hepatic neoplasia in companion animals is warranted.

In the authors' clinic, a renal mass in a dog was treated percutaneously with microwave ablation.[65] In that dog, a solitary left renal nodule (1.1 cm × 1.2 cm × 1.4 cm) was identified cytologically as carcinoma, and a microwave ablation antenna was placed into the nodule; no complications were encountered, and that dog remains alive nearly three years post-ablation.[65]

Laser Ablation

Similar to RF and microwave ablation, laser energy results in electromagnetic heating to result in coagulative necrosis of tumor cells.[3] With laser-based thermal ablation, tissue-specific chromophores in cells optimally absorb laser energy at specific wavelengths, and this absorbed energy subsequently is converted into heat within the chromophores and diffuses via conduction to adjacent tissues.[13] The depth of laser penetration and conduction of heat influence the zone of ablation via this modality.[13] Equipment required for laser ablation includes imaging guidance, a power source, laser medium, and reflecting mirrors.[13] The most commonly used laser device is Nd-YAG, which generates a wavelength of 1064 nm.[13,38]

Several case series have documented the use of laser ablation as a treatment modality in companion animals with luminal obstructive disease.[79–83] In the largest study to date, 38 dogs with obstruction or potential obstruction secondary to transitional cell carcinoma (TCC) were treated with near-infrared diode laser ablation.[80] Several complications were encountered with the laser ablation procedure and included stranguria, stenosis at the cystourethral junction, TCC seeding of the lower urinary tract and urethrostomy site, and urethral penetration.[80] Although median survival time in that group of dogs was 380 days, there are tremendous risks with this procedure (eg, urethral penetration and seeding abdominal structures), and it remains to be determined whether the potential benefit outweighs these risks.[80] In a separate study, a carbon dioxide laser was used in conjunction with chemotherapy to treat eight dogs with TCC of the lower urinary tract.[79] The investigators of that study determined that better resolution of clinical signs was achieved when laser ablation was used adjunctively to chemotherapy relative to when chemotherapy was administered alone.[79] In addition, laser ablation has been utilized for treatment of *Spirocerca lupi*–associated esophageal sarcoma in dogs of two separate studies.[81,82] In those studies, laser ablation was successful as a palliative treatment option with lower morbidity and shorter hospitalization times compared with traditional surgical management of these tumors.[81,82] A tracheal osteochondroma has also been ablated successfully in a dog using a diode laser.[83]

Ultrasound Ablation

High-intensity focused ultrasound (HIFU) is a newer ablative modality that uses an extracorporeal ultrasound probe with piezoelectric transducer that emits a focused beam of sound energy to target lesions.[13] Mechanical vibration of the focused sound waves subsequently is converted into heat within the tissue, and coagulative necrosis ensues.[13] Although the mechanism of cytotoxicity via HIFU ablation is predominantly thermal in nature, mechanical cell injury can occur when cavitations (formed secondary to the high-intensity acoustic pulses) in tissues grow rapidly and then collapse, subsequently releasing shock waves into surrounding tissues.[12] Temperature increases rapidly within the target tissue following intense pulses that last 3 seconds or less, and an elliptical region (sonication) of necrosis forms with a long axis parallel to the ultrasound beam.[13] In the frequency range of 0.8 MHz to 5 MHz, the ultrasound wavelength in tissue is approximately 2 mm to 0.3 mm, such that small regions of high intensity can be created at a distance from the source within the focal plane.[84]

Equipment required for HIFU ablation includes imaging guidance (such as MR or ultrasound), a transducer, signal generator, amplifier, matching circuitry, power meter, and potentially a method of transducer cooling.[84] Four types of devices have been designed to optimize HIFU ablation treatment to wide-ranging applications: extracorporeal, transrectal, interstitial, and percutaneous; some investigators propose classifying interstitial ultrasound ablation separately from HIFU due to the more direct and invasive application of energy via an applicator placed within the target tissue with this modality.[1,12,84–86] Indications for use of extracorporeal HIFU devices include superficial and benign tumors not surrounded by bone or air (such as uterine fibroids and leiomyomas).[12,87,88] Indications for use of transrectal HIFU devices include prostate tumors.[12,89] Indications for use of interstitial ultrasound ablation devices include biliary and esophageal tumors.[12,89] Indications for use of percutaneous HIFU devices include deeper tumors, although clinical applicability is limited at this time.[12,90,91]

One advantage of HIFU involves the focused zone of ablation that is produced with minimal collateral damage, with tissue in the ultrasound propagation path largely unaffected.[13,84] Also, ablation via HIFU can be noninvasive and does not require transcutaneous insertion of probes into the target tissue, unlike other thermal ablation techniques.[84] The transducer can be placed either outside the body on skin (for treatment of liver, kidney, breast, uterine, pancreatic, brain, and bone tumors) or within the rectum (for treatment of prostate tumors).[84] Limitations of HIFU include a potential ineffectiveness in treatment of deeper lesions due to ultrasound penetrance through tissues, potential for injury of tissues (such as skin burns, peripheral nerve damage, and intestinal injury) due to scatter and reflection of HIFU waves, and limited use in regions that are subject to respiratory motion (due to lack of precision) or are deep to bone (due to sonic shadowing).[12,90,91] Additionally, ultrasound propagation is limited by coagulation, desiccation, and vapor formation, such that careful planning is required to ensure adequate tumor coverage of the ablative treatment.[12,92] Ultimately, however, HIFU poses an attractive option for thermal energy–based tissue ablation in that it offers the least invasive of all techniques, and the HIFU ablation field is rapidly evolving with the onset of multiple recent studies and novel equipment and techniques for use.[84]

The use of ultrasound ablation has been described in the treatment of several canine solid tumors.[93,94] MR-guided focused ultrasound (MRgFUS) has been used to treat a hepatocellular carcinoma in a dog.[93] Four separate MRgFUS treatments were performed over an 8-week period in this dog; 3 weeks after the fourth treatment, the tumor was surgically excised.[93] The MRgFUS technique was shown to have high precision in targeting of the tumor.[93] In a separate study, 11 dogs underwent HIFU for the treatment of solid tumors, several of which were TCC.[94] In many of those dogs, clinical signs improved; in particular, HIFU resulted in cessation of bleeding in four dogs with hemorrhagic tumors.[94]

Cryoablation

In contrast to the hyperthermic energy–based ablation techniques, cryoablation uses cold injury to produce cytotoxic effects. Cryoablation systems utilize the Joule-Thomson effect.[13,24] In this process, as the liquefied gas cryogen (typically argon) moves from an internal feed line into an internal expansion chamber, it creates a heat sink at the distal end of the cryoprobe that cools the probe to temperatures of −160°C or colder.[3,24,69] Heat is transferred from the tissue into the cryoprobe via passive thermal diffusion.[24] After a period of freezing, cryoprobe warming and thawing of the tissue generally are performed through the same system by using high-pressure helium.[95] The required temperature for cell death with cryoablation is between −20°C and −40°C, and this temperature must be present 1 cm beyond the tumor periphery in order to result in complete tumor ablation.[69,96,97] Different zones and mechanisms of cryoablative injury have been documented, including direct cell injury, vascular injury and ischemia, apoptosis, and immunomodulation.[69,98] Direct injury occurs at the center of the cryoablative lesion, where ice forms from the extracellular space inwards with subsequent osmotic cell shrinkage and ice crystal formation within cells, leading to coagulative necrosis at the center of the cryoablative lesion.[69] Vascular injury also occurs at the center of the cryoablative zone with endothelial cell damage, platelet aggregation and microthrombosis, vasoconstriction, and increased vascular permeability; subsequent ischemia results in further coagulative necrosis.[69] Reversible damage occurs in more peripheral zones of sublethal cold temperatures, and apoptosis of cells occurs in this region.[24,69,99] Also, complex immunomodulation with mechanisms that both increase and reduce antitumor immunity can be induced by cryoablation.[69]

Equipment required for cryoablation includes imaging guidance (ultrasound to monitor ice ball formation in real time or CT or MR to monitor change in tissue contrast), compressed argon gas for cooling, possible helium gas for thawing (some more recent systems do not require helium gas), cryoprobes, thermal sensors, and a console to control the circulation of high-pressure gases through the cryoprobes.[13] Tumor size influences the number and distribution of cryoprobes that should be used; in general, probes should be placed within 1 cm of the tumor margin and no greater than 2 cm apart from other probes.[13,100] Performing multiple freeze-thaw cycles results in greater cellular death, but benefit is limited beyond two freeze-thaw cycles.[13,95,101]

One advantage of cryoablation is that the expanding ice ball (ablation zone) is easily visualized with ultrasound, CT, and MR imaging, thereby enabling more precise monitoring of treatment than with many heat-based ablation modalities.[24,102,103] Another advantage of cryoablation is that, due to an anesthetic effect associated with cooling of tissues and nerves, it tends to be less painful compared with heat-based thermal ablation modalities; therefore, cryoablation does not require general anesthesia for many human patients.[95] An additional benefit of cryoablation is that each cryoprobe can act independently, thereby allowing for an individualized treatment protocol given the individual tumor size, shape, and location.[95] Although cryoablation results in small vessel thrombosis, larger vessels are generally spared, which allows surrounding tissues to remain viable but also allows for potential tumor lysis syndrome and heat-sink effects.[13] After the ice ball melts, the ablation zone is reperfused, and this results in a rapid release of cellular debris into the systemic circulation; thus, systemic complications can be seen with cryoablation (cryoshock) that are rare with heat-based ablation.[24,104,105] Moreover, as opposed to RF and microwave ablation, cryoablation devices do not provide a zone of direct or active cooling, and subsequently, the cryoprobe's surface area limits cooling efficiency.[24] Thus, multiple cryoprobes generally are needed to treat tumors, and ablation times generally are longer than those used with microwave or RF ablation.[24,106] Other potential disadvantages of cryoablation include relatively small ablation zones compared with other modalities and a possibly increased risk for hemorrhagic complications due to a lack of large vessel thrombosis and coagulation.[12,13,95,107–109] Moreover, the brittle nature of frozen tissues can result in fracture of the organ if excessive torque or cryoprobe displacement occurs, subsequently causing hemorrhage.[95,110]

In companion animals, tumors of the head have been targeted most commonly with cryoablation. Long-term control of a nasal adenocarcinoma has been described in one dog.[111] Additionally, cryoablation was combined with transarterial embolization and systemic chemotherapy to cause partial tumor remission in a dog with a maxillary fibrosarcoma.[112]

ENERGY-BASED ABLATION—NONTHERMAL

Irreversible electroporation uses repeated pulses of short duration (microseconds to milliseconds), high-voltage, electrical current (up to 3 kV/cm) transmitted through electrodes to cause irreversible cellular membrane damage and apoptosis; thus, the cause of cell death is not associated with heat production.[1,3,12,113] Because of the very short duration of IRE treatment pulses, precision is important and adjustments during treatments are not possible.[12] Irreversible electroporation ablation zones generally are sharp with clear demarcations between ablated and nonablated tissue, which is valuable in attaining precise control of the ablation zone.[12,114–116] Equipment required for IRE includes imaging guidance (such as ultrasound), IRE electrodes, a pulse generator, and circuit.

Advantages of IRE include the precisely controlled nature of the ablation zone with minimal collateral tissue damage, short treatment times, and the reduced influence of heat-sinks (such as large vessels) on the ablation zone compared with thermal ablation treatments.[3,12,117] Disadvantages of IRE include high cost, complexity, and invasiveness of IRE procedures compared with other ablation modalities, because multiple applicators with precise parallel alignment/positioning are needed.[3,12,118] Another disadvantage of IRE is the typical delay (up to several minutes) in imaging characteristics associated with IRE when using ultrasound, although when characteristic imaging findings of IRE are visualized, fewer artifacts (such as microbubble formation) may be present relative to imaging with thermal ablation.[12,13,119] Furthermore, the possible need for general anesthesia with paralytics should be considered when performing IRE due to muscle contraction and cardiac arrhythmias that can develop subsequent to alterations in ion transport.[3,12,120,121] There also is a lack of coagulation around IRE electrode insertion sites, which may increase the risk of hemorrhage complications.[3]

The clinical application of IRE in veterinary patients has been reported infrequently.[122–125] In the first described case, IRE was used to treat an intracranial glioma.[122] This treatment resulted in tumor volume reduction and improvement of intracranial hypertension; due to the positive effect of IRE, this dog was able to undergo radiation therapy for further treatment.[122] More recently, IRE was used to treat seven dogs with glioma; in six of seven dogs, no direct neurotoxicity was noted.[124] Additionally, performance scales were improved post-treatment with IRE, and objective tumor responses were noted in four of five dogs with quantifiable target lesions.[124] Lastly, a dog with a soft tissue sarcoma located near the femur and adjacent to the sciatic nerve and femoral arteries has been treated with IRE.[123] In this dog, complete remission was noted 6 weeks post-ablation, and a marked improvement in clinical signs occurred.[123]

REFERENCES

1. Ahmed M, Solbiati L, Brace CL, et al. Image-guided tumor ablation: standardization of terminology and reporting criteria—a 10-year update. J Vasc Interv Radiol 2014;25:1691–705.
2. Goldberg SN, Grassi CJ, Cardella JF, et al. Image-guided tumor ablation: standardization of terminology and reporting criteria. J Vasc Interv Radiol 2009;20: S377–90.
3. Ahmed M, Brace CL, Lee FT Jr, et al. Principles of and advances in percutaneous ablation. Radiology 2011;258:351–69.
4. Dodd GD, Soulen MC, Kane RA, et al. Minimally invasive treatment of malignant hepatic tumors: at the threshold of a major breakthrough. Radiographics 2000; 20:9–27.
5. Goldberg SN, Gazelle GS, Mueller PR. Thermal ablation therapy for focal malignancy: a unified approach to underlying principles, techniques, and diagnostic imaging guidance. Am J Roentgenol 2000;174:323–31.
6. Herbold T, Wahba R, Bangard C, et al. The laparoscopic approach for radiofrequency ablation of hepatocellular carcinoma—indication, technique and results. Langenbecks Arch Surg 2013;398:47–53.
7. Vavra P, Dostalik J, Zacharoulis D, et al. Endoscopic radiofrequency ablation in colorectal cancer: initial clinical results of a new bipolar radiofrequency ablation device. Dis Colon Rectum 2009;52:355–8.
8. Cornelis F, Balageas P, Le Bras Y, et al. Radiologically-guided thermal ablation of renal tumours. Diagn Interv Imaging 2012;93:246–61.
9. Santambrogio R, Barabino M, Bruno S, et al. Long-term outcome of laparoscopic ablation therapies for unresectable hepatocellular carcinoma: a single European center experience of 426 patients. Surg Endosc 2016;30:2103–13.
10. Lakhtakia S, Seo DW. Endoscopic ultrasonography-guided tumor ablation. Dig Endosc 2017;29:486–94.
11. Scheffer HJ, Nielsen K, de Jong MC, et al. Irreversible electroporation for nonthermal tumor ablation in the clinical setting: a systematic review of safety and efficacy. J Vasc Interv Radiol 2014;25:997–1011.
12. Knavel EM, Brace CL. Tumor ablation: common modalities and general practices. Tech Vasc Interv Radiol 2013;16:192–200.

13. Saldanha DF, Khiatani VL, Carrillo TC, et al. Current tumor ablation technologies: basic science and device review. Semin Intervent Radiol 2010;27(3):247–54.
14. Faroja M, Ahmed M, Appelbaum L, et al. Irreversible electroporation ablation: is all the damage nonthermal? Radiology 2013;266:462–70.
15. Cressman EN, Jahangir DA. Dual mode single agent thermochemical ablation by simultaneous release of heat energy and acid: hydrolysis of electrophiles. Int J Hyperthermia 2013;29:71–8.
16. Georgiades C, Rodriguez R. Renal tumor ablation. Tech Vasc Interv Radiol 2013;16:230–8.
17. Shimada K, Sakamoto Y, Esaki M, et al. Role of the width of the surgical margin in a hepatectomy for small hepatocellular carcinomas eligible for percutaneous local ablative therapy. Am J Surg 2008;195:775–81.
18. Lencioni R, Cioni D, Crocetti L, et al. Early-stage hepatocellular carcinoma in patients with cirrhosis: long-term results of percutaneous image-guided radiofrequency ablation. Radiology 2005;234:961–7.
19. Gervais DA, McGovern FJ, Arellano RS, et al. Radiofrequency ablation of renal cell carcinoma: part 1, Indications, results, and role in patient management over a 6-year period and ablation of 100 tumors. Am J Roentgenol 2005;185:64–71.
20. Lencioni R, Crocetti L, Cioni R, et al. Response to radiofrequency ablation of pulmonary tumours: a prospective, intention-to-treat, multicentre clinical trial (the RAPTURE study). Lancet Oncol 2008;9:621–8.
21. Hiraki T, Gobara H, Iishi T, et al. Percutaneous radiofrequency ablation for clinical stage I non–small cell lung cancer: results in 20 nonsurgical candidates. J Thorac Cardiovasc Surg 2007;134:1306–12.
22. Callstrom MR, Charboneau JW. Image-guided palliation of painful metastases using percutaneous ablation. Tech Vasc Interv Radiol 2007;10:120–31.
23. Gillams A, Cassoni A, Conway G, et al. Radiofrequency ablation of neuroendocrine liver metastases—the Middlesex experience. Abdom Imaging 2005;30:435–41.
24. Hinshaw JL, Lubner MG, Ziemlewicz TJ, et al. Percutaneous tumor ablation tools: microwave, radiofrequency, or cryoablation—what should you use and why? Radiographics 2014;34:1344–62.
25. Kawano M. An experimental study of percutaneous absolute ethanol injection therapy for small hepatocellular carcinoma: effects of absolute ethanol on the healthy canine liver. Gastroenterol Jpn 1989;24:663–9.
26. Shiina S, Tagawa K, Unuma T, et al. Percutaneous ethanol injection therapy for hepatocellular carcinoma. A histopathologic study. Cancer 1991;68:1524–30.
27. Giovannini M, Seitz JF. Ultrasound-guided percutaneous alcohol injection of small liver metastases. Results in 40 patients. Cancer 1994;73:294–7.
28. Long CD, Goldstein RE, Hornof WJ, et al. Percutaneous ultrasound-guided chemical parathyroid ablation for treatment of primary hyperparathyroidism in dogs. J Am Vet Med Assoc 1999;215:217–21.
29. Wells AL, Long CD, Hornof WJ, et al. Use of percutaneous ethanol injection for treatment of bilateral hyperplastic thyroid nodules in cats. J Am Vet Med Assoc 2001;218:1293–7.
30. Rasor L, Pollard R, Feldman EC. Retrospective evaluation of three treatment methods for primary hyperparathyroidism in dogs. J Am Anim Hosp Assoc 2007;43:70–7.
31. Guttin T, Knox VW 4th, Diroff JS. Outcomes for dogs with primary hyperparathyroidism following treatment with percutaneous ultrasound-guided ethanol

ablation of presumed functional parathyroid nodules: 27 cases (2008–2011). J Am Vet Med Assoc 2015;247:771–7.
32. Agut A, Soler M, Laredo FG, et al. Imageing diagnosis-ultrasound guided ethanol sclerotherapy for a simple renal cyst. Vet Radiol Ultrasound 2008; 49:65–7.
33. Sadler RA, Fields EL, Whittemore JC. Attempted ultrasound-guided ethanol ablation of a suspected pancreatic pseudocyst in a dog. Can Vet J 2016;57: 1169.
34. Nikfarjam M, Muralidharan V, Christophi C. Mechanisms of focal heat destruction of liver tumors. J Surg Res 2005;127:208–23.
35. McGahan JP, Dodd GD III. Radiofrequency ablation of the liver: current status. Am J Roentgenol 2001;176:3–16.
36. Hsu TH, Fidler ME, Gill IS. Radiofrequency ablation of the kidney: acute and chronic histology in porcine model. Urology 2000;56:872–5.
37. Siperstein AE, Rogers SJ, Hansen PD, et al. Laparoscopic thermal ablation of hepatic neuroendocrine tumor metastases. Surgery 1997;122:1147–55.
38. Nikfarjam M, Christophi C. Interstitial laser thermotherapy for liver tumours. Br J Surg 2003;90:1033–47.
39. Hong K, Georgiades C. Radiofrequency ablation: mechanism of action and devices. J Vasc Interv Radiol 2010;21:S179–86.
40. McGahan JP, Gu W-Z, Brock JM, et al. Hepatic ablation using bipolar radiofrequency electrocautery. Acad Radiol 1996;3:418–22.
41. Ritz J-P, Lehmann KS, Reissfelder C, et al. Bipolar radiofrequency ablation of liver metastases during laparotomy. First clinical experiences with a new multipolar ablation concept. Int J Colorectal Dis 2006;21:25–32.
42. Schramm W, Yang D, Haemmerich D. Contribution of direct heating, thermal conduction and perfusion during radiofrequency and microwave ablation. Engineering in Medicine and Biology Society, 2006 EMBS 2006 28th Annual International Conference of the IEEE. New York, August 31-September 3, 2006. p. 5013–5016.
43. Haemmerich D, Pilcher TA. Convective cooling affects cardiac catheter cryoablation and radiofrequency ablation in opposite directions. Engineering in Medicine and Biology Society, 2007 EMBS 2007 29th Annual International Conference of the IEEE. Lyon, France, August 23-26, 2007. p. 1499–1502.
44. Pereira PL, Trübenbach J, Schenk M, et al. Radiofrequency ablation: in vivo comparison of four commercially available devices in pig livers. Radiology 2004;232:482–90.
45. Livraghi T, Solbiati L, Meloni MF, et al. Treatment of focal liver tumors with percutaneous radio-frequency ablation: complications encountered in a multicenter study. Radiology 2003;226:441–51.
46. Rhim H, Dodd GD III, Chintapalli KN, et al. Radiofrequency thermal ablation of abdominal tumors: lessons learned from complications. Radiographics 2004;24: 41–52.
47. Steinke K, Gananadha S, King J, et al. Dispersive pad site burns with modern radiofrequency ablation equipment. Surg Laparosc Endosc Percutan Tech 2003;13:366–71.
48. Ahmed M, Liu Z, Humphries S, et al. Computer modeling of the combined effects of perfusion, electrical conductivity, and thermal conductivity on tissue heating patterns in radiofrequency tumor ablation. Int J Hyperthermia 2008; 24:577–88.

49. Liu Z, Ahmed M, Weinstein Y, et al. Characterization of the RF ablation-induced 'oven effect': the importance of background tissue thermal conductivity on tissue heating. Int J Hyperthermia 2006;22:327–42.
50. Solazzo SA, Liu Z, Lobo SM, et al. Radiofrequency ablation: importance of background tissue electrical conductivity—an agar phantom and computer modeling study. Radiology 2005;236:495–502.
51. Goldberg SN, Gazelle GS, Compton CC, et al. Radiofrequency tissue ablation in the rabbit lung: efficacy and complications. Acad Radiol 1995;2:776–84.
52. Morrison PR, VanSonnenberg E, Shankar S, et al. Radiofrequency ablation of thoracic lesions: part 1, experiments in the normal porcine thorax. Am J Roentgenol 2005;184:375–80.
53. Goldberg SN, Gazelle GS, Solbiati L, et al. Radiofrequency tissue ablation: increased lesion diameter with a perfusion electrode. Acad Radiol 1996;3:636–44.
54. Goldberg SN, Solbiati L, Hahn PF, et al. Large-volume tissue ablation with radio frequency by using a clustered, internally cooled electrode technique: laboratory and clinical experience in liver metastases. Radiology 1998;209:371–9.
55. Laeseke PF, Sampson LA, Haemmerich D, et al. Multiple-electrode radiofrequency ablation creates confluent areas of necrosis: in vivo porcine liver results. Radiology 2006;241:116–24.
56. Laeseke PF, Sampson LA, Haemmerich D, et al. Multiple-electrode radiofrequency ablation: simultaneous production of separate zones of coagulation in an in vivo porcine liver model. J Vasc Interv Radiol 2005;16:1727–35.
57. Laeseke PF, Sampson LA, Frey TM, et al. Multiple-electrode radiofrequency ablation: comparison with a conventional cluster electrode in an in vivo porcine kidney model. J Vasc Interv Radiol 2007;18:1005–10.
58. Brace C, Laeseke P, Sampson L, et al. Radiofrequency ablation with a high-power generator: device efficacy in an in vivo porcine liver model. Int J Hyperthermia 2007;23:387–94.
59. Pollard RE, Long CD, Nelson RW, et al. Percutaneous ultrasonographically guided radiofrequency heat ablation for treatment of primary hyperparathyroidism in dogs. J Am Vet Med Assoc 2001;218:1106–10.
60. Mallery KF, Pollard RE, Nelson RW, et al. Percutaneous ultrasound-guided radiofrequency heat ablation for treatment of hyperthyroidism in cats. J Am Vet Med Assoc 2003;223:1602–7.
61. Bucy D, Pollard R, Nelson R. Analysis of factors affecting outcome of ultrasound-guided radiofrequency heat ablation for treatment of primary hyperparathyroidism in dogs. Vet Radiol Ultrasound 2017;58:83–9.
62. Dear J, Kass P, Della Maggiore A, et al. Association of hypercalcemia before treatment with hypocalcemia after treatment in dogs with primary hyperparathyroidism. J Vet Intern Med 2017;31:349–54.
63. Leal RO, Frau Pascual L, Hernandez J. The use of percutaneous ultrasound-guided radiofrequency heat ablation for treatment of primary hyperparathyroidism in eight dogs: outcome and complications. Vet Sci 2018;5 [pii:E91].
64. Ahrar K, Price RE, Wallace MJ, et al. Percutaneous radiofrequency ablation of lung tumors in a large animal model. J Vasc Interv Radiol 2003;14:1037–43.
65. Culp WTN, Johnson EG, Palm CA, et al. Use of thermal ablation techniques in the treatment of canine urogenital neoplasia, in Proceedings. Veterinary Interventional Radiology and Interventional Endoscopy Society Meeting. Cabo San Lucas, Mexico, June 22-24, 2017.

66. Bertram JM, Yang D, Converse MC, et al. A review of coaxial-based interstitial antennas for hepatic microwave ablation. Crit Rev Biomed Eng 2006;34: 187–213.
67. Brace CL. Microwave tissue ablation: biophysics, technology, and applications. Crit Rev Biomed Eng 2010;38:65–78.
68. Brace CL. Radiofrequency and microwave ablation of the liver, lung, kidney, and bone: what are the differences? Curr Probl Diagn Radiol 2009;38:135–43.
69. Chu KF, Dupuy DE. Thermal ablation of tumours: biological mechanisms and advances in therapy. Nat Rev Cancer 2014;14:199.
70. Lubner MG, Brace CL, Hinshaw JL, et al. Microwave tumor ablation: mechanism of action, clinical results, and devices. J Vasc Interv Radiol 2010;21:S192–203.
71. Andreano A, Brace CL. A comparison of direct heating during radiofrequency and microwave ablation in ex vivo liver. Cardiovasc Intervent Radiol 2013;36: 505–11.
72. Yang D, Converse MC, Mahvi DM, et al. Measurement and analysis of tissue temperature during microwave liver ablation. IEEE Trans Biomed Eng 2007; 54:150–5.
73. Brace CL, Laeseke PF, Sampson LA, et al. Microwave ablation with a single small-gauge triaxial antenna: in vivo porcine liver model. Radiology 2007;242: 435–40.
74. Wright AS, Lee FT, Mahvi DM. Hepatic microwave ablation with multiple antennae results in synergistically larger zones of coagulation necrosis. Ann Surg Oncol 2003;10:275–83.
75. Knavel EM, Hinshaw JL, Lubner MG, et al. High-powered gas-cooled microwave ablation: shaft cooling creates an effective stick function without altering the ablation zone. Am J Roentgenol 2012;198:W260–5.
76. Li X, Zhang L, Fan W, et al. Comparison of microwave ablation and multipolar radiofrequency ablation, both using a pair of internally cooled interstitial applicators: results in ex vivo porcine livers. Int J Hyperthermia 2011;27:240–8.
77. Yang T, Case JB, Boston S, et al. Microwave ablation for treatment of hepatic neoplasia in five dogs. J Am Vet Med Assoc 2017;250:79–85.
78. Mazzaccari K, Boston SE, Toskich BB, et al. Video-assisted microwave ablation for the treatment of a metastatic lung lesion in a dog with appendicular osteosarcoma and hypertrophic osteopathy. Vet Surg 2017;46:1161–5.
79. Upton ML, Tangner C, Payton ME. Evaluation of carbon dioxide laser ablation combined with mitoxantrone and piroxicam treatment in dogs with transitional cell carcinoma. J Am Vet Med Assoc 2006;228:549–52.
80. Cerf DJ, Lindquist EC. Palliative ultrasound-guided endoscopic diode laser ablation of transitional cell carcinomas of the lower urinary tract in dogs. J Am Vet Med Assoc 2012;240:51–60.
81. Yas E, Kelmer G, Shipov A, et al. Successful transendoscopic oesophageal mass ablation in two dogs with Spirocerca lupi associated oesophageal sarcoma. J Small Anim Pract 2013;54:495–8.
82. Shipov A, Kelmer G, Lavy E, et al. Long-term outcome of transendoscopic oesophageal mass ablation in dogs with Spirocerca lupi-associated oesophageal sarcoma. Vet Rec 2015;177:365.
83. Bottero E, Cagnasso A, Gianella P. Diode laser ablation of a tracheal osteochondroma in a dog. J Small Anim Pract 2016;57:382–5.
84. ter Haar G. HIFU tissue ablation: concept and devices. Therapeutic ultrasound. Basel, Switzerland: Springer; 2016. p. 3–20.

85. Deardorff DL, Diederich CJ. Axial control of thermal coagulation using a multi-element interstitial ultrasound applicator with internal cooling. IEEE Trans Ultrason Ferroelectr Freq Control 2000;47:170–8.
86. Kinsey AM, Tyreus PD, Rieke V, et al. Interstitial ultrasound applicators with dynamic angular control for thermal ablation of tumors under MR-guidance. Engineering in Medicine and Biology Society, 2004 IEMBS 2004 26th Annual International Conference of the IEEE. San Francisco, California, September 1-5, 2004. p. 2496–2499.
87. Ren X-L, Zhou X-D, Yan R-L, et al. Sonographically guided extracorporeal ablation of uterine fibroids with high-intensity focused ultrasound: midterm results. J Ultrasound Med 2009;28:100–3.
88. Taran F, Tempany C, Regan L, et al. Magnetic resonance-guided focused ultrasound (MRgFUS) compared with abdominal hysterectomy for treatment of uterine leiomyomas. Ultrasound Obstet Gynecol 2009;34:572–8.
89. Zhou Y-F. High intensity focused ultrasound in clinical tumor ablation. World J Clin Oncol 2011;2:8.
90. Kim Y-S, Rhim H, Choi MJ, et al. High-intensity focused ultrasound therapy: an overview for radiologists. Korean J Radiol 2008;9:291–302.
91. Li J-J, Xu G-L, Gu M-F, et al. Complications of high intensity focused ultrasound in patients with recurrent and metastatic abdominal tumors. World J Gastroenterol 2007;13:2747.
92. Roberts WW, Hall TL, Ives K, et al. Pulsed cavitational ultrasound: a noninvasive technology for controlled tissue ablation (histotripsy) in the rabbit kidney. J Urol 2006;175:734–8.
93. Kopelman D, Inbar Y, Hanannel A, et al. Magnetic resonance-guided focused ultrasound surgery (MRgFUS). Four ablation treatments of a single canine hepatocellular adenoma. HPB (Oxford) 2006;8:292–8.
94. Ryu M-O, Lee S-H, Ahn J-O, et al. Treatment of solid tumors in dogs using veterinary high-intensity focused ultrasound: a retrospective clinical study. Vet J 2018;234:126–9.
95. Erinjeri JP, Clark TW. Cryoablation: mechanism of action and devices. J Vasc Interv Radiol 2010;21:S187–91.
96. Mala T. Cryoablation of liver tumours–a review of mechanisms, techniques and clinical outcome. Minim Invasive Ther Allied Technol 2006;15:9–17.
97. Mala T, Samset E, Aurdal L, et al. Magnetic resonance imaging-estimated three-dimensional temperature distribution in liver cryolesions: a study of cryolesion characteristics assumed necessary for tumor ablation. Cryobiology 2001;43:268–75.
98. Hoffmann NE, Bischof JC. The cryobiology of cryosurgical injury. Urology 2002;60:40–9.
99. Gage AA, Baust J. Mechanisms of tissue injury in cryosurgery. Cryobiology 1998;37:171–86.
100. Wang H, Littrup PJ, Duan Y, et al. Thoracic masses treated with percutaneous cryotherapy: initial experience with more than 200 procedures. Radiology 2005;235:289–98.
101. Hinshaw JL, Lee FT Jr. Cryoablation for liver cancer. Tech Vasc Interv Radiol 2007;10:47–57.
102. Weber SM, Lee FT Jr, Warner TF, et al. Hepatic cryoablation: US monitoring of extent of necrosis in normal pig liver. Radiology 1998;207:73–7.
103. Lee FT Jr, Chosy SG, Littrup PJ, et al. CT-monitored percutaneous cryoablation in a pig liver model: pilot study. Radiology 1999;211:687–92.

104. Jansen MC, van Hillegersberg R, Schoots IG, et al. Cryoablation induces greater inflammatory and coagulative responses than radiofrequency ablation or laser induced thermotherapy in a rat liver model. Surgery 2010;147:686–95.
105. Chapman WC, Debelak JP, Pinson CW, et al. Hepatic cryoablation, but not radiofrequency ablation, results in lung inflammation. Ann Surg 2000;231:752.
106. Littrup PJ, Jallad B, Vorugu V, et al. Lethal isotherms of cryoablation in a phantom study: effects of heat load, probe size, and number. J Vasc Interv Radiol 2009;20:1343–51.
107. Lee FT Jr, Mahvi DM, Chosy SG, et al. Hepatic cryosurgery with intraoperative US guidance. Radiology 1997;202:624–32.
108. Yang Y, Wang C, Lu Y, et al. Outcomes of ultrasound-guided percutaneous argon-helium cryoablation of hepatocellular carcinoma. J Hepato-Biliary-Pancreatic Sci 2012;19:674–84.
109. Seifert JK, Morris DL. World survey on the complications of hepatic and prostate cryotherapy. World J Surg 1999;23:109–14.
110. Hruby G, Edelstein A, Karpf J, et al. Risk factors associated with renal parenchymal fracture during laparoscopic cryoablation. BJU Int 2008;102:723–6.
111. Murphy S, Lawrence J, Schmiedt C, et al. Image-guided transnasal cryoablation of a recurrent nasal adenocarcinoma in a dog. J Small Anim Pract 2011;52:329–33.
112. Weisse C BA, Solomon S. Combined transarterial embolization, systemic cyclophosphamide, and cryotherapy ablation for "Hi-Lo" maxillary fibrosarcoma in a dog. Proceedings: 8th Annual Meeting, Veterinary Endoscopy Society. San Pedro, Belize, May 5-7, 2011.
113. Golberg A, Yarmush ML. Nonthermal irreversible electroporation: fundamentals, applications, and challenges. IEEE Trans Biomed Eng 2013;60:707–14.
114. Lee EW, Thai S, Kee ST. Irreversible electroporation: a novel image-guided cancer therapy. Gut Liver 2010;4:S99.
115. Lee EW, Chen C, Prieto VE, et al. Advanced hepatic ablation technique for creating complete cell death: irreversible electroporation. Radiology 2010;255:426–33.
116. Lee EW, Loh CT, Kee ST. Imaging guided percutaneous irreversible electroporation: ultrasound and immunohistological correlation. Technol Cancer Res Treat 2007;6:287–93.
117. Onik G, Mikus P, Rubinsky B. Irreversible electroporation: implications for prostate ablation. Technol Cancer Res Treat 2007;6:295–300.
118. Adeyanju O, Al-Angari H, Sahakian A. The optimization of needle electrode number and placement for irreversible electroporation of hepatocellular carcinoma. Radiol Oncol 2012;46:126–35.
119. Schmidt CR, Shires P, Mootoo M. Real-time ultrasound imaging of irreversible electroporation in a porcine liver model adequately characterizes the zone of cellular necrosis. HPB (Oxford) 2012;14:98–102.
120. Deodhar A, Dickfeld T, Single GW, et al. Irreversible electroporation near the heart: ventricular arrhythmias can be prevented with ECG synchronization. Am J Roentgenol 2011;196:W330–5.
121. Thomson KR, Cheung W, Ellis SJ, et al. Investigation of the safety of irreversible electroporation in humans. J Vasc Interv Radiol 2011;22:611–21.
122. Garcia P, Pancotto T, Rossmeisl J Jr, et al. Non-thermal irreversible electroporation (N-TIRE) and adjuvant fractionated radiotherapeutic multimodal therapy for intracranial malignant glioma in a canine patient. Technol Cancer Res Treat 2011;10:73–83.

123. Neal RE III, Rossmeisl JH Jr, Garcia PA, et al. Successful treatment of a large soft tissue sarcoma with irreversible electroporation. J Clin Oncol 2011;29: e372–7.
124. Rossmeisl JH, Garcia PA, Pancotto TE, et al. Safety and feasibility of the NanoKnife system for irreversible electroporation ablative treatment of canine spontaneous intracranial gliomas. J Neurosurg 2015;123:1008–25.
125. Latouche EL, Arena CB, Ivey JW, et al. High-frequency irreversible electroporation for intracranial meningioma: a feasibility study in a spontaneous canine tumor model. Technol Cancer Res Treat 2018;17.

Electrochemotherapy in Veterinary Oncology

State-of-the-Art and Perspectives

Enrico Pierluigi Spugnini, DVM, PhD[a,*], Alfonso Baldi, MD[b]

KEYWORDS

- Biphasic pulses • Bleomycin • Carcinoma • Cisplatin • Electroporation
- Mast cell tumor • Pets • Sarcoma

KEY POINTS

- The cell membrane is the major obstacle to be overcome by chemotherapy agents in order to reach their biological targets. This is especially true for lipophobic agents like bleomycin.
- Electroporation is a technique that greatly increases the uptake of such drugs by tumors. The combination of permeabilizing pulses and chemotherapy is called electrochemotherapy (ECT).
- ECT has been successfully used in combination with bleomycin and cisplatin to treat solid tumors such as carcinoma, sarcoma, and hematologic malignancies such as mast cell tumor.
- Novel applications include the treatment of visceral tumors under ultrasonographic guidance and the delivery of molecular compounds such as oligonucleotides, plasmids, and small proteins.

INTRODUCTION

Achieving local tumor control in veterinary patients with cancer affected by solid neoplasms represents one of the major challenges for veterinary oncologists, frequently due to late referrals or rapid tumor growth.[1–4] This clinical presentation often prevents the achievement of local control with surgery alone, needing a multimodality approach involving adjuvant therapies, such as chemotherapy, radiotherapy, or electrochemotherapy (ECT).[1–5]

Disclosure Statement: E.P. Spugnini and A. Baldi are stockholders of Biopulse srl.
[a] Biopulse srl, Via Toledo 256, Naples 80132, Italy; [b] Department of Environmental, Biological and Pharmaceutical Sciences and Technologies, Campania University "Luigi Vanvitelli", Via Vivaldi, 43, Caserta 81100, Italy
* Corresponding author.
E-mail address: info@enricospugnini.net

Vet Clin Small Anim 49 (2019) 967–979
https://doi.org/10.1016/j.cvsm.2019.04.006 vetsmall.theclinics.com
0195-5616/19/

Chemotherapy can be adopted as a strategy to reduce the tumor volume, thus permitting a wide excision, or can be used, in selected histotypes, as a tool to decrease the probability of local recurrence after surgery.[3] Finally, its major application is to reduce the chances of distant dissemination.[3] Radiation therapy is the cornerstone of combined approach to solid tumors, usually as an adjuvant therapy or as palliation for inoperable neoplasms.[1–3] ECT has been extensively investigated over the past 15 years as an additional treatment modality for local control of solid neoplasms, evidencing high rates of responses with limited side effects.[5–8] It involves the combination of chemotherapy agents (mostly lipophobic molecules) with the application of permeabilizing electric pulses that promote the uptake of these drugs by cancer cells.[5–8] This therapy is rapidly becoming popular among the veterinary community because of its favorable characteristics: ease of administration, effectiveness, low morbidity, and relative inexpensiveness.[5–8]

TECHNICAL ASPECTS OF ELECTROCHEMOTHERAPY

Electroporation is the creation of aqueous pathways (electropores) in the cell membrane following the exposition to short intensive electric fields having appropriate waveforms. This temporary permeabilization permits free transit of molecules, ions, and water between the 2 sides of the cell membrane (**Fig. 1**).[9,10] After the exposure to the permeabilizing pulses, the cell has 2 possible fates: (1) reversal of the process and return to the previous steady state, and (2) impossibility to reverse the ion fluxes and activation of the caspase apoptotic or necrotic pathways with progression to

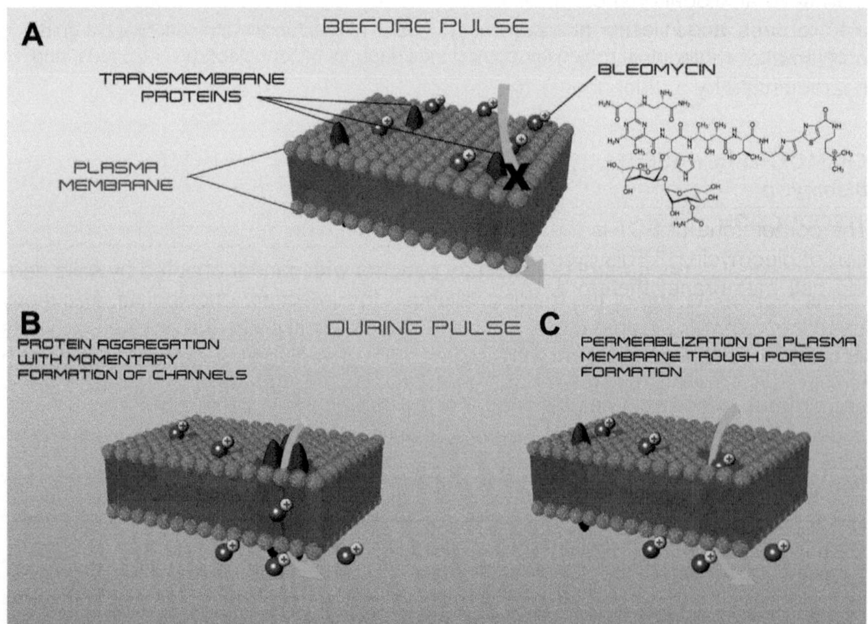

Fig. 1. Mechanisms of drug perfusion following electroporation. (*A*) Cytoplasmic membrane before the application of permeabilizing pulses: the lipophobic drug cannot enter the cell without the intervention of a transmembrane carrier. (*B*) The permeabilizing pulses induce aggregation of the transmembrane proteins and/or (*C*) formation of pores in the lipid bilayer of the membrane.

cellular death. The crossroad between the 2 destinies is the ability to pump the calcium ions outside the membrane and sequester them within the endoplasmic or the sarcoplasmic reticulum.[9,11] The first phenomenon is defined as reversible electroporation; the latter is named irreversible electroporation.[11] Electroporation can be structured, for convenience purposes, in 5 phases: induction, expansion, stabilization, resealing, and memory effect.[12] Another effect of cell exposure to permeabilizing electric fields is the transient clustering of transmembrane proteins, with the formation of pseudotunnels that contribute to the cross-flow of material.[13] Electroporation has been defined as a threshold phenomenon occurring when the permeabilizing pulses exceed the value of the transmembrane potential ($\Delta\phi m$) accordingly to the formula: $\Delta\phi m = 1.5 \times E_{ext} \times r \times \cos\Theta$ (Θ = polar angle at the membrane with respect to the E_{ext}, the external electrical field).[14,15] This physical model is too crude for ECT of neoplasms. In fact, even if shown to be qualitatively acceptable, it does not consider the cellular heterogeneity within of neoplastic tissue, the presence of neoplastic foci, or the variable content of connective tissue, as well as the different orientation of the cancer cells in terms of field polarity, parameters that would prevent an unopposed permeabilization.[15] For these factors, ECT trains are split into 2 perpendicular trains of 4 pulses or administered as trains of biphasic pulses.[16–18] Length, number, and shape of the pulses are key factors for a successful electroporation. Further experiments elucidated the phenomenon of electroporation, showing 2 phases of relevant clinical application: (1) an early phase of pore induction, and (2) a later phase of pore enlargement.[19,20] These early pores are called "transient electropores," which, after the disappearance of the electric field, shrink in size and stabilize to form the so-called long-lasting electropores.[20] In terms of uptake, large molecules (greater than several kilodaltons) can cross the cell membrane mostly through the transient electropores, and in lesser quantity, through the protein pseudotunnels.[21] Conversely, only smaller molecules can transit through the "long-lasting electropores" that are characterized by a much longer half-life.

CHEMOTHERAPY AGENTS USED IN VETERINARY ELECTROCHEMOTHERAPY

Bleomycin

The cornerstone of ECT is the combination of electrical pulses with the administration of bleomycin.[5–8] This drug is lipophobic and uses protein receptors to penetrate the cell membrane; therefore, the uptake is slow and quantitatively limited under normal conditions.[5–8] The loss of this membrane receptor by tumor cells is the main mechanism of chemoresistance against bleomycin. A way to bypass this obstacle is the permeabilization of the cell membrane by using electric pulses that can promote bleomycin captation by a factor of 700-fold.[5–8] **Fig. 1** shows the 2 proposed mechanisms of membrane permeabilization following application of electric pulses.

The mechanism of action of bleomycin is the fragmentation of DNA, under normal conditions, which results in G2-M phase arrest of the neoplastic cell cycle. When used in combination with ECT, the number of DNA lesions is dramatically increased, leading to apoptosis.[5–8]

Cisplatin

Cisplatin and its analogues interact with cancer cells through binding with DNA bases,[5–8] leading to cross-linking of DNA that causes cell death. Electroporation enhances the transmembrane passage of this drug by a factor of 4 to 8, thus increasing the number of cross-links.[5–8] This property of ECT has allowed its topical use in cats, which are notoriously intolerant to this agent. Presently, cisplatin is the second most extensively adopted drug for ECT.

Doxorubicin

Doxorubicin belongs to the anthracycline class. Mechanisms of action include various interactions with tumor DNA, such as base intercalation, DNA strand breakage, and topoisomerase II inhibition. Other mechanisms consist of DNA polymerase activity inhibition, altered regulation of gene expression, and release of free radicals.[22] Preclinical studies inferred that ECT could improve doxorubicin efficacy in in vitro and in vivo models.[22] This agent has been also adopted for ECT palliation in pets affected by mammary cancer with acceptable results (Enrico Pierluigi Spugnini, personal observation).

Mitoxantrone

Mitoxantrone is a synthetic anthracycline analogue with much less cardiotoxicity than the other members of the family, and its mechanisms are similar to doxorubicin. It diffuses through the cell membrane according to the composition of the lipid bilayer. ECT has been shown to increase its efficacy in human and veterinary patients.[23]

CLINICAL ELECTROCHEMOTHERAPY PROTOCOLS IN VETERINARY ONCOLOGY

There are 3 major considerations that differentiate veterinary ECT from human ECT:

1. In humans, it is mostly limited to the palliation of cancer cutaneous metastases or for the treatment of primary skin tumors. In veterinary oncology, ECT is adopted as first-line treatment of solid tumors and of the treatment of selected visceral neoplasms.
2. Although in humans, ECT is frequently administered under local anesthesia, in veterinary applications, ECT is performed with the patients under heavy sedation or general anesthesia.
3. Veterinary ECT can be palliative, adjuvant, or neoadjuvant and can be administered simultaneously with surgery (intraoperative ECT).

The protocols involve patient sedation using a combination of different drugs, including butorphanol, medetomidine, acepromazine, methadone, and ketamine, as per standardized induction protocols.[24] After the induction, propofol or barbiturates are intravenously administered for greater the depth of anesthesia. In cases of intraoperative ECT, the patient is generally maintained with gases such as isoflurane or sevoflurane.[24] With the patient properly sedated, the chemotherapy agents are administered systemically and/or locally. As a general rule, bleomycin is given as an intravenous bolus at the concentration of 20 to 30 mg/m^2 (or mitoxantrone at the dose of 5 mg/m^2).[5–8,24] Locally, cisplatin can be injected within tumor or in tumor beds at the concentration of 0.5 to 1 mg/mm^3 or, alternatively, bleomycin at the concentration of 1.5 mg/mm^3. Administration of the 2 agents has been successfully combined to increase therapeutic efficacy. Subsequently, following a given time interval (usually 5 minutes), sequences of 8 permeabilizing pulses are administered. **Fig. 2** summarizes an ECT session in a veterinary patient. The 2 most popular waveforms are square and biphasic.[5–8,24] The permeabilizing protocols can vary in terms of electrical shapes, voltage, amperage, frequency, and interpulse duration.[5–8,24] The authors' previous setting adopted a train of 8 biphasic pulses lasting 50 + 50 microseconds each, with 1-ms interpulse intervals, delivered in trains of 1300 V/cm (800 V/cm for intraoperatory ECT), 1-Hz frequency, using caliper or needle array electrodes. Currently, the

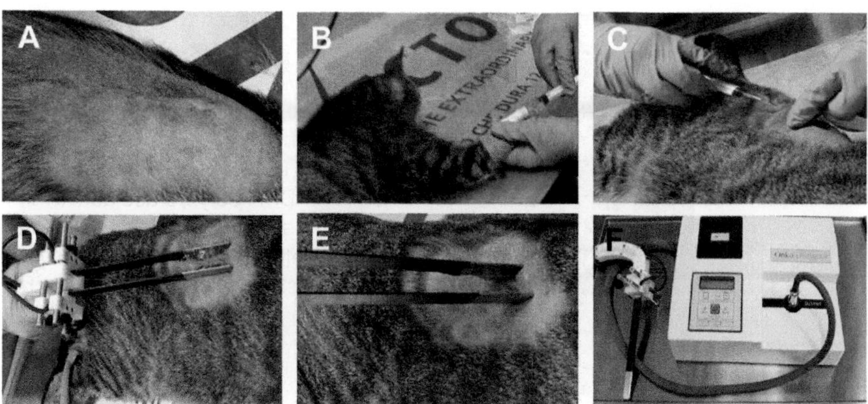

Fig. 2. Different phases of an ECT session. (*A*) The patient is shaved to expose the underlying scar of an incompletely excised fibrosarcoma. (*B*) After sedation, the patient is treated with a bolus of bleomycin. (*C*) The surgical scar is injected with cisplatin. (*D*) Electrical pulses are administered with the larger surface of a plate electrode. (*E*) Electrical pulses are administered with the smaller surface of a plate electrode. (*F*) An overview of an ECT instrument.

authors reduced the interpulse to a 300-μs interpulse (total treatment time per train 3.2 ms) and adopted an amperage dampener that significantly reduced the morbidity.[8] Contact of the external electrodes to the lesions and electrical conduction is improved using electroconductive gel. The treatment is repeated at 2-week intervals. In cases of postoperative ECT, the number of sessions is limited to 2 treatments, whereas in the case of direct ablation of gross disease, ECT is administered until a complete response is reached or tumor progression occurs.

Protocol for Ultrasound-Guided Electrochemotherapy for Intracavitary Tumors

After the induction of patient sedation, bleomycin is administered intravenously, and then paired needles with electrical shielding are inserted within the tumor using ultrasonographic guidance. Imaging assistance allows for avoidance of necrotic and hemorrhagic foci, and Doppler technique consents to avoid major vessels. At this time, 5 series of biphasic electric pulses are delivered to the tumor with a starting voltage of 800 V and modified according to the tissue conductivity.[25] This protocol combines the Joule effect (direct thermal ablation) with the effects of ECT. Treatment is repeated until tumor coverage is achieved. The sessions are repeated every 2 weeks until a tumor response is observed (**Fig. 3**).

CLINICAL RESULTS OBTAINED BY ELECTROCHEMOTHERAPY IN VETERINARY ONCOLOGY: SOLID TUMORS

Mesenchymal Tumors

Feline soft tissue sarcoma

Feline patients have a special record in veterinary ECT, being the very first pets to be enrolled in a clinical trial. In the late 1990s, a group of cats with recurring soft tissue sarcomas following adjuvant cobalt radiation therapy and surgical ablation was enrolled in a compassionate ECT study and compared with untreated controls.[26] This trial reported a single responder with partial remission, likely as a consequence of acquired chemoresistance by relapsing tumors. The need for additional preliminary investigations resulted in 2 studies enrolling pets with various neoplasms (including several

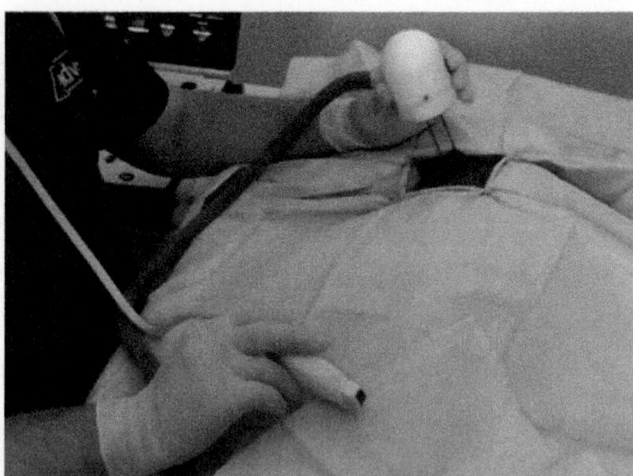

Fig. 3. An ultrasonography-guided ECT in a canine patient; the impulses are delivered through needle array electrode.

soft tissue sarcomas), directly targeted using ECT. Different from other histotypes, mesenchymal tumors evidenced a lower response rate and rare complete remissions.[27,28] Preliminary observation in a cat with an incompletely excised hemangiopericytoma receiving 2 postoperative sessions of ECT resulted in long-term control.[29] The necessity for a different approach to further ameliorate the effectiveness of ECT in sarcomas led to the adoption of adjuvant ECT (both intraoperatively and postoperatively) following surgical tumor excision. A cohort of feline patients was enrolled to receive intraoperative or postoperative ECT using local injection with bleomycin. These cats were matched against a cohort treated with surgery alone.[30] A total of 72 cats were assigned to the 3 experimental groups. Results evidenced that ECT led to extended local tumor control and survival, independently by its modality of administration. Numerous prognostic factors, including previous treatments and tumor size, were identified in this study, and side effects were limited to local inflammation and occasional wound dehiscence.[30] Notably, a cat with a previously radiated sarcoma experienced a radiation recall following ECT.[31] Over the years, perfecting of ECT protocols has allowed the clinical recovery of chemotherapy drugs with narrow therapeutic indices. An early case involved the treatment of a cat with bilateral facial rhabdomyosarcoma using cisplatin-based adjuvant ECT.[32] The swift transmembrane translation of the drug during ECT deters the toxicities (fatal pulmonary edema) reported in felines receiving cisplatin. Last, a broader confirmatory study further investigated the use of cisplatin with adjuvant ECT for feline sarcoma. A total of 64 cats with sarcomas were recruited and treated with ECT, and their responses were compared with a control group of 14 patients receiving surgery alone.[33] ECT resulted in increased local control with a mean time to recurrence of 666 days versus 180 of controls.

Canine soft tissue sarcoma

In dogs, the use of adjuvant ECT for the treatment of incompletely excised soft tissue sarcomas was described in a cohort of 22 dogs treated with intralesional bleomycin at the tumor site.[34] The protocol was well tolerated and resulted in a median time to recurrence of 730 days. Negligible side effects were noted. A case report described the effectiveness of neoadjuvant ECT in a dog with an inoperable high-grade soft tissue sarcoma by shrinking the tumor mass to an operable size. Neoadjuvant ECT allowed the removal of the residual tumor and the sterilization of the surgical field resulting in long-term tumor control.[35] A very recent investigation from the authors' group used the combination of systemic bleomycin with local administration of cisplatin in a cohort of 30 dogs for the treatment of incompletely excised soft tissue sarcomas. At the time of this writing, 26 dogs had no evidence of recurrence; 3 dogs had recurrence, and 1 dog had both local recurrence and pulmonary metastases. Median estimated time to recurrence was 857 days. ECT using a combination of bleomycin and cisplatin appears to be well tolerated and highly effective in the treatment of incompletely resected soft tissue sarcomas in dogs and is the current standard protocol in the authors' group.[36]

Unusual mesenchymal neoplasms: canine fibromatosis

Canine fibromatosis is a rare neoplasm of the soft tissues. It is characterized as rapidly growing and invasive and is prone to scar tissue–like recurrence. Because of growth patterns and tumor locations, these lesions pose a clinical challenge. One report describes the positive outcome of a Great Dane diagnosed with recurring fibromatosis after incomplete surgical excision. The dog achieved complete remission after 4 courses of ECT and died 3 years later of unrelated disease.[37]

Epithelial Tumors

Canine perianal and anal sac tumors

Canine hepatoid glands tumors, especially adenomas, are exquisitely responsive to ECT. The treatment can be used to treat large perianal neoplasms that do not regress following castration. In selected cases, the authors performed ECT with spinal anesthesia with good patient tolerability. The first report using cisplatin-based ECT for the treatment of large perianal tumors in dogs reported an overall response rate of 82% with 41% achieving complete response.[38] A subsequent report described the use of bleomycin-based ECT for these neoplasms with a total of 91% responders and 83% attaining complete response.[39] Considering the involvement of deep underlying tissues by these tumors (especially those involving the anal sacs) and the frequent ulceration and bleeding that could affect proper drug distribution, an adjuvant approach has been recently proposed for these aggressive neoplasms combined with surgical excision.[40] For invasive anal sac carcinoma, especially those extending to the abdominal cavity, an ultrasound approach is deemed more appropriate. These strategies are the proof of concept that ECT can be successfully adopted in sensitive tissues, such as the anus, allowing tumor control and preservation of function with conservative surgery.

Feline head and neck carcinoma

White cats are extremely prone to sun-induced malignancies, in particular, squamous cell carcinoma (SCC), affecting the nasal planum, the eyelid, and the head.[41] Patients are often diagnosed with these tumors in an advanced condition that precludes radical excision. Therefore, these tumors are generally treated with radiation therapy.[42] ECT has been successfully proposed as an alternate therapy for these tumors. The proof of concept has been a preliminary investigation treating a small cohort of 9 cats with intralesional bleomycin and ECT. Seven of the cats (77.7%) had a complete response of various durations.[43] Subsequent work adopted the systemic administration of bleomycin within an ECT protocol, again reporting a good control rate with preservation of the anatomic structures.[44] A larger cohort of feline patients with advanced SCC of the head and neck was treated with systemic bleomycin potentiated by permeabilizing electric pulses (ECT) and matched against a control group receiving bleomycin alone. The ECT group had a significantly better outcome than the control. Median times to progression were 30.5 and 3.9 months, respectively.[45] Generally speaking, side effects are confined to local inflammation; however, cats with advanced nasal planum SCC (ie, T4 stage) can develop significant scar tissue that can potentially result in anosmia (E.P. Spugnini, personal observation). This study verified the ability of ECT to attack extensive carcinomatous lesions, even in challenging areas, such as the eyelids and the peri-ocular area. **Fig. 4** shows the outcome of a cat with ocular SCC successfully treated with ECT.

Miscellaneous skin tumors

Cutaneous tumors are generally treated with surgery. ECT is currently limited to the treatment of inoperable tumors, tumors with regional metastatic cascade, or tumors affecting areas where a conservative strategy could not be pursued.

Scientific literature reports the ECT treatment of an apocrine gland carcinoma with cervical lymph node metastases, a ganglioneuroblastoma of the footpad, and a trichoblastoma of the digit. The dog with the apocrine gland carcinoma was treated with systemic mitoxantrone-based ECT that resulted in tumor control in excess of 6 months.[23] The cat with the ganglioneuroblastoma was treated with 3 sessions of ECT and achieved a complete remission in excess of 450 days.[46] The digital trichoblastoma was successfully treated with 3 sessions of ECT using systemic bleomycin. The tumor volume decreased throughout the ECT sessions, with a complete response reached after 81 days. The patient achieved a disease-free interval of 700 days.[47]

CLINICAL RESULTS OBTAINED BY ELECTROCHEMOTHERAPY IN VETERINARY ONCOLOGY: ROUND CELL TUMORS

Canine Melanoma

Melanoma was among the first round cell tumors to be treated with ECT. A small study investigated intralesional bleomycin–based ECT in a group of 10 dogs, which resulted in a response rate of 80%, and 40% of responders was controlled in excess of 1 year.[48] A factor that promoted a longer response was the tumor location in soft areas of the oral cavity, where the lack of bone allowed a more homogeneous drug distribution. Remarkably, complete responders showed persistent vitiligo-like discolorations at the tumor sites, possibly secondary to ECT-induced triggering of an immune response. More recently, a case report described the successful palliation of an anal melanoma in a dog, whereby ECT allowed preservation of the anal functionality for 3 months.[49]

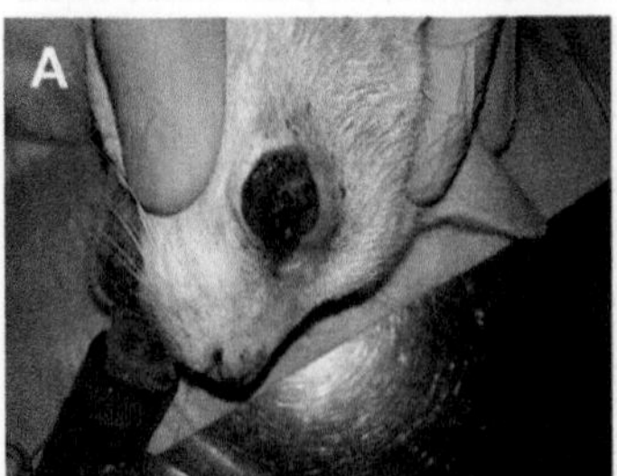

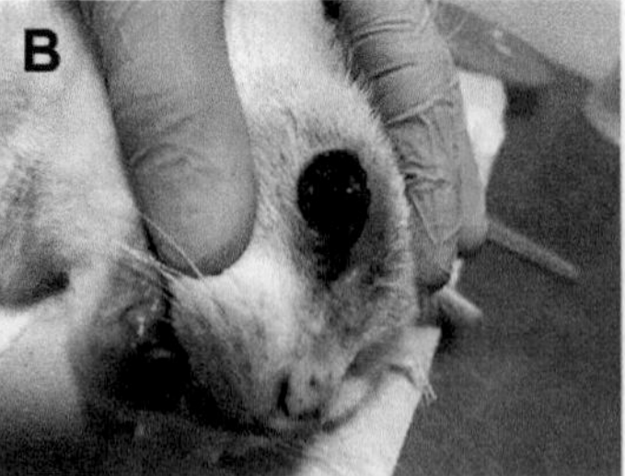

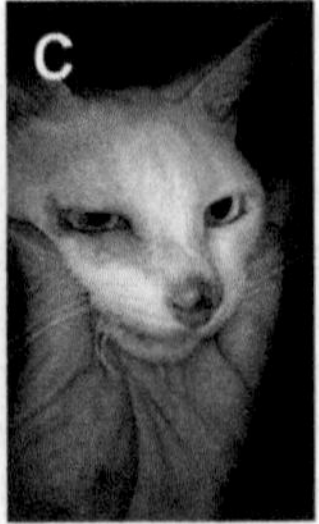

Fig. 4. Outcome of a sun-induced palpebral SCC in a cat treated with ECT. (*A*) Patient at presentation. (*B*) Patient after 1 session of ECT: the mass is reduced and appears less vascularized. (*C*) Patient after 2 sessions of ECT, showing complete resolution of the palpebral neoplasm. (*Courtesy of* D. Santos dos Anjos, DVM, MSc, PhD student (Unesp-Jaboticabal), Brazil, Mexico.)

Canine Mast Cell Tumors

Mast cell tumors (MCTs) are among the most common neoplasms in veterinary medicine and may be difficult to control because of growth rate, location, and high content of histamine and other vasoactive substances.[50] ECT can be used to directly attack these tumors or as an adjuvant following surgical excision. The first article described the successful use of locally administered bleomycin-based ECT in a cohort of 28 dogs with incompletely excised mast cell neoplasms.[51] Another study compared the results of directly attacking MCTs with ECT to surgery, inferring that ECT could be a potential alternative to surgery.[52] A third prospective study treated 37 dogs with incompletely excised grade II and grade III MCTs using cisplatin-based ECT and showed a 78% response rate with minimal side effects.[53] However, another report describes the use of ECT in dogs with MCTs as either first-line therapy or an adjuvant to surgery. In this retrospective study, 51 dogs with MCTs were classified in the following treatment groups (ECT-only, 15 cases; intraoperative ECT, 11 cases; ECT adjuvant to surgery, 14 cases; surgery followed by ECT, 11 cases).[54] In this study, the intraoperative group of dogs showed the best disease-free interval. Pooled, these observations showed that ECT is a very effective and pliable technique that can be used alone or in combination with other therapies.

Canine and Feline Lymphoma

ECT literature for lymphoma in pets is limited to a single article assessing the potential of bleomycin-based ECT in the treatment of localized canine and feline lymphoma.[55] A total of 6 patients were recruited in this study, having clinical responses that ranged from 1 week up to 3 years. ECT was well tolerated, and side effects were limited despite the treatment of sensitive tissues, such as the nasal cavity and the retrobulbar space. Feline patients with nasal or retrobulbar lymphoma were the best responders in terms of degree and duration of response. The authors' group is mostly adopting this approach for the palliation of chemoresistant oral lymphoma.

Sticker Sarcoma

Sticker sarcoma is a transmissible venereal tumor (TVT) that is sexually transmitted within the canine population. This neoplasm is successfully treated with vincristine. Rarely, chemoresistance has been reported, and doxorubicin is suggested as second-line treatment. Alternatively, radiation therapy has been successfully used for local control. A clinical report describes the possible use of ECT as a rescue, reporting 3 chemoresistant TVT cases that successfully responded to intralesional bleomycin and electroporation.[56]

IMAGING-BASED ELECTROCHEMOTHERAPY

The frontier of ECT is now its application in the treatment of visceral and intracavitary neoplasms. The first application of ultrasound-assisted ECT has been the treatment of a clear cell thymoma in a cat.[25] The patient was treated under general anesthesia with systemic bleomycin, and then permeabilizing electric pulses were administered through a specifically designed ecoreflective electrode. The tumor had a long-term partial response that resulted in a 14+ months' survival. Another novel field of ECT application is the treatment of nasal cavity tumors. A recent article describes the use of a single-needle electrode to treat deeply sited neoplasms.[57] A total of 11 dogs with miscellaneous nasal tumors were treated using ECT, with 91% of patients responding. Overall survival rates of 60% at 1 year and 30% at 2 years were reported. Endoscopic ECT has been successfully attempted on 2 canine patients with rectal neoplasms (adenocarcinoma and lymphoma), achieving good tumor control. These therapeutic avenues are currently being investigated, but the preliminary reports show promise as novel technologies are developed and field tested.[58]

SUMMARY

ECT combines the use of some standard chemotherapy agents with electroporation to promote their efficacy. It allows the use of lipophobic drugs with narrow therapeutic indices to obtain high response rates. while sparing the patient from toxicosis. In veterinary oncology, this approach is becoming a first-line therapy for various cancer histotypes, because of its high efficacy and low toxicity.[59] An additional advantage of this approach is the possibility of repeated courses of ECT in case of recurrence. Care must be exerted in selecting adequate patients for this therapy in order to avoid undesirable complications. In particular, patients with bulky neoplasms might be prone to toxicosis secondary to the massive destruction of neoplastic tissues (ie, tumor lysis syndrome, thromboembolism, disseminated intravascular coagulation) or to delayed wound healing, cheloids, and local necrosis.

ACKNOWLEDGMENTS

The authors thank Dr Christine Merrick for the critical revision of their article.

REFERENCES

1. Bray JP. Soft tissue sarcoma in the dog—part 2: surgical margins, controversies and a comparative review. J Small Anim Pract 2017;58:63–72.
2. Bray JP. Soft tissue sarcoma in the dog—part 1: a current review. J Small Anim Pract 2016;57:510–9.
3. Hohenhaus AE, Kelsey JL, Haddad J, et al. Canine cutaneous and subcutaneous soft tissue sarcoma: an evidence-based review of case management. J Am Anim Hosp Assoc 2016;52:77–89.
4. Bacon NJ, Dernell WS, Ehrhart N, et al. Evaluation of primary re-excision after recent inadequate resection of soft tissue sarcomas in dogs: 41 cases (1999-2004). J Am Vet Med Assoc 2007;230:548–54.
5. Spugnini EP, Azzarito T, Fais S, et al. Electrochemotherapy as first line cancer treatment: experiences from veterinary medicine in developing novel protocols. Curr Cancer Drug Targets 2016;16:43–52.
6. Spugnini EP, Fanciulli M, Citro G, et al. Preclinical models in electrochemotherapy: the role of veterinary patients. Future Oncol 2012;8:829–37.
7. Spugnini EP, Fais S, Azzarito T, et al. Novel instruments for the implementation of electrochemotherapy protocols: from bench side to veterinary clinic. J Cell Physiol 2017;232:490–5.
8. Spugnini EP, Melillo A, Quagliuolo L, et al. Definition of novel electrochemotherapy parameters and validation of their in vitro and in vivo effectiveness. J Cell Physiol 2014;229:1177–81.
9. Dotsinky I, Mudrov N, Mudrov T. Technical aspects of electrochemotherapy. In: Spugnini EP, Baldi A, editors. Electroporation in laboratory and clinical investigations. New York: Nova Science; 2012. p. 45–61.
10. Liu L, Marti GP, Wei X, et al. Age-dependent impairment of HIF-1alpha expression in diabetic mice: correction with electroporation-facilitated gene therapy increases wound healing, angiogenesis, and circulating angiogenic cells. J Cell Physiol 2008;217:319–27.

11. Gissel H, Raphael C, Gehl J. Electroporation and cellular physiology. In: Kee SJ, Gehl J, Lee EW, editors. Clinical aspects of electroporation. New York: Springer; 2011. p. 9–17.
12. Teissie J, Golzio M, Rols MP. Mechanisms of cell membrane electropermeabilization: a minireview of our present (lack of?) knowledge. Biochim Biophys Acta 2005;1724:270–80.
13. Spugnini EP, Arancia G, Porrello A, et al. Ultrastructural modifications of cell membranes induced by "electroporation" on melanoma xenografts. Microsc Res Tech 2007;70:1041–50.
14. Mir LM, Orlowski S, Belehradek J Jr, et al. Biomedical applications of electric pulses with special emphasis on antitumor electrochemotherapy. Bioelectrochem Bioenerg 1995;38:203–7.
15. Orlowski S, Mir LM. Cell electropermeabilization: a new tool for biochemical and pharmacological studies. Biochim Biophys Acta 1993;1154:51–63.
16. Sersa G, Cemezar M, Semrov D, et al. Changing electrode orientation improves the efficacy of electrochemotherapy of solid tumors in mice. Bioelectrochem Bioenerg 1996;39:61–6.
17. Daskalov I, Mudrov N, Peycheva E. Exploring new instrumentation parameters for electrochemotherapy. Attacking tumors with bursts of biphasic pulses instead of single pulses. IEEE Eng Med Biol Mag 1999;18:62–6.
18. Peycheva E, Daskalov I. Electrochemotherapy of skin tumours: comparison of two electroporation protocols. J BUON 2004;9:47–50.
19. Kinosita K, Ashikawa I, Saita N, et al. Electroporation of cell membrane visualized under a pulsed-laser fluorescence microscope. Biophys J 1988;53:1015–9.
20. Hibino M, Shigemori M, Itoh H, et al. Membrane conductance of an electroporated cell analyzed by submicrosecond imaging of transmembrane potential. Biophys J 1991;59:209–20.
21. Glogauer M, McCulloch CA. Introduction of large molecules into viable fibroblasts by electroporation: optimization of loading and identification of labeled cellular compartments. Exp Cell Res 1992;200:227–34.
22. Meschini S, Condello M, Lista P, et al. Electroporation adopting trains of biphasic pulses enhances in vitro and in vivo the cytotoxic effect of doxorubicin on multidrug resistant colon adenocarcinoma cells (LoVo). Eur J Cancer 2012;48:2236–43.
23. Spugnini EP, Dotsinsky I, Mudrov N, et al. Successful rescue of an apocrine gland carcinoma metastatic to the cervical lymph nodes by mitoxantrone coupled with trains of permeabilizing electrical pulses (electrochemotherapy). In Vivo 2008;22:51–3.
24. Spugnini EP, Baldi A. Electrochemotherapy in veterinary oncology: from rescue to first line therapy. Methods Mol Biol 2014;1121:247–56.
25. Spugnini EP, Menicagli F, Pettorali M, et al. Ultrasound guided electrochemotherapy for the treatment of a clear cell thymoma in a cat. Open Vet J 2017;7:57–60.
26. Mir LM, Devauchelle P, Quintin-Colonna F, et al. First clinical trial of cat soft-tissue sarcomas treatment by electrochemotherapy. Br J Cancer 1997;76:1617–22.
27. Tozon N, Sersa G, Cemazar M. Electrochemotherapy: potentiation of local antitumour effectiveness of cisplatin in dogs and cats. Anticancer Res 2001;21:2483–8.
28. Spugnini EP, Porrello A. Potentiation of chemotherapy in companion animals with spontaneous large neoplasms by application of biphasic electric pulses. J Exp Clin Cancer Res 2003;22:571–80.
29. Baldi A, Spugnini EP. Thoracic haemangiopericytoma in a cat. Vet Rec 2006;159:598–600.

30. Spugnini EP, Baldi A, Vincenzi B, et al. Intraoperative versus postoperative electrochemotherapy in high grade soft tissue sarcomas: a preliminary study in a spontaneous feline model. Cancer Chemother Pharmacol 2007;59:375–81.
31. Spugnini EP, Dotsinsky I, Mudrov N, et al. Electrochemotherapy-induced radiation recall in a cat. In Vivo 2008;22:751–3.
32. Spugnini EP, Filipponi M, Romani L, et al. Electrochemotherapy treatment for bilateral pleomorphic rhabdomyosarcoma in a cat. J Small Anim Pract 2010;51:330–2.
33. Spugnini EP, Renaud SM, Buglioni S, et al. Electrochemotherapy with cisplatin enhances local control after surgical ablation of fibrosarcoma in cats: an approach to improve the therapeutic index of highly toxic chemotherapy drugs. J Transl Med 2011;9:152.
34. Spugnini EP, Vincenzi B, Citro G, et al. Adjuvant electrochemotherapy for the treatment of incompletely excised spontaneous canine sarcomas. In Vivo 2007;21:819–22.
35. Spugnini EP, Vincenzi B, Betti G, et al. Surgery and electrochemotherapy of a high-grade soft tissue sarcoma in a dog. Vet Rec 2008;162:186–8.
36. Spugnini EP, Vincenzi B, Amadio B, et al. Adjuvant electrochemotherapy with bleomycin and cisplatin combination for canine soft tissue sarcomas: a study of 30 cases. Open Vet J 2019;9:88–93.
37. Spugnini EP, Di Tosto G, Salemme S, et al. Electrochemotherapy for the treatment of recurring aponeurotic fibromatosis in a dog. Can Vet J 2013;54:606–9.
38. Tozon N, Kodre V, Sersa G, et al. Effective treatment of perianal tumors in dogs with electrochemotherapy. Anticancer Res 2005;25:839–45.
39. Spugnini EP, Dotsinsky I, Mudrov N, et al. Biphasic pulses enhance bleomycin efficacy in a spontaneous canine perianal tumors model. J Exp Clin Cancer Res 2007;26:483–7.
40. Spugnini EP, Dotsinsky I, Mudrov N, et al. Adjuvant electrochemotherapy for incompletely excised anal sac carcinoma in a dog. In Vivo 2008;22:47–9.
41. Thomson M. Squamous cell carcinoma of the nasal planum in cats and dogs. Clin Tech Small Anim Pract 2007;22:42–5.
42. Gasymova E, Meier V, Guscetti F, et al. Retrospective clinical study on outcome in cats with nasal planum squamous cell carcinoma treated with an accelerated radiation protocol. BMC Vet Res 2017;13:86.
43. Spugnini EP, Vincenzi B, Citro G, et al. Electrochemotherapy for the treatment of squamous cell carcinoma in cats: a preliminary report. Vet J 2009;179:117–20.
44. Tozon N, Pavlin D, Sersa G, et al. Electrochemotherapy with intravenous bleomycin injection: an observational study in superficial squamous cell carcinoma in cats. J Feline Med Surg 2014;16:291–9.
45. Spugnini EP, Pizzuto M, Filipponi M, et al. Electroporation enhances bleomycin efficacy in cats with periocular carcinoma and advanced squamous cell carcinoma of the head. J Vet Intern Med 2015;29:1368–75.
46. Spugnini EP, Citro G, Dotsinsky I, et al. Ganglioneuroblastoma in a cat: a rare neoplasm treated with electrochemotherapy. Vet J 2008;178:291–3.
47. Dos Anjos DS, Rossi YA, Magalhães LF, et al. Digital trichoblastoma treated with electrochemotherapy in a dog. Vet Rec 2018;6:e000671.
48. Spugnini EP, Dragonetti E, Vincenzi B, et al. Pulse-mediated chemotherapy enhances local control and survival in a spontaneous canine model of primary mucosal melanoma. Melanoma Res 2006;16:23–7.
49. Spugnini EP, Filipponi M, Romani L, et al. Local control and distant metastasis after electrochemotherapy of a canine anal melanoma. In Vivo 2007;21:897–9.

50. Sledge DG, Webster J, Kiupel M. Canine cutaneous mast cell tumors: a combined clinical and pathologic approach to diagnosis, prognosis, and treatment selection. Vet J 2016;215:43–54.
51. Spugnini EP, Vincenzi B, Baldi F, et al. Adjuvant electrochemotherapy for the treatment of incompletely resected canine mast cell tumors. Anticancer Res 2006;26:4585–9.
52. Kodre V, Cemazar M, Pecar J, et al. Electrochemotherapy compared to surgery for treatment of canine mast cell tumours. In Vivo 2009;23:55–62.
53. Spugnini EP, Vincenzi B, Citro G, et al. Evaluation of Cisplatin as an electrochemotherapy agent for the treatment of incompletely excised mast cell tumors in dogs. J Vet Intern Med 2011;25:407–11.
54. Lowe R, Gavazza A, Impellizeri JA, et al. The treatment of canine mast cell tumours with electrochemotherapy with or without surgical excision. Vet Comp Oncol 2017;15:775–84.
55. Spugnini EP, Citro G, Mellone P, et al. Electrochemotherapy for localized lymphoma: a preliminary study in companion animals. J Exp Clin Cancer Res 2007;26:343–6.
56. Spugnini EP, Dotsinsky I, Mudrov N, et al. Biphasic pulses enhance bleomycin efficacy in a spontaneous canine genital tumor model of chemoresistance: Sticker sarcoma. J Exp Clin Cancer Res 2008;27:58.
57. Maglietti F, Tellado M, Olaiz N, et al. Minimally invasive electrochemotherapy procedure for treating nasal duct tumors in dogs using a single needle electrode. Radiol Oncol 2017;51:422–30.
58. Forde PF, Sadadcharam M, Bourke MG, et al. Preclinical evaluation of an endoscopic electroporation system. Endoscopy 2016;48:477–83.
59. Spugnini EP, Baldi F, Mellone P, et al. Patterns of tumor response in canine and feline cancer patients treated with electrochemotherapy: preclinical data for the standardization of this treatment in pets and humans. J Transl Med 2007;5:48.

Printed and bound by CPI Group (UK) Ltd, Croydon, CR0 4YY

03/10/2024

01040483-0001